Sozialwissenschaftliche Gesundheitsforschung

Reihe herausgegeben von
Andreas Hanses, Dresden, Deutschland
Henning Schmidt-Semisch, Bremen, Deutschland

Sozialwissenschaftliche Gesundheitsforschung untersucht gesellschaftliche Verhältnisse auf der Makro-, Meso- und Mikroebene in ihren Auswirkungen auf Gesundheit und Krankheit. Im Fokus der Betrachtung stehen die staatlichen und sozialen, die kulturellen und gemeinschaftlichen, die individuellen und biographischen Be- und Verarbeitungen von Gesundheit und Krankheit sowie von gesundheitlichen Risiken und Krisen. Dabei nimmt eine sozialwissenschaftliche Gesundheitsforschung sowohl die sozialen und psychosozialen Wechselwirkungen zwischen Gesundheit und Gesellschaft in den Blick als auch das Verhältnis von individuellem Handeln und gesellschaftlichen Rahmenbedingungen. Besondere Bedeutung kommt hier den gesellschaftlichen und diskursiven Aushandlungsprozessen von Gesundheit und Krankheit und den damit verbundenen sozialen Konstruktionen von Normalität und Abweichung zu. In der Reihe erscheinen gleichermaßen theoretisch wie auch empirisch orientierte Bände.

Weitere Bände in der Reihe http://www.springer.com/series/15849

Tom John Wolff

The Touristic Use of Ayahuasca in Peru

Expectations, Experiences, Meanings and Subjective Effects

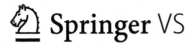

Tom John Wolff
Bremen, Germany

The book is based on a dissertation at the Institute for Public Health and Nursing Sciences at the University of Bremen. The book does not contain the chapter 'Data and Supplements', which is part of the original dissertation.

ISSN 2523-854X	ISSN 2523-8558 (electronic)
Sozialwissenschaftliche Gesundheitsforschung
ISBN 978-3-658-29372-7	ISBN 978-3-658-29373-4 (eBook)
https://doi.org/10.1007/978-3-658-29373-4

© The Editor(s) (if applicable) and The Author(s), under exclusive license to Springer Fachmedien Wiesbaden GmbH, part of Springer Nature 2020

This work is subject to copyright. All rights are solely and exclusively licensed by the Publisher, whether the whole or part of the material is concerned, specifically the rights of translation, reprinting, reuse of illustrations, recitation, broadcasting, reproduction on microfilms or in any other physical way, and transmission or information storage and retrieval, electronic adaptation, computer software, or by similar or dissimilar methodology now known or hereafter developed.

The use of general descriptive names, registered names, trademarks, service marks, etc. in this publication does not imply, even in the absence of a specific statement, that such names are exempt from the relevant protective laws and regulations and therefore free for general use.

The publisher, the authors and the editors are safe to assume that the advice and information in this book are believed to be true and accurate at the date of publication. Neither the publisher nor the authors or the editors give a warranty, expressed or implied, with respect to the material contained herein or for any errors or omissions that may have been made. The publisher remains neutral with regard to jurisdictional claims in published maps and institutional affiliations.

This Springer VS imprint is published by the registered company Springer Fachmedien Wiesbaden GmbH part of Springer Nature.
The registered company address is: Abraham-Lincoln-Str. 46, 65189 Wiesbaden, Germany

Acknowledgement

I would like to express my gratitude to those who have supported me during completing this book:

Dr. Mónica Silva González, who is my beloved wife and partner in this life. She made it all possible, encouraged me and supported this work in every possible way.

Luna M. A. Wolff, who accepted the great changes that our life in Peru brought to her. She took my work as a matter of course.

Carl N. V. Wolff, for his playful lightness and love.

Prof. Dr. Torsten Passie for his trust in me, his guidance, motivation and constructive critique. Thank you for your persistent food for thought and insightful comments throughout the dissertation process that allowed me to reflect on the research topic and gain a broader perspective.

Prof. Dr. Henning Schmidt-Semisch, for his openness and support, which made this research officially possible at the University of Bremen.

Dr. Craig McMahan who read large parts and corrected many spelling mistakes. He suffered humorously from some colo(u)rful wordings as well as the extensive use of British spelling.

Dr. Simon Ruffell and MSc Nigel Netzband for their collaboration and support during the Iquitos study.

Lara Charlotte and Ashley Avery who openly received me and opened the doors of their healing centre Garden of Peace near Tarapoto for this research.

Hegner Paredes Melendez, who walks this strenuous way of being an Amazonian healer. I thank him for his kindness and willingness to open his world to my curiosity.

My professional colleagues, who provided valuable intellectual exchange and advice.

The lovely people who shared their very personal experiences for this research.

Notes

All digital numbers are written in continental style; the decimal place is represented by a comma, not a dot.

Interviews have been sound recoreded and transcribed without any major streamlining or correction of grammar. Few comments for better understanding or grammatical completions have been added in square brackets. Unintelligible parts of phrases have been marked with [?]. Sentences not finished by interviewees and pauses have been marked with 3 full stops ... Some conversational sounds have also been transcribed when recognised as important for the understanding of a phrase, e.g. [laughs].

Direct citations of participants from interviews are coded by the number of the interviewee followed by the numbers of the finding location in the transcript of the interview. Example: (2: 17-19) refers to the paragraphs 17 to 19 of the transcript from the second interviewee. Transcript paragraphs were automatically numbered by the application MAXQDA2018, which was used for the analyses of qualitative material.

For statistical calculations, the applications SPSS 23 and Microsoft Excel were used. This book was written using Microsoft Word 2019

Contents

1 Introduction 1
    1.1   Why be interested as mental health professional 2

2 Traditional Settings 7
    2.1   Church Settings 9
    2.2   Healer settings 10

3 Ayahuasca tourism 11
    3.1   Touristic settings 11
    3.2   Relation between tourism and ayahuasca 13
    3.3   "Western" ayahuasca users 17
    3.4   Explicit research on "western" ayahuasca tourists 19

4 Spirituality 23

5 Neo-shamanism 25

6 Historical approaches on DMT 29
    6.1   Interest in psychoactive substances and research 32

7 Phenomenology of psychedelic experiences 39
    7.1   Psychotoxic base-syndrome 39
    7.2   Stages of the inebriation syndrome of H. Leuner 40
    7.3   Progressive phases of the inebriation syndrome 41
    7.4   Depth stages of the psychedelic inebriation of Masters & Houston .. 42
    7.5   Basic Perinatal Matrices and depth stages after Stanislav Grof 45
    7.6   Transphenomenal dynamic control systems 46
    7.7   Systems of condensed experience 47

8 Ritual elements that influence psychedelic experiences 49
    8.1   Set, setting and substance 49
    8.2   Elements of ayahuasca rituals 58

9 Research about DMT and ayahuasca ... 63
- 9.1 Pharmacological and botanical research on ayahuasca ... 64
- 9.2 Interaction theory ... 67
- 9.3 Physiological effects ... 68
- 9.4 Psychological effects ... 69
- 9.5 Psychological scales ... 80

10 Health and health theories ... 83
- 10.1 Loads, demands and consequences ... 84
- 10.2 Stress ... 85
- 10.3 Salutogesis und SOC ... 98
- 10.4 Subjective health and disease theories ... 101

11 The empirical research ... 111
- 11.1 The research field of the healing centre Garden of Peace ... 111

12 Main questions and general research ideas ... 127
- 12.1 Why qualitative methods? ... 128

13 General design ... 131
- 13.1 Ethics and confidentiality ... 132
- 13.2 Quality criteria for qualitative research ... 133

14 Motivational structure for the ingestion of ayahuasca in the Internet ... 137
- 14.1 Research questions of the first study ... 137
- 14.2 Location and associated institutions of the first study ... 137
- 14.3 Ethics and confidentiality regarding the first study ... 138
- 14.4 Data collection of the first study ... 138
- 14.5 Analysis methods ... 140
- 14.6 Demographic summary ... 140

15 Phenomenological analysis of experiences of ayahuasca ... 141
- 15.1 Research question and methodical considerations ... 141
- 15.2 Case Selection ... 142
- 15.3 Reliability ... 143
- 15.4 Data collection ... 145
- 15.5 Methodological considerations about narrative interviews ... 147
- 15.6 Preparation of the narrative interviews ... 148
- 15.7 Constructing the coding frame ... 148
- 15.8 Analysis of the data ... 149

| 15.9 | Participants and demographics | 149 |
| 15.10 | Answering the research question about ayahuasca phenomenology | 152 |

16 Expectations, motivation, experiences, meaning and subjective effects 157
16.1	Research questions	157
16.2	Location and associated institutions	157
16.3	Design	157
16.4	Methods of the quantitative data collection	158
16.5	Methods of qualitative data collection	159
16.6	Data collection	164
16.7	Demographic summary	165
16.8	Psychometric Questionnaires	166
16.9	SOC-29: Sense of coherence questionnnaire	167
16.10	Methods of data collection and analysis	169

17 Results, conclusions and discussion 177
17.1	Motivational structure	177
17.2	Phenomenological analysis of subjective experiences	179
17.3	Hypothetic psychological working model during flooding and plateau	189
17.4	Process model of ayahuasca-tourism experiences	192
17.5	Summary and conclusions about demographics	202
17.6	Discussion of quantitative results	204
17.7	Discussion of qualitative results	210
17.8	Stress-theoretical considerations	232
17.9	Model of supply and demand interaction in ayahuasca tourism	234

18 Limitations 237

19 Closing words 241

References 247

Tables

Table 1: Synopsis of setting elements in substance supported psychotherapy from different authors (adapteded and modified from Abegleen, 1996; Leuner, 1987; Metzner, 1994; Hess, 2008).................................. 50

Table 2: Classification and considerations of setting elements in substance supported psychotherapy and ayahuasca ceremonies (adapted and extended from Hess, 2008)... 51

Table 3 List of process levels of the stress reaction in humans in transactional stress models.. 87

Table 4: Timetable of a 10-days-retreat at the centre Garden of Peace (Tarapoto, Peru).. 164

Table 5: Comparison of demographic data of the three samples 203

Table 6: List of themes and frequencies of expectation about personal treatment in 20 participants of ayahuasca retreats of the Garden of Peace centre (Tarapoto, Peru).. 212

Table 7: Distribution of motivational elements (motivational subcategories) in 20 participants of ayahuasca retreats at the Garden of Peace centre (Tarapoto, Peru) 214

Figures

Figure 1: Schematic presentation of the complex interaction between set, setting, substance and experience 58
Figure 2: Schematic presentation of loads, demands and demand consequences from a health psychological perspective (adapted from Schröder, 1996) 85
Figure 3: Schematic presentation of the transactional stress model of Lazarus (Lazarus & Folkman 1984; Lazarus, 1999; Yong Wah Goh et al. 2010) 90
Figure 4: Schematic presentation of aspects of human regulation activity (adapted from Schröder, 1997) 94
Figure 5: General components of the model of Salutogenesis 99
Figure 6: Schematic presentation of the folk model of the mind (adapted from D'Andrade, 1995) 108
Figure 7: Schematic presentation of the mutual influence of subjective theory, perceived interaction process between individual and environment in healers and clients 110
Figure 8: Age distribution of the Iquitos sample (study about the phenomenology of the ayahuasca experience) 151
Figure 9: Coding frame part 1 - Preparation, physical symptoms, phantasies, visions, received messages, cognitive reactions and attribution of meaning reported after a shamanic ayahuasca ceremony in the Amazon region (Iquitos, Peru) in narrative interviews of 9 foreign participants using qualitative content analyses (taken from Wolff et al. 2019. All rights reserved) 153
Figure 10: Coding frame part 2 - Recognized meaning of psychedelic content and emotional reactions reported after a shamanic ayahuasca ceremony in the Amazon region (Iquitos, Peru) in narrative interviews of 9 foreign participants using qualitative content analyses (taken from Wolff et al. 2019. All rights reserved) 154
Figure 11: Coding frame part 3 - Appraisal to the process, role of ritual singing and of the shaman, reactions of the individual reported after a shamanic ayahuasca ceremony in the Amazon region (Iquitos, Peru) in narrative interviews of 9 foreign participants

     using qualitative content analyses (taken from Wolff et al. 2019.
     All rights reserved) 155
Figure 12: Schematic presentation of the data collection design of the study
     about expectations, motivations, experiences, meaning and some
     effects of subjects participating in ayahuasca retreats in Peru 158
Figure 13: Schematic presentation of an amplification circle between
     subjective psychedelic perceptions and reactions (modulated by
     external, therapeutic and other stimuli) 191
Figure 14: 'El Supay – Temple', oil on canvas, copyright permission
     granted by © José Luis Vasques Gonzales 198
Figure 15: Schematic presentation of the interaction and feedback between
     physical sickness and the activation of psychological themes 201
Figure 16: Known-group validities of the original and new OAV scales
     (taken from Studerus et al., 2010, copyright permission granted.
     All rights reserved) 209
Figure 17: Graphic presentation of the 5D ASC ayahuasca-profile,
     found in the Tarapoto sample 210
Figure 18: Schematic presentation of a theoretical circle of subjective
     confirmation of the "spiritual world" among tourists consuming
     ayahuasca in shamanic South American jungle settings 225
Figure 19: Schematic presentation of mutual expectations between demand
     side and supply side, which shape ayahuasca tourism 236

Abbreviations, acronyms, foreign terms

ASC	Altered state of consciousness
5D-ASC	Extended Questionnaire for measuring ASCs. The current German version which is based on the APZ from A. Dittrich and two revisions is called 5D-ABZ. Earlier versions are called OAV and OVAV. The most recent version includes Auditory Alterations (AA) and Reduction of Vigilance (RV).
Agua de florida	Spanish: flower water. Often, a cheap industrial made perfume of this brand is used to clear the air of ceremonial spaces. Sometimes, it is spat over the client during ceremony. Some *curanderos* produce their own *agua de florida* from natural ingediences.
Ajo sacha	*Mansoa alliacea*
Ayahuasca	*Banisteriopis caapi* or the psychoactive tee made from B. caapi and other plant ingredients
Ayahuasquero	Spanish: healer who works with ayahuasca
BC	Bootstrap confidence interval
Bobinsana	*Calliandra angustifolia*
BPM	Basic perinatal matrices
Chacapa	Leaf-bundle rattle made from Pariana bush or other plants
Chacruna	*Psychotria viridis*
Chaliponga	*Diplopterys cabrerana*
Chiric sanango	*Brunfelsia grandiflora*
Chuplada	Spanish: sucking - special healing-technique of some curanderos of the Amazon
COEX	System of condensed experiences
Curandero	Spanish: healer
Dieta	Spanish: diet. In traditional Amazonian medicine, the treatment can include a diet with partial or full retreat from social activities and certain types of food. Sometimes, patients or healers search the isolation in the jungle for their *dieta*. It often includes the renunciation from salt, all kinds of spices, sour and bitter tasts and a

	varying list of food, such as meat (especially pork), fermented food, Alcohol, etc. Often, the reduced board contains mostly unsalted rice and *platanos* (cooking banana). During the dieta, patients can ingest prescribed plant medicines for healing or healers ingest those plant extracts for broadening their knowledge, communicate with the spirits of those plants and learn their special songs.
DMT or N,N-DMT	N,N-Dimethyltryptamine
Ícaro or ikaro	Quechua language: medical song. *Ícaros* are the "language" through which the Upper-Amazonian healers believe to communicate with the spiritual world. A healer often has different songs for different spiritual entities, e.g. different plant spirits, and for different purposes during the ceremony. It is said and widely believed that they influence the psychedelic and physical experience of participants who have drunk ayahuasca or other psychedelic substances, e.g. the San Pedro Cactus.
IQR	Interquartile range
LSD	Lysergic acid diethylamide
Maloka	Ceremonial rotunda
MAOI	Monoamine oxidase inhibitor
Mapacho	Cigarette, usually made from black tobacco, *nicotiana rustica*
Maraca	Gourd rattle with seeds
Mucura	*Petivera alliacea*
OAV	Another abbreviation for the 5D-ASC questionnaire
QCA	Qualitative content analysis
Palo santo	Peruvian incense wood from *bursera graveolens*
Shipibo-Conibo	An indigenous people, consisting of two closely related groups, living along the Ucayali river of the Peruvian Amazon rainforest
Chiric sanango	*Brunfelsia grandiflora*
Soplada	Spanish: blowing - frequent technique of curanderos of the Amazon
SD	Standard deviation
Std err	Standard error = SD/square-root(N)
Tabaquero	Spanish: Amazonian folk healer, focussed on the use of tobacco
tdySt	Transphenomenal dynamic control system

Vegetalistas	Spanish: plant healers of the Amazon region. They often use so-called master plants and ayahuasca.
Vegetalismo	Spanish: vegetalism. A healing and belief system of the Amazon region, which emphasises spirits and entities of plants and natural sources, which would interact with humans and the environment. They can be contacted and invited to heal or to harm.
Yagé	In Columbia, the word *yagé* is widly used instead of *ayahuasca*.

Das, was den Indianer den "Aya-huasca-Trank" lieben macht, sind, abgesehen von den Traumgesichten, die auf sein persönliches Glück Bezug habenden Bilder, die sein inneres Auge während des narkotischen Zustandes schaut.
Louis Lewin, Phantastica (1924, p. 148)

1 Introduction

The following book is concerned with the complex phenomenon of contemporary ayahuasca practice in Peru. It focusses on expectations, experiences, meaning and subjective effects of persons participating in cross-cultural ayahuasca tourism. The purpose is not an evaluation of traditional ayahuasca therapy but a psychological, explorative, hypotheses-generating investigation as well as documentation of psychological aspects of contemporary ayahuasca-tourism in the Upper Amazon. For this purpose, the reader is introduced into the field of Peruvian ayahuasca healing-practices and ayahuasca tourism in South America. An overview about the relevant research literature, as well as the research questions, methods and analysis procedures of three empirical studies, are presented. Results and limitations are extensively discussed.

First, an online-questionnaire study was performed, in order to explore the distribution of motivational elements among ayahuasca interested individuals already known from the previous literature as well as to collect demographic data and explore the accessibility and openness of the ayahuasca scene towards scientific research. Introspective and spiritual purposes were identified as the main aspects in the motivation to ingest ayahuasca in members of social media in the Internet. The motivation of members of social ayahuasca networks in the Internet seems not to be monodimensional but a composite of different aspects of which a subconglomerate of psychospiritual reasons and individual self-development seems to be the most dominant. The findings support motivational differences to local ayahuasca shaman clients in the Upper Amazon region that have been previously described in the ethnologic literature. Further studies could develop standardised instruments for the investigation of the motivation of the ingestion of (psychedelic) drugs in particular settings as well as explore a possible connection between the motivation and outcomes.

Second, a qualitative, data-driven study among foreign participants of traditional Peruvian ayahuasca ceremonies in the Amazon rain forest explored phenomenological categories of the experience during ayahuasca ingestion. What distinguishes this study from previous phenomenological approaches is that qualitative data were collected immediately after the ayahuasca ceremony and not weeks, months or years later. The coding frame, extracted from narrative interviews by Qualitative Content Analysis, is presented and discussed. The study suggests that psychodynamic processes, for example, possible activation of emotional conflicts, can take place spontaneously during ayahuasca intake in this particular setting. Some participants attributed symbolic meaning to the visionary content, which was more likely to take place in psychotherapeutically motivated clients. The specific setting influence as well as corresponding expectations of the participants in native wisdom could have considerable influence on experiences and interpretations, such as communication with entities as well as receiving personal teachings.

Third, a concept-driven qualitative study, was designed. Ayahuasca tourists were accompanied through participant observation and interviewed six weeks after completing a typical ayahuasca retreat in a Peruvian healing centre in the Amazon rain forest. Half-structured guideline interviews and Qualitative Content Analysis was used to extract personal meaning, experiences, subjective effects and integration experiences. The qualitative main part was accompanied by quantitative mental-health related data collected at baseline, post-1, post-2 as well as quantitative data of altered states of consciousness collected after ayahuasca ceremonies. A great variety of findings among the investigated individuals are presented and discussed. Subjective improvements include greater self-understanding, personal guidance, clarification of desires, self-esteem, self-care and self-love. Improvements of ailments are not consistent among participants. A minority experienced integration crises or aggravation of psychological issues. A process model of ayahuasca tourism was proposed: Attitude and motivation forming phase; Ingestion phase (turning inwards, flooding phase, plateau, peak points and release); reflection and attenuation phase, integration phase. Subjective operating concepts about ayahuasca include a catalysator function for psychological insight as well as magical elements.

1.1 Why be interested as mental health professional

This book will examine the experiences and subjective health and healing concepts of western clients of Amazonian ethno-therapy in South America. In general, there are several arguments for the relevance of investigations of health-related concepts that were provided by Flick (1998):

- Subjective ideas about health and illness determine our health-related behaviour and decisions substantially. That is why health related subjective theories are highly relevant for the success of all kinds of health services.
- The gap between the theories of physicians and psychotherapists and those of their patients is one of the main reasons for non-compliance and therapy breakup (Flick, 1998; Jing et al., 2008).
- Subjective theories about disease, health and healing are also most relevant with the coping of disease.

- For the modern medicine that orients itself towards the patients and not exclusively towards the diseases, the subjective concepts of health and disease are central.
- An aim of western psychotherapy is the recognition of implicit subjective theories that affect perception, interpretation and action in order to make them accessible to conscious decisions and a possible change.
- Specific target groups have specific needs and concepts about health and disease. This influences the process of informed consent and affects the compliance.
- The transformation of health conceptions could be an indicator for the evaluation of health education.
- The development of scientific models about should start with the investigation of subjective constructs of everyday life, especially when there has not been done much research in that particular field (Schütz, 1971).
- The reconstruction of subjective ideas helps to investigate the existing concepts of health and disease and the process of their progression.
  Ethno-therapy tourists can be seen as an increasing medical "target group".

They often have a distinct profile of motivational elements, expectations and ideas about healing, as shown later. The successful present situation of internationally recognized ethno-therapeutic offers in South America, especially in Peru, has developed almost completely outside the official medical systems, which largely refused the integration of present folk medicine practices. Because the treatments of traditional or traditionalized jungle therapy contain strong medical interventions like purging therapy, diets and psychedelic plant potion intake with sometimes dangerous ingredients that need a profound formation of the therapist, they affect public health issues and should not be ignored. Also, the countless numbers of individual reports that appear in the social media and attract new seekers should be reason enough to investigate this phenomenon of specialized tourism with fair curiosity. The use of the hallucinogenic or visionary Amazonian jungle beverage "ayahuasca" is spreading into the alternative western psychotherapy and esoteric scenes. Many people from the so-called "first world" come to South America to have a "shamanic" ayahuasca experience. Previous research has found that those visitors do not fit the profile of hedonistic drug users. Here I take a closer look at their motivations, expectations and subjective working theories about ayahuasca related healing. The interest in traditional Amazonian medicine through help seekers, tourists and researchers from abroad affects the local folk medicine practice economically and in form and content. With this study the author also wants to provide relevant information for the perspective of cultural anthropology on the processes of alternative medicine and ethno-tourism.

1.1.1 New interest in substance supported psychotherapy and ethno-medicine

This work is also related to the new interest in psychedelics within its multi-tension field between laymen´s use and the search for professional therapeutic use. On one side, there are often undifferentiated and highly emotionalized condemnation reflexes, suspicion and legal prosecution of its application, which culminated in the political expression "global war on drugs" and the still on-going obstruction and suppression of research. On the other side, an undifferentiated glorification and belief of global salvation or defiant insistence for the private right of self-determination on inebriation is observed. In between, there has grown a new research interest in the actual benefits and risks of hallucinogenic compounds for the treatment of specific diseases, e.g. drug addiction (Ross, 2012; Bogenschutz & Pommy, 2012; Hendricks, 2014; Krebs & Johansen, 2012) and some depressive and anxiety disorders (Vollenweider & Kometer, 2010). Others said to have found a large effect of 3,4,-methylenedioxymethamphetamine (MDMA) assisted psychotherapy on chronic PTSD (Chabrol & Oehen, 2013). Therapeutic potential seems to have been found from the beginning but was stopped when this substance became included within a larger drug subculture. Now, there seems to be evidence to discuss MDMA as a medicine again, along with other substances such as heroine and amphetamine (Sessa & Nutt, 2015; ClinicalTrials.gov, 2018).

Gasser et al. (2014a) found in a well-controlled study that the application of LSD in a 'methodologically rigorous medically supervised psychotherapeutic setting' can reduce anxiety in patients who face life-threatening diseases. A prospective follow-up with 10 individuals after one year showed that the effects of reduced anxiety were sustained. In the qualitative part of the study, participants 'consistently reported insightful, cathartic and interpersonal experiences, accompanied by a reduction in anxiety (77,8%) and a rise in quality of life (66,7%). Evaluations of subjective experiences suggest facilitated access to emotions, confrontation of previously unknown anxieties, worries, resources and intense emotional peak experiences à la Maslow as major psychological working mechanisms. The experiences created led to a restructuring of the person's emotional trust, situational understanding, habits and world view.' (Gasser et al., 2014b).

These examples are presented here in order to show that there is a new general research interest in psychedelics and its potential therapeutic use. A simple literature research at the online database PubMed on the 28.04.2016 showed 179 articles under the search term ayahuasca (http://www.ncbi.nlm.nih.gov/pubmed). Eight of them were placed within in the first four months of the same year 2016. 23 articles where published in 2015. A detailed literature research (provided in 2014 for the period from 1960 until 2014 in the data bases of PubMed, Scopus, Science Direct, Scielo and Web of Science) showed that the number of scientific, first time published articles under the term ayahuasca were 312. Upon the first period of 35 years from 1960 until 1995, there appeared only 31 articles. From 1995 until the present, the number increased rapidly so that only in the year 2012 the number of 41 articles were published and in 2014 and 33 articles (Castelan Filipe, 2015, p. 33).

1.1.2 Non-European medicines and its relationships to the western medicine

Beside the historic and new western attempts of substance-assisted psychotherapy, there are traditional approaches in other parts of the world, which have been subsumed under the rather Eurocentric term "ethno-medicine". The WHO defines traditional medicine as followed:

> 'Traditional medicine has a long history. It is the sum total of the knowledge, skills and practices based on the theories, beliefs and experiences indigenous to different cultures, whether explicable or not, used in the maintenance of health, as well as in the prevention, diagnosis, improvement or treatment of physical and mental illnesses. The terms complementary/alternative/non-conventional medicine are used interchangeably with traditional medicine in some countries.' (WHO, 2000)

Further, a footnote says:

> 'The term complementary and alternative medicine is used in some countries to refer to a broad set of health care practices that are not part of the country's own tradition and are not integrated into the dominant health care system' (WHO, 2000)

The Canadian evaluation researcher Brian Rush (2016) quotes in an unpublished report that in the developing countries with low income, 75%-85% of the patients with serious psychic diseases are not reached through the health systems (Demyttenaere et al., 1996). Behind the interest to do more research in the psychedelic medicine of the Amazon, lays the fact that in many countries there is a huge gap between the high load of the mental health and the lack of therapeutic help for psychic diseases and addictions. In places which have possibilities for help, it often does not reach the needs because of different reasons (McKenzie et al., 2004). This is especially the case in regions with indigene population. That is why Rush quotes Incayawar, who emphasizes that the cooperation of the modern Psychiatry with the local healing tradition is required (Incayawar, 2007). Sobiecki (2014a; 2014b) supposes that 72% of the black population of Africa hold traditional healers as their main medical supply source.

It could be the aim of the international research community to look for effective interventions, which work within the cultural field in which they shall be implemented.

1.1.3 Some attempts to connect both in the South Americas

Some psychotherapists and institutions use ayahuasca and other South American traditional interventions as part of their therapeutic program (Dörfler, 2015). The Takiwasi centre in Tarapoto (Peru) is the internationally most well-known. It offers detoxification and long-term cessation therapy for drug addicts. It combines a therapeutic community, group-therapy, ayahuasca and other traditional and semi-traditional medicine and complementary medicine interventions. Bouso & Riba (2014) found evidences for the effectiveness on alcohol and drug dependency treatment. Retrospective studies have shown that, t hrough the religious use of ayahuasca within the Santo Daime and UDV churches in Brasil and the U.S., alcohol and drug abstinence could be reached from dependent individuals (Grob et al., 1996; Labate et al.; 2013; Fábregas et al., 2010; Halpern et al., 2008).

The Hoasca Project was the first biochemical investigation on long-term ayahuasca consumers such as in the Brazilian ayahuasca churches (McKenna et al., 1998). Besides other results, an increase in the number of binding sides on platelet cells, which mediate the serotonin uptake was found (Callaway et al., 1994). This might be relevant for evidences of anti-depressive and anxiolytic effects (Osório et al., 2015).

Loizaga-Velder & Loizaga Pazzi (2014) found in a qualitative study that participants of ayahuasca-based treatment consider the combination of ayahuasca experiences with known elements of addiction treatments such as group therapy, art therapy, and psychosocial counselling important for psychodynamic insight, inner cleaning, peak experience and development of visions. Another qualitative study shows that patients from different countries and contexts see therapeutic potential and benefit in the ayahuasca-based treatment (Loizaga-Velder & Verres, 2014).

2 Traditional Settings

The use of natural psychoactive substances has been identified as a strategy to induce altered states of consciousness that can be found in several cultures (Dittrich & Scharfetter, 1987). In 90% out of 488 observed ethnicities, altered states of consciousness were institutionally integrated part of their societies (Bourguignon, 1973).

Within the wide Amazonian area, the use of hallucinogenic plants is an integrated part of the traditional medicine and folk-psychotherapy (McKenna, 2007). Many indigenous people consider ayahuasca as a sacred and most important medicine provided by nature (Presser-Velder, 2012). The use of this brew, which nowadays mostly contains N,N-dimethyltryptamine (DMT) and harmala-alkaloids as monoamine oxidase inhibiter (MAOI), is traditionally embedded in ritualized oral ingestion. The MAOI is provided from species of Banisteriopsis (B. caapi, B. muricata). It is a rife vine in the Amazonian area. The DMT comes from leafs of Psychotria viridis or Diplopterys cabrerana. Various recipes and rituals from different groups have been reported and the change of rituals over the time has been documented (Luna, 2006; Ott, 1994).

For the indigenous shamanic beliefs, ayahuasca has been used for 'foreseeing the future, sending messages to other groups, contacting distant relatives, determining if wives were unfaithful, determining plans of the enemy, identifying sorcerers and practicing love magic' (Luna, 2004, p. 378-382), also to enter unseen realms and other realities (Luna, 2010, p. 2) and to communicate with spirits in order to gain protection, perform witchcraft and sorcery against others and to achieve ecstasy (de Rios, 1972). Ayahuasca often has been experienced as a personalized entity, which acts as a plant teacher to the shaman (Luna, 1986b, p. 60).

For the Amazonian area of the Napo river, 'it is also evident, that the ayahuasca shamanism was fully developed in the Napo before the DMT admixtures were ever introduced, and eventually evolved into practices with DMT admixtures as it spread' (Highpine, 2012). Many other plants are traditionally known to be admixture to the Banisteriopsis caapi vine and 'most of these "admixtures" are not added to enhance the psychoactive effect of ayahuasca; rather they are mixed with ayahuasca in order to understand and communicate with those plants. Ayahuasca has a traditional supportive role for other plant medicines.' (ibid., 2012).

Unlike the popular forms of ritualized collective intake and purging, for some tribes it is or was common that only the shaman drinks the ayahuasca brew because its intake is considered to be unpleasant and left to the professional healer (Schultes, 1983, p. 140). 'The "medicine" with psychic properties that enables the medicine–man easily through hallucinations to see or converse with malevolent spirits from whom come all illness and death are usually far more important in native cultures than those medicines with purely physical properties' (Schultes, 1983, pp. 140-141). Others have ritualized dances (colombian Tucanoans) or use Banisteriopsis for enhancing hunting skills (Waorani) (Miller-Weisberger, 2000). For the first part of the 20th century, Louis Lewin mentioned the use of 'Banisteria caapi' by 'the Guahibo, Tukano, e.g. Coreguáje and Táma, the Zaparo, Uaupé Yekuaná, Baré, Baniva, Mandavaka, Tariana, Cioni, Jibáros, Kolorados, Cayapas and others.' (Lewin, 1924, p. 141). He reported that the strongly cooked brew would be drunk solely. The sorcerer instead, would ingest another recipe, which would contain other plants such as 'Jahi, Yaje or Yahe' (ibid., p. 142). They would use this for finding causes of diseases, for healing, or to hex enemies. Note, that nowadays Yagé is the widely used name for the psychedelic ayahuasca brew in Colombia. Lewin continued, that the Jabáros tribe would have performed "Natema"-celebrations up to 8 days on which B. caapi would have been ingested collectively by men, women and adolescents. But they also would have drunk it alone for all kinds of reasons and the desire to experience trance (ibid., p. 142). The use of B. caapi would have been connected with religious ideas because the delusions of the senses would have been perceived as real (ibid., p. 144).

For the traditional "indian" societies of some Amazonian areas, it was mentioned by Schultes that the medicine–man often would not know a lot about plants in general. He would concentrate on the ritualized or magical use of his sacred plants, which are mostly psychoactive or hallucinogenic. For the phyto-therapeutic medicine (plant-medicine), most tribes also had what we would call a medical doctor who usually did not use those plants in a magical or shamanic way but had a greater knowledge about curative plant use in general. Those 'botanists of the society', as Schultes called them, usually worked cooperative with the payés or medicine–men although they seemed to have a lower rank than medicine-men (Schulte, 1983, pp.146-147).

Differences in the aetiological systems of urban and rural healers have been documented for Central America (Zacharias, 2005) and indicate a change and adjustment to new surroundings, circumstances and patient's needs.

Unlike most western academic healing theories, the separation between spiritual, religious practice on one side and medical, therapeutic on the other may not have existed for most of the indigenous users. Everything seems to be part of a holistic sacred cosmology in which magic, religion and healing are one. It seems to be that this combination provides one of the attractions for western ayahuasca seekers, particularly, as described later, if seen in regard of the characteristics of neo-shamanism.

2.1 Church Settings

Another big group of ayahuasca users are the syncretic ayahuasca religions, mostly found in Brazil. There is the Santo Daime church, which was founded in the 1930s by Mestre Irineu (Raimundo Irineu Serra) in the state Acre and the smaller União do Vegetal (UDV) which was founded in the year 1961 by Mestre Gabriel (José Gabriel da Costa). Various branches of the Santo Daime have spread over South America and have reached North America, Europe and Asia (Labate & Jungaberle, 2011; Labate & MacRae, 2010). The religious use is legal in Brazil, Netherlands, Japan and partly the USA. The brew is ritually consumed, sometimes with more than 100 followers. It is considered a sacrament similar to the Christian churches. There are some differences between these two religious groups. The Santo Daime ritual can last four to twelve hours and it contains collective singing and dancing. There are hymns and a synchronized dance (bailado), accompanied by strong percussion and melodic instruments. In the UDV ritual, which lasts up to four hours, the participants remain seated most of the time. The music is performed by single participants and comes from stereo devices. Participants direct questions to the preacher and there are also some periods of silence (Barbosa et al., 2005). Barbosa et al. conducted a mixed methods psychological investigation on 28 first time ayahuasca users in an urban ritual context of the Santo Daime and Unidão do Vegetal Churches in Brazil. 64,3% of them believed in reincarnation and 57,1% had a so-called metaphysical religiosity (concerning supernatural beings, parallel dimensions, cosmic energy, eastern esoteric or spiritual concepts such as chakras, yoga and meditation practice). Only 3,6% described themselves as agnostics. 42,9% of them were motivated through the expectation of self-knowledge and 28,6% of spiritual latencies (search for awakening hidden spiritual attributes like e.g. "the superior self"). Curiosity about the effects of ayahuasca was mentioned as motivational factor from 25% and healing (psychosocial problems) was only mentioned from 21,4%. 17,9% were looking for improvement in equilibrium, general well-being and behaviour (Barbosa et al., 2005). Although the sample size was rather little for generalized interpretations, the authors concluded out of their socio-demographic data that, 'despite the Amazonian origins of Santo Daime and UDV among the working classes, the religious use of ayahuasca in south-eastern Brazilian large cities seems to be a predominantly middle and educated social class phenomenon' (ibid, p. 197). The findings, especially the low curiosity factor of the motivation for ayahuasca, would corroborate the hypothesis of the search for new ways of life and spiritual values and alternatives to materialistic and utilitarian values in parts of the urban Brazilian middle class.

2.2 Healer settings

There are many mestizo curanderos (Spanish: healer) throughout South America who provide ayahuasca for a range of health related and psychotherapeutic problems. The Spanish word mestizo refers to a South American population of descendants of mainly white and indigene ancestors. Usually those healers get paid for their services. The use of ayahuasca-ritual therapy depends strongly on the area and the economic and educational level of the participants. Often it belongs to the rather low socio-economic parts of society. Nevertheless, it is an integrated and accepted part of indigene and mestizos healing practice (Incayawar, 2007) and is engaged in the diagnosis and treatment of medical, psychological and psychosomatic diseases as alternative or additional to the physician´s treatment. The mestizo ayahuasca-shamans are sometimes called vegetalistas or ayahuasqueros. They have in common that important elements of their healing practices are a continuation of the shamanism of native groups, e.g. they often claim to receive knowledge directly from spirits and plants and they often claim to collaborate with some of the spirits. Sometimes those spirits are called doctors or doctorcitos and they would manipulate the client's body directly for healing purposes. They also use special healing songs (ícaros) during their rituals and many consider the diet as important part for preparation and healing. Christian elements and saints have been woven into the mestizo shamanism (Luna, 2003, p. 20-23; Luna, 1986b, pp. 14-15, 16, 31-32, 141; Kamppinen 1989, p. 114; Fotiou, 2012, pp. 16-20). For many mestizo customers the curanderism dos not conflict with their Catholic religion or with scientifically-based medical services.

The boundary between the local or traditional mestizo ayahuasca healing practices and new influences like elements of western or Asiatic ideas, religions and relaxation practices is often blurred nowadays, especially when the clientele changes.

3 Ayahuasca tourism

3.1 Touristic settings

Since the 1980s, non-religious ayahuasca groups were established. Ayahuasca spread to the cities and was internationally recognized from a larger audience (Barbosa et al., 2012).

Ayahuasca-tourism in Peru hGrunwelas developed to become a professional business in the last 20 years (Grunwell, 1998) due to a Western demand for personal insights and guidance, emotional catharsis, spiritual confirmation and epiphany, psychosomatic healing and "adventurous experience" (De Rios, 1994; Kristensen, 1998; Winkelman 2005; Fotiou, 2010; Schmid, 2010; Losonczy & Mesturini, 2010; Hudson, 2011; Fiedler, 2011; Wolff, 2018).

One hotspot of western ayahuasca tourism is the town Iquitos located in the northern Peruvian jungle (Fotiou, 2010, p. 121). Touristic areas, which were traditionally less involved in the Amazonian ayahuasca practice have discovered its economic potential and offer it to western tourists. One example is the well-known Andean city Cusco.

Nowadays, more and more "healing centres" and lodges appear, which mostly cater to urban and western travellers and offer their ayahuasca rituals on the Internet. They are more or less professionalized and commercialized. Often a combination of ayahuasca-shamanism and other activities is offered, like visits to local communities, sites, lectures and longer ayahuasca seminars (Znamenski, 2007, pp.155-157; Holman, 2011, p. 68). These professional lodges usually offer "all inclusive" accommodation. Shamans who run such centres do not necessarily stand in only one tradition of a particular native group any more. There are also several westerners who offer ayahuasca and some centres are owned by westerners. The ayahuasca tourism in South America grown for 10 or 20 years. But the situation on the traditional medicine health market in Peru is vastly unregulated.

The government of Peru has brought out the Resolutión Ministerial 836 del INC on the 24th of June 2008 that declares the traditional use of ayahuasca to be a Cultural Heritage of the Nation. It declares:

> 'Que, mediante el documento del visto la Dirección de Estudio y Registro Cultural en el Perú Contemporáneo solicita la declaración como Patrimonio Cultural de la Nación a los conocimientos y usos tradicionales asociados al ayahuasca y practicados por las

comunidades nativas amazónicas, conforme al Expediente elaborado por doña Rosa A. Giove Nakazawa del Centro Takiwasi – Tarapoto y presenado por la Gerencia Regional de San Martín;
Que la planta Banisteriopsis caapi es una especie vegetal que cuenta con una extraordinaria historia cultural, en virtud de sus cualidades psicotrópicas y a que se usa en un brebaje asociado a la planta conocida como chakruna psicodria-viridis;
Que dicha planta es conocida por el mundo indígena amazónico como una planta sabia o maestra que enseña a los iniciados los fundamentos mismos del mundo y sus componentes. Los efectos de su consumo constituyen la entrada al mundo espiritual y a sus secretos, es así que en torno al ritual del ayahuasca se ha estructurado la medicina tradicional amazónica en algún momento de sus vidas, e indispensable para quienes asumen el papel de portadores privilegiados de estas culturas, se trate de los encargados de la comunicación con el mundo espiritual o de los que lo expresen plásticamente; ...
Que, por la información de sustento se desprende que la práctica de sesiones rituales de ayahuasca constituye uno de los pilares fundamentales de la identidad de los pueblos amazónicos y que su uso ancestral en los rituales tradicionales, garantizando continuidad cultural, está vinculado a las virtudes terapéuticas de la planta; ...'
(Resolución Ministerial 836 del INC, 2008)

Translation: That through the seen document the Directorate of Study and Cultural registry in Contemporary Peru requests a declaration as Cultural Patrimony of the Nation the knowledge and traditional uses associated with ayahuasca and practiced by native Amazon communities, according to the dossier prepared by Dona Rosa A. Giove Nakazawa of the Takiwasi Centre - Tarapoto and presented by Regional Management San Martin;
Banisteriopsis caapi is a plant species that has an extraordinary cultural history, by virtue of its psychotropic qualities and used in a concoction known as associated with psicotria-viridis chacruna plant;
That this plant is known by the indigenous Amazonian world as a wise teacher who teaches the initiates the very foundations of the world and its components. The effects of consumption are the entrance to the spiritual world and its secrets, so at some point in their lives traditional Amazonian medicine has structured around the ritual of ayahuasca, and indispensable for those who assume the role of carriers privileged of these cultures, dealing with those responsible for communication with the spirit world or those who express plastically; ...
That the supporting information shows that the practice of ritual ayahuasca sessions constitutes one of the fundamental pillars of the identity of Amazonian peoples and their ancestral use in traditional rituals, guaranteeing cultural continuity, it is linked to the therapeutic virtues of the plant; ...

Due to the increasing shaman-touristic interest the number of shamans and healing centres grows. This can be seen in the increasing number of English web pages and prices in USD on the Internet. A simple research in the Peruvian Google search engine (https://www.google.com.pe) on the 8th of March 2016 with the two words "ayahuasca" and "retreat" brought about 223000 hits and the same search on the 23 of October 2018 brought 562000 hits.

The anthropologist, Evgenia Fotiou, who has done her fieldwork from 2003 until 2005 reported that not only the number of western shaman tourists has probably doubled after her stay in Iquitos (Fotiou, 2010, pp. 122-123) but also the interest of young local mestizos in becoming a shaman had increased. Most of them are reported not to be an apprentice for a couple of years but start their business after few months of apprenticeship. They often claim to have apprenticed with an indigenous shaman (Fotiou, 2010, pp. 305-306). In the case of Iquitos, the ayahuasca was urbanized and mixed with Christianity a long time before the western interest appeared. Shamanism was a mestizo profession before (Fotiou, 2010, ibid.). It is consumed within its cultural Amazonian and mestizo origin and nowadays also in a commodified globalized context. Ayahuasca rituals are offered in worldwide Facebook groups in North America and Europe and it is present in real and virtual marketplaces such as the mercado de Belén in Iquitos, Cuzcos's mercado San Pedro, and BouncingBearBotanicals.com (own observations, 2016; Hudson, 2011). 'Its fetishization is strong' (ibid.). The image of the indigene shaman is popular and may be an archetypical invitation that leads quickly to associations and wishes. Contractors and agencies of shaman tours might seize wishes for imagined authenticity. Besides the issue of therapeutic quality and responsibility, shaman tourism 'benefits financially from its association with the icon of the shaman' (ibid.). Some believe that the tourism destroys the authentic use of ayahuasca through commercialization of the Amazonian spirituality. Others are reported to think that indigenous ecotourism could provide a future to indigenous cultures (Zografos, 2005). Shamanism is and probably has always been a profession not only related to foreign tourists but also to local clients (Ott, 2011, p. 114).

3.2 Relation between tourism and ayahuasca

There are on-going discussions in closed ayahuasca internet-groups of Facebook about the question, what a real shaman is. Some western people request advice in finding an "authentic" shaman. The search for authentic experience and phenomena of constructed authenticity, which are known to the sociological and social-psychological tourism research since Groffmann (1959) and MacCannell (1973), can be observed very well in the field of the ayahuasca tourism scene: 'It is found that tourists try to enter back regions of the places they visit because these regions are associated with intimacy of relations and authenticity of experience. It is also found that tourist settings are arranged to produce the impression that a back region has been entered even when this is not the case' (MacCannel, 1973).

Experiences of the ayahuasca rituals seem to suit well for such "back regions" because the experiences are strong and extraordinary and, because of being strongly internal experiences, they might be easily believed not to be arranged to produce the impression of authenticity. Ayahuasca tourists often search for what they naïvely imagine to be the authentic shamanism (Herbert, 2010, pp. 1-2; Fotiou, 2010, p. 136). They often do not recognize its historical, economic, cultural development and its belief systems because they search for something else that they believe has to be pure and not yet contaminated with western influences. Shamans in the view of western ayahuasca tourists should be indigenous or at least trained by indigenous shaman from the jungle (Holman, 2011, 69-70). On the other hand, ayahuasca shamanism is publicized in line with a universal wisdom or shamanism, 'which does not belong to the Indians; they are only the caretakers of that knowledge. The new shamans, according to their prophesies, are us, …' (The tour operator Alex Madrigal in Znamenski, 2007, p. 161). Suppliers of ayahuasca experiences react to the romantic desire for a specific western imagination of authenticity and universal connection with adaptation and purgation of ambiguous and unpalatable elements of their rituals (Peluso & Alexiades, 2006, p. 73). Christian elements, which are often a normal part of local mestizo shaman tradition in Peru, are less present or disappear in ayahuasca rituals, which are adjusted for western tourists (Fotiou, 2010, p. 138). Christian element might be experienced from tourists as impurity of the presented shamanism. Local people usually do not put such importance on the location of the ceremony. Western participants rather like ceremonies in nature (Fotiou, 2010, p. 137) and in a traditional appearing architecture. Also, the appearance of the shaman himself seems most important to western tourists. Shamans do usually not wear native or traditionalized clothing when they conduct ceremonies for local people, while western tourists take such as a sign of authenticity (Fotiou 2010, p. 137-138). An anecdote told by Carlos Tanner, a US-citizen and founder of the Ayahuasca Foundation that offers ayahuasca treatment and formations near Iquitos, might serve as an example. During an ayahuasca conference held in Iquitos a couple of years ago, the local shamans were put in an uncomfortable competition when they were asked to present themselves to the public to point out their individual advantage, knowing that the number of paying participants would depend on this presentation in comparison to the other shamans. While they were sitting and waiting for the people to sign, one of them wore a big feather crown. A long line of attendees formed at his table to sign for his ceremonies. (Carlos Tanner in a personal talk, October 3, 2016 in Lima).

Ayahuasca tourists tend to believe to take part in an indigenous spiritual tradition that would provide a pure connection to a global or universal wisdom. This also reflects in in the alignment of local shamans, f.e. by talking about chakras, by offering reiki, yoga or meditation.

The common practice to sing their personal ícaros during the ayahuasca rituals changes as well. The Colombian mestizo shaman Lucho Flores from the southern town Mocoa e.g. sings his songs during his ayahuasca rituals in Spanish and accompanies himself with the guitar (personal field observation), others sell their songs on CDs to the tourists (Fotiou, 2012, p.19). Besides their local knowledge successful shamans have reinterpreted and adapted the rituals to a multitude of expectations and languages.

> 'Al mismo tiempo, la "occidentalización" de la demanda suscita paradójicamente una estandarización creciente de la acción ritual a través de la yuxtaposición casi obligatoria de las secuencias ritualizadas que acompañan la ingesta de ayahuasca y que funcionan como metonimias de distintos pueblos y culturas: cabaña de sudación, ejercicios de yoga y de relajación, ayunas y dietas, cantos y danzas de proveniencia étnica variada, círculos de palabra que recuerdan la psicoterapia de grupo.'
> (Losonczy & Mesturini, 2010)

> Translation: At the same time, the 'westernization' of demand paradoxically raises an increasing standardization of ritual action through the almost obligatory juxtaposition of ritualized sequences that accompany the intake of ayahuasca and function as metonymy of different people and cultures: sweat lodge, yoga exercises and relaxation exercises, fasting and diets, songs and dances from a variety of ethnic backgrounds, circles reminiscent of group-psychotherapy.

The costs for ceremony participation can vary greatly between locals and tourists, like for almost everything else in Peru. A full day in a jungle lodge or healing centre costs between 50 – 300 USD. The participation in a ceremony only costs between 20 and 50 USD. There are also differences between locals and foreign tourists in the judging criteria over the quality of the healer. Foreign clientele desire that the knowledge of the healer is from indigenous origin. For locals the indisputable proof of the shamanic power is the ability to handle conflicts of mutual attacks and witchcraft among specialists in the area (Losonczy & Mesturini, 2010).

MacCannel believed that modern tourism couldn't provide authentic experiences at all, although this might be what tourists always actually seek for – not unsimilar to religious pilgrims. Greenwood (1977) expressed that objects, services and cultural properties would lose sense due to their commercialization: 'That is the final perversity. The commoditization of culture does not require the consent of the participants; it can be done by anyone. Once set in motion, the process seems irreversible and its very subtlety prevents the affected people from taking any clearcut action to stop it' (Greenwood, 1977).

Later authors gather a differentiated position on the problem of authenticity and tourism from the early views: Authenticity is emerged through a continuing process of mediation. It is not a fixed cultural trait, which is only there before tourism appears and destroys it. Artificial products can gain authentication as well in a gradual process. This was named "emergent authenticity" by Cohen (1988) according to the term 'emergent ethnicity' for ethnic realms from Yancey (et al., 1976). One example is mentioned by Cohen: The Disneyland which can change to be an authentic product of US-American culture. May be similar processes happen with the use of ayahuasca in non-traditional settings (such as "New-Age"-, urban-, European, north American, Christian and Islam settings), as well as with adapted or new rituals and with shamans who apparently act outside a fixed traditional use or come from another cultural background and "invent" or "find" their own style of authenticity. Philip Pearce (1988) - as mentioned in Vester (1993) - found that the amount of authenticity is not a primary trait of touristic occurrences. Because it is a category of perception, that depends from expectations, experience and the desires of the tourist. The front or backstage character of the touristic scenery and the acting protagonists can differ in their grade of authenticity. For touristic satisfaction authenticity is not always wanted nor necessary.

For this study some of the above-mentioned categories like the expectations and wants of the interviewed persons will be examined in the field of ayahuasca tourism. But the analyse of the perception of authenticity will not be the main issue. Nevertheless, the construction and perception of authenticity could be an important element of the shamanic healing practice and should be kept in mind.

The post-touristic position of Urry (1990) indicates that post touristic proposals do not claim to give an authentic cultural heritage, a natural landscape nor a natural exotic way of living. In this view authenticity cannot be discovered nor can it be reconstructed but only constructed or invented. The results can be found in playful touristic presentations of history and culture. The "post tourist" (Feifer, 1985) on the other side will not be disappointed if he finds inauthenticity because he does not have the naive hope to find authenticity within a touristic action (Urry, 1990). Some positions show critical points of view against tourism and its inauthenticity, 'hyper reality' (Eco, 1986), 'simulations' (Baudrillard, 1988) and 'pseudo-event' character (Boorstin, 1964). Vester (1933) asks to bear in mind that without the touristic commercialisation of cultural heritages many traditions would be already forgotten and 'hence the (re-)invention of culture – which has been criticised as inauthentic – makes the problematisation of its authenticity possible' (ibid.).

The use of the term ayahuasca tourism may indicate a subordination of touristic motives (which must be defined) to the non-local participants of ayahuasca rituals as well as the suppliers. There can be found different definitions of tourism, but the World Tourism Organization (UNWTO) defines tourism as followed: 'Tourism is a social, cultural and economic phenomenon which entails the movement of people to countries or places outside their usual environment for personal or business/professional purposes. These people are called visitors (which may be either tourists or excursionists; residents or non- residents) and tourism has to do with their activities, some of which involve tourism expenditure.' (UNWTO, 2014)

This is a demand-side definition. It mainly refers to the transportation outside the usual environment and the personal or professional motivation of the traveller. The definition exceeds the restrictions to only recreational purposes or visiting relatives or friends. Another definition from the supply-side could be: 'Tourism is a composite of activities, services, and industries that deliver a travel experience: transportation, accommodations, eating and drinking establishments, shops, entertainment, activity facilities, and other hospitality services available for individuals or groups that are traveling away from home. It encompasses all providers of visitor and visitor-related services. Tourism is the entire world industry of travel, hotels, transportation, and all other components that, including promotion, serve the needs and wants of travellers. Finally, tourism is the sum total of tourist expenditures within the borders of a nation or a political subdivision or a transportation-centred economic area of contiguous states or nations' (Goeldner & Brent Ritchie, 2003).

In order to avoid the motivational limitations of a touristic definition of the ayahuasca phenomenon, Tupper (2009) recommended the expression 'cross-cultural vegetalismo' for European and North American who travel to South America in order to consume ayahuasca as well as South American ayahuasqueros who travel in the opposite direction to provide ayahuasca rituals abroad. But this term also has its limitations because not all ayahuasca motivated travellers take part in cross-cultural ayahuasca rituals, but some visitors take part in rituals with North American or European providers or some might drink it alone in their hotel room.

3.3 "Western" ayahuasca users

A wider western audience took notice the first time of ayahuasca with the Yage Letters, published in 1963, from the beat–poets William S. Burroughs and Allen Ginsberg. The letters describe Burroughs search of Yagé from Mexico to South America and are accompanied by other anecdotes. In the end Ginsberg chronicles his own experiments with the brew. Burroughs could be seen as the first known western ayahuasca tourist in history.

Many travellers from Europe and North America seek specifically for this experience. Why do they go for such a long journey, pay a lot of money and have partly unpleasant sensations within the ritual such as vomiting, vertigo, hallucinations and loss of control in a strange environment? This question leads directly to ask for their motivations, underlying working theories about ayahuasca, health and healing concept as well as expectations for the ayahuasca event itself. As Beyer

(2012b, p. 3) mentions that the western ayahuasca seekers differ profoundly from local mestizos and native shamans in their mental concepts and the way in which illness and salutogenesis is perceived. Their etiological and nosological concepts are often based in alternative medicine and popular psychology. They bring their own different assumptions about the healing potential and healing mechanisms of ayahuasca. For locals of the Upper Amazon, diseases are primary not a matter of individual pathology but a relational problem, whereas for the North American and European visitors it is the opposite. Such relational causes could be, e.g. 'the seducer of an unfaithful spouse, the secret dealings of a business rival, the location and nature of the malignant darts within the patient's body' (ibid.). For traditional ayahuasca healers and local patients the visionary potion seems to have been primarily a diagnostic tool to search causes and treatment. Ayahuasca and did not cure directly. (ibid.). In the case of western ayahuasca seekers they often look and find causes of illness through internal attributions, whereas traditionally they are mostly externally attributed (Fotiou, 2012, pp. 7-8). The idea to initiate healing of psychological wounds, cleansing and life changing transformative processes through the ayahuasca experience seem to be common leading themes of the western ayahuasca tourism on both sides, the tourists as well as the supplier. Healing centres often focus on cleansing and transformative therapeutic work and the tourists are prepared in this direction (Fotiou, 2010, p. 239, 241, 259; Beyer, 2009, p. 353; Beyer, 2012b, p. 3).

The motivational factors, which have been identified in previous studies, are presented later in detail, but here it can be said that according to Holman (2010, pp. 8-9) there is traditional, anecdotic and scientific evidences that indicates that in fact ayahuasca can play a helpful role in western psychotherapy, like other mind-altering substances or practices too. 'Though ayahuasca's medical qualities are much celebrated, its visionary effects are central to its appeal' (Hudson, 2011). 'Shamans in the Upper Amazon do not drink ayahuasca to heal; they drink ayahuasca to get information – to screen the disease and search treatment' (Beyer, 2009).

There are also multiple health issues on the touristic use of psychedelic substances. For whom and in which situation is this useful and for whom and in which circumstances not? In a substance supported psychotherapy, the responsible therapist will carefully decide together with his patient if and when the right point in therapy has come to enhance the process. He will consider contraindications. He will accompany the patient before and after the psychedelic or psycholytic experiences and give assistance during the experience. He will medically ensure the right dose and quality of the substance due to his formation, guidelines and official supply for the substance. In the case of shaman tourists, these points are either not controlled or have to be solved individually by the participants through personal information seeking from Internet or laymen. It is interesting to know which kind of psychotherapeutic embedding ayahuasca tourists have.

One hypothesis could point to the differential indication. It seems likely that all kinds of mind-altering experiences such as holotropic breathing, consumption of psychedelic substances, trance inducing therapies are rather difficult for patients with a low level of ego-structure and instability of emotion such as borderline personality disorder or multiple or early traumatization but helpful for patients on a neurotic level with inner conflicts.

3.4 Explicit research on "western" ayahuasca tourists

Some authors seem to have a rather mono-causal perspective on the motivation of western visitors to consume ayahuasca. The seeking for the extraordinary experience, which cannot be provided by their own cultures, has been identified from Marlene Dobkin de Rios (1994) and Grunwell (1998) as the main motivation. Fotiou, who has done culture-anthropologic fieldwork for years around the Peruvian jungle town Iquitos, quotes de Rios with the proposition that 'the empty self … which is soothed and made cohesive by becoming filled up by consuming food, consumer products and experiences' would be the reason for this interest. She responds to it with the comment that 'such a perspective does not leave any room for the possibility that westerners might have meaningful or engaging ayahuasca experiences' (Fotiou, 2010, p. 126). But, she herself sees the common theme behind al kinds of motivations in the general attraction of 'anything that is perceived as the antithesis of western civilisation: pre-industrial, pre-modern, natural, exotic, spiritual, sacred, traditional and timeless' (Fotiou, 2010, ibid.). The attraction to shamanism as an expression of rebellion against the western consumerist culture would be 'traced to modernity, and is consistent with romanticism and Western individualism' (Fotiou, 2010, p. 303). It would contain the misconception that the offered shamanism 'is perceived as ancient and representing a time when people lived in harmony with nature and each other' (Fotiou, 2010, p. 304).

Kristensen (1998) provides a description about ayahuasca and the ritual elements he took part in. He applied a survey to 10 North American ayahuasca tourists who had made the journey (1998, p. 10). For him, it was difficult to access people who are willing to speak about their experiences. The analysis showed four main reasons for the interest in ayahuasca: self-exploration and spiritual growth, curiosity, physical and emotional healing, and the desire for a vacation to an exotic location. The age margin was between 31 and 60 years. All of them were white Americans. The majority had at least a middle-class income and were experienced in self-help or personal growth, meditation as well as other hallucinogenic experiences (ibid,

p. 16). From his own field exploration, he reports that European and North American participants often come with questions of 'personal growth or spiritual nature' (ibid., p. 9) and the shaman struggled with such matters as he was 'accustomed to providing answers to more practical matters such as illness, money, and relationship problems' (ibid, p. 10).

Winkelman (2005) used an ethnographic approach and took part in a 11-day ayahuasca retreat in the Amazonian jungle and conducted 16 informal interviews during the course about motivations and benefits in order to find out whether participants can be described as typical hedonistic motivated drug tourists "or as people pursuing spiritual and therapeutic opportunities." Winkelman mentions that the term 'drug tourism' was brought up by de Rios (1994) and that she described an Amazonian 'charlatan psychiatry' which was invented by no authentic folk healers who 'are common drug dealers dressed for deception' (de Rios, 1994) in order to fulfil the demand for empty-self treatment through hedonistic drug-dilettantism. Winkelman wanted to give an initial empirical answer to this question. Every participant paid around 3000 USD for this two-week event. Their age differed between 27 and 71 years by mean of 44,8 (data from 15 participants). As a principal reason for the participation the wishes for establishing spiritual awareness, relations and personal spiritual development were found. For many of them 'this included emotional healing and, for some, assistance in dealing with substance abuse' (Winkelman 2005, p. 211). Another reason was the desire for personal direction and to engage in a personal evolution. Only one person mentioned hedonistic reasons, i.e. the visual effects produced by ayahuasca (ibid.). The achieved benefits were from the following categories: Self-awareness and personal development, insights into one's life, access to deeper levels of the self and strengthening the higher self (ibid., p. 212). Transpersonal concerns and personal insight and development were reported as main motivational categories as well as benefits. The hypothesis of a general hedonistic drug tourism motivation cannot be maintained for the sample (ibid, p. 215).

In a German qualitative study with 15 Europeans about their self-treatment with ayahuasca, participants it was concluded that their use could be described as 'transhedonistic' rather than hedonistic because they feel confident that it may involve enjoyments but also challenging and unpleasant experiences. Most of the interviewed persons had a very conscious and reflected view on ayahuasca. They understood the ritualized consumption as "inner work" about personal problems. Their healing motivation had often been loaded with religious or sacral aspects. The prevalence of drug use was still higher than the German average but often lowered through the ayahuasca consumption as said in the interviews. Some of the participants had non or almost no pre-experience with psychoactive drugs. They understood the brew as a medicine or sacrament. Ayahuasca was used as an unspecific treatment for a wide range of diseases. The subjective functional theories where mostly psychosomatically or psychologically orientated, enriched with mystical and magical elements. The use of ayahuasca had the purpose of "inner cleaning" and introspective discovering of the true reasons for diseases, which would lie in internal spiritual-psychological matters – even for physical problems. Subjective effects were also unspecifically positive. Within such ritualized contexts, the use of ayahuasca has not increased an uncontrolled handling with other psychoactive drugs nor were subjective health conditions or health behaviour lowered (Schmid, 2010).

Another content analysis study interviewed 21 ayahuasca users in Holland three times between 2003 and 2012) about their motives to consume ayahuasca within the religious context of the Santo Daime Church. Religious and spiritual motives were the most important as well as attempts of self-treatment. Additional motivations were the wish for social interactions and for new and extraordinary experiences through psychoactive substances. 'Hedonistic motives, an intention to improve performance, or motives based on underlying pathologies or disorders were negligible' (Fiedler et al, 2011).

Kjellgren et al. (2009) found in a semi-structured study with 25 anonymous questionnaire responders that ayahuasca-processes derived from retrospective trip reports include the following stages: 1. Motivation and aim (previous the ingestion), 2. Contractile frightening state, 3. Sudden transformation of the experience, 4. Limitless expansive state with transpersonal experiences, 5. Reflections, 6. Changed worldview and new orientation to life. The last feeds back towards stage 1 in the model. They see psychotherapeutic potential.

3.4.1 Types of western ayahuasca users

Attempts have been made to categorize the use of ayahuasca of non–locals. There is the practical three–categories typology of Holman (2010, pp. 187-210), which was distilled from qualitative interviews:

1. Tourists who come to South America with the main purpose of consuming ayahuasca. Other touristic motivations like local culture, nature and people are of minor interest. They usually spend larger amounts of money for their ayahuasca experiences, which they have often planned in advance specifically for this and often stay in the "healing centre" or lodge all the time.

2. Tourists who do not come with the exclusive motivation for ayahuasca. They usually want to travel around and take part in different activities of which ayahuasca is only one besides others. These types are more interested in the experimental experiences than in a specific shaman healing.

3. Tourists who come across the opportunity individually on the street. They are not part of any organized ayahuasca seminar but take part in ayahuasca offers from different shamans.

Schmid (2014, pp. 89-90) describes seven types of European ayahuasca users regarding their motivation:

> '1. Only loosely connected to an ayahuasca network or church, the "event type" uses ayahuasca only occasionally (e.g., often by attending in workshop-like settings or within an organized trip to South America). Often, they only attend a few rituals a year or have only one trip to a "healing camp."
> 2. The "therapy type" is either searching for an alternative cure for a specific medical disease as a complement to scientific medical treatment or for 'Psycholytic therapy" as a complement to classical psychotherapy. Ayahuasca is considered a therapeutic device for all kinds of maladies. When the intended curative effects fail to occur, the therapy types often transform into a spiritual or religious type. Remarkably, when people become more spiritual, they also become healthier.
> 3. The "seeker type" is an individual searching for a philosophy, concepts of identity, or an affirmation of his or her reality. This frequently unresolved search is not limited to psychoactive substances, but may also include meditation, yoga, Buddhism and many other schools of thought. Often a seeker is a postmodern rationalist.
> 4. The "healer type" is often a "gifted" person who thinks of him or herself as having the power and mission to cure or help other people by facilitating ayahuasca sessions for them. This usually happens after they have had a healing experience with ayahuasca or had revelations about their future as a "healer".
> 5. The "spiritual type" is on a search for individual transpersonal or spiritual experiences. The religious type differs from the spiritual one by using ayahuasca within a stable committed community of ayahuasca users, like a church, and is therefore often more willing to accept dogmatic world views.
> 6. The "substance user type" is often experienced with a large number of psychoactive drugs. He consumes ayahuasca in a way that is very similar to his use of other kinds of psychoactive substances (LSD, magic mushrooms, etc.). He may be driven by recreational motives or sheer curiosity.
> 7. Being different is part of the "alternative type", a category that is often an expression of ecological orientation sometimes combined with non-conformist personalities. Often these persons are engaged in activities like saving the rainforest or fighting for the rights of indigenous people.'

4 Spirituality

The term spirituality is often used and widely accepted within the international ayahuasca scenes, but it is often unclear what exactly is meant. (The same applies to the word healing.)

However, there is no generally accepted scientific definition for the word. The term has greatly expanded from a narrow Christian definition throughout recent history. Broad consensus seems to be that spirituality is a rather multi-dimensional construct. It is known that religiosity can be operationalized more easily than spirituality. Both have something in common but are not the same.

Religiosity, for example, can be understood as a personal attitude that is a collective term for religious awareness and behaviour and is mostly geared towards an organized system of beliefs, practice and symbols in order to come near a higher power. Whereas 'spirituality is a personal, meaningful attitude that represents transcendent self-reflection. It may or may not involve religious thinking' (Gisinger et al., 2007).

Typical dimensions recognized as aspects of spirituality are 'the search for meaning and the capacity for self-transcendence (surrender to values and persons); self-acceptance and self-development; positive social relationships; intensive experience of the beauty and sacredness of nature; general oneness (connectedness) with people, nature and the cosmos; connectedness with God (theistic), the Absolute (pantheistic) or a deity (polytheistic); mindfulness and other meditation experiences, premonitions, experiencing "psycho-cosmic energy".' (Grom, 2011, p.15; see also Bucher, 2007; MacDonald et al., 1995; Zwingmann, 2004).

There are structural definitions as well as procedural definitions. The first ones try to grasp spirituality as a cognitive schema (higher power, science, etc.), as abilities (cognitive, intellectual, emotional, behavioural, social), as a system of beliefs and attitudes, or as a personality dimension. The others see spirituality as a dynamic process involving individual behaviour as well as complex phenomena of human development. Spirituality can be understood here as motivation, as a process of self-transcendence, as the search for meaning and goals, as relationship to the sacred and as a process of self-actualization (Skrzypińska, 2014).

© The Editor(s) (if applicable) and The Author(s), under exclusive license to Springer Fachmedien Wiesbaden GmbH, part of Springer Nature 2020
T. J. Wolff, *The Touristic Use of Ayahuasca in Peru*, Sozialwissenschaftliche Gesundheitsforschung, https://doi.org/10.1007/978-3-658-29373-4_4

5 Neo-shamanism

The first contact with American shamanism was made through the European discovery of America and the early knowledge and appraisal was provided from Christian missionaries. Native practitioners were accused of messing with demons or being confused about the devil's influence (Narby & Huxley, 2001, pp.1). European discoverers and merchants described them as jugglers, sorcerers, wizards and conjurers or in other pejorative terms (ibid, p.2). The early Ethnography saw indigenous people as savages and primitives and believed them to belong to inferior societies (ibid., p. 2). Later this general view was challenged and revised by scientists like Frank Boas (*1858 – +1942), Knud Rasmussen (*1879 – +1933) and Claude Levi-Strauss (*1908 – +2009). In the year 1951, Mircea Eliade (*1907 – +1986) published his influential book Le Chamanisme et les techniques archaïques de l'extase (French: Shamanism: Archaic Techniques of Ecstasy). He compared the knowledge about healing practices cross-culturally and described shamanism mainly as a religious phenomenon of Siberia and Central Asia by defining it through its archaic techniques of ecstasy and the shaman's magical flight (Eliade, 1964, p. 5; Morris, 2006, p. 17). But, he also implicitly noted the existence of North and South American shamanism as well as South-East Asian shamanism, Oceania shamanism and Indo-European shamanism (Eliade, 1964, pp. 288-427; Morris, p. 17). The term shaman referred originally to the spirit-mediums of the eastern Siberian Evenki (Tungus) people (ibid, p. 16). Shamanism now is a generalisation and a modern construct.

During the 1970s and 1980s, the US-American author and anthropologist Carlos Aranha Castaneda (*1925 – +1998) became internationally popular for writing best sellers about his alleged field studies about Yaqui Indian esoteric practices and his formation as a shaman. For some years his books were recognized by the academic community but soon rejected as fiction literature (de Mille, 1976; 2000). Nevertheless, his writings had a huge impact. He elated millions for the neo-shamanic practices of self-enhancement and plant psychedelics and is one of the fathers of the neo-shamanism and the New-Age movement. Another important author was Joan Halifax who wrote an anthology about visionary shamanic experiences in her book 'Shamanic Voices – a survey of visionary narratives' (1979). Since the 1960s, the development of neo-shamanism was embedded into the interest for non-western spirituality, the search for existential alternatives, anti-capitalism, the critical distance or avoidance of the institutional Christian religions, environmental protection movement, feminism, human potential movement and drug cultures (Lindquist, 1997, p. 53; Morris, 2006, p.34). Since then, neo-shamanic practices of westerners have often become a syncretic mixture of different esoteric traditions and practices and reflect the personal biography of the search for meaning.

General elements of neo-shamanism are (Lademann-Priemer, 2000):

- Self-healing through the shamanic experience
- Ecological criticism against the modern western society
- Personal spiritual experiences
- The use of techniques of ecstasy
- Self-empowerment

The neo-shamanic scene is not homogeneous in its beliefs, theories and methods. While in Europe, the US-American Michael Harner was one of the central figures. The range seems a bit wider in North America. Harner represented a modern pan-cultural core-shamanism, which would use the same indigenous techniques and would reach the same spiritual sources. The experiences would be real and comparable with those of no-literate cultures. Only the cultural pattern around would differ (Harner, 1990, p. XIV).

Many neo-shamans see themselves in opposition to the main culture and society in which they live. It is often identified as an unhealthy, destructive and alienating environment. They withdraw themselves from this environment, and one of the key motives of neo-shamanism is the reconnection with the nature. Traditional shaman healers were an integrated part of their society, shared with their social environment the cultural consensus of a nature endowed with spirits and wisdom and had a social role, engagement and responsibility within this society.

They seek for individual experiences that provide and integrate the understanding of the ir own person and the world through inner visions and helping forces. Neo-shamanism focuses on the enhancement of well-being, self-actualisation, self empowerment and rapid results. ‚Healing' does not necessarily emphasize the curing of ailments (Morris, 2006, p. 36). Health and disease always have a dimension of a transpersonal sense in this view. One of the main characteristics - that at the same time strongly distinguishes between neo-shamanism and traditional shamanism - is the idea that everybody can be a shaman.

The spirits and power animals tend to be rather benign in neo-shamanism, and there is less engagement in sorcery with malevolent spirits than in traditional shamanism like the one from the Inuit and Evenki people (Jakobsen, 1999, p. 186).

The following statements have been identified as core ideas of neo-shamanism as they have been investigated in Scandinavian New-shamanism circles (Lindquist, 1997, pp. 53-121):

- Individual nature: Every person can have shamanic experiences, but this ability can be hidden because of cultural pattern. It can be rediscovered.
- No-ordinary reality, spirit helpers and power animals: The neo-shaman practitioner seeks for the authentic experience of another reality that lies behind or parallel to the ordinary reality. It contains entities, spirits or ghosts, which can be asked for help. They show themselves, e.g. as power animals. Such animals are associated with certain properties and serve as symbols for it. In opposition to some traditional shaman concepts in which those spirits were known to the whole community, modern neo-shaman power animals are personal and belong to each individual.
- Imagination and spiritual journey: Imagination is used to make the non-ordinary world visible and accessible. The journey often starts with the visualisation of other places that can be entered. Later the imaginations of the journey can be shared as narrative and thus get the character of real personal experience, which has transformative power.
- Healing: Besides the exploration of altered states of consciousness, the shaman also heals and gives advice to the sick person. Spiritual intruders have to be identified and removed, lost power animals and parts of the soul have to be found and brought back.

Neo-shamanism has been criticised as a romantic projection and a European desire for a perfect world or paradise. It would differ strongly from indigenous life and thinking. Parts of neo-shamanism would be steeped in progressive thought and mania of feasibility, even when denied. It would be reduced to its technique for ecstasy and to its market share. It would be a failing attempt to flee western thinking. In ancient tribes, it would have been a burden to be a shaman. People would not have paid to voluntarily enter the spiritual world or to become a shaman themselves. They would rather have paid the shaman for doing this unpleasant and dangerous job. The shamans or healers would have been representatives of their people with a social responsibility for their community. In opposition to that, neo-shamans would experiment for themselves. They would use the native shamanism as a quarry for their individual needs without taking social responsibility (Lademann-Priemer, 2000).

In the western view, the shaman has changed over the decades from being a charlatan, witchdoctor, psychotic and devil-worshipper to a visionary ecologist, mystic and global warrior for the good (Morris, 2006, p. 36).

Criteria for neo-shamanism can be found in samples of ayahuasca tourists as well as the western owners of such healing centres, even if the leader of such group retreats might often be a local person from South America.

6 Historical approaches on DMT

The Amazonian ayahuasca brews are known under many names: caapi, yahé, kaji, mihi, dapa, natema, shuri, kamalampi, pinde, vegetal, daime, hoasca, la purge, etc., but nowadays the most common name is ayahuasca from the northern Quechua language. 72 indigenous groups are known to use ayahuasca, and 42 different indigenous names have been reported (Luna, 1986a,b).

Marlene Dobkin de Rios (1972) states that ayahuasca was widely used by the native people of South America for healing, sorcery, magical and religious reasons and divination. But there is no secured knowledge about a pre-Columbian history of ayahuasca. The outstanding importance of ayahuasca within native medicine in the earlier history was also emphasised by Schultes (1983), when he writes: 'It is true that, in this whole region the "medicines" par excellence – and those which are administered not to the patient but usually to the medicine–man – are the hallucinogens' (Schultes, 1983, p. 140). Several native myths exist, which relate the creation of ayahuasca with the origin of the people (Reichel-Dolmatoff, 1972). What is known for sure is that ayahuasca use was already widely spread when first anthropologists discovered it in the mid 19th century. The old world took notice of American hallucinogenic practices in the 17th century when the Church became concerned about it.

One of the early chroniclers of pre-Columbian religion practices in central Mexico was the cleric, Hernando Ruiz de Alarcón, who wrote his most important 'Treatise on the Heathen Superstitions: That Today Live Among the Indians Native to This New Spain' in 1629. He believed that their healers were talking to the devils, using the psychoactive potion ololiuhqui and the Peyote cactus for diagnosing diseases or witchcraft. The use of visionary plants was forbidden by the Inquisition in 'Edict of Faith concerning the Illicit Use of Peyote' since 1620. There it says:

> 'Being as it is impossible that the said herb and any other herb can have the virtue or natural property that they ascribe to it for the stated effects nor can any herb cause imaginary illusions, phantasms, and other representations in which are based the foundations of such said predictions and divinations, and when using them the person sees them out of suggestion and with the assistance of the devil, the chief author of these vile illusions, who uses them in order to introduce and trick the simple minds of these Indians to their natural inclination toward idolatry and, by the way, deceive many other persons who are little fearful of God and the faith, ... We are obligated by our

office to attack this herb ... we are in agreement to issue this present edict of faith and warn that under the penalty of Major Excommunication ... and many other penalties both physical and corporal that from here onward no person of any status or condition whatsoever can use, grow, or make use of the said herb of Peyote. Nor can anyone use any other herb for the same effects or for any similar effects under any other name, nor should anyone make or order that the Indians or any other person should take this herb or any like it.' (Inquisition in Mexico, 1620).

The Jesuit Franz, Xavier Veigl published 1798 a monograph about his observations and conclusions about the West Amazonian territory where he worked as a missionary. He referred directly to ayahuasca:

'Unter die schädlichen Gewächse darf ich wohl voraus die sogenannte Hayac-huasca, das ist, den bittern Ried, oder vielmehr Strick, setzen, weil man sich dessen einzig zu Aberglauben und Zaubereien bedienet. Dieses Gewächs ist von der Art des schon gemeldeten Bejuco, wächst aber wie ein breites, doch rindenartiges Band, an den höchsten Bäumen hinauf. Die Indier trinken immerzu den daraus (weis nicht mit was Feyerlichkeit) zugerichteten Saft, und kommen dadurch auf einige Zeit völlig von Sinnen.' (Veigl, 1798, p. 189)

Translation: Among the harmful plants I am with no doubt allowed the so called Hayac-huasca, that is, the bitter reed, or rather rope, to place, because one only uses it for superstition and sorcery. This plant is from the kind of the before reported Bejuco, but grows like a wide, yet bark-like belt, up onto the highest trees. The Indians drink incessantly from this (do not know with what solemnity/festiveness) concocted juice, and thus come for some time completely out of senses.

This source shows that the ritualized use of ayahuasca was already common in the Upper Amazonian area, and it had a present role in native societies as Veigl observed it in the 17th century.

From the very early times, archaeological evidences such as snuffing trays, tubes, pottery vessels, vegetable powders show that hallucinogenic plant use was already well established between 1500 and 2000 B.C. in the Ecuadorian region of the Amazon but also relates to other psychoactive substances like tobacco, coca, vilka snuff derivated from Anadenanthera species (McKenna, 1999). Until the present, there is no preserved botanical material or other iconographic evidences, which support the widely-spread hypothesis of the prehistoric history of today's oral ayahuasca practice.

The oldest known snuff trays in South America are made from whalebone and tubes from bird bone. They were excavated by Junius Bird (1943) and Frederic Engel from the central Peruvian costal sides of Huaca Prieta and Asia. Bird himself dated the tray and tube approximately 1200 B.C. (Torres, 1996, p. 298-299). Another evidence for the early ritualistic use of hallucinogenic plants is found in the remains of the pre-Peruvian Chavin culture (1000-300 B.C.). Potions and inhalants made from the mescaline-containing cactus San-Pedro were part of the Chavin culture. Stone figures and decorations at important public places such as the so-called Old Temple of Chavin indicate this importance. Representations of San Pedro are also found on several ceramics from this period. The temple at the costal site of Garagay from approximately 1200-100 B.C. shows two figures which are included in an offering scene, holding a San Pedro spine (ibid. p. 300-301).

The site of Tiwanaku – located in the Bolivian highlands, 30 km south of lake Titicaca – was a centre of the Tiwanaku empire between approximately 500-1000 A.D.. Many highly decorated snuff trays and tubes from this culture have been found as grave goods in the region of this ancient empire. Torres et al. (1991) published a mass-spectrometric analysis, which had been performed on two snuff samples which were found as grave goods for an approximately 45-year-old male at San Pedro de Atacama in Chile. The grave was dated approximately 780 A.D. The snuff samples contained bufotenine (N-dimethyltryptamine), DMT (dimethyltryptamine), and 5-MeO-DMT (5-methoxydimethyltryptamine). Bufotenine suggests that the source of the DMT-containing powder was any of several plants in the genus, Anadenanthera. Small pouches, which contained seeds, have been found in other burials in the Solcor 3 cemetery. They belonged to the same period and 'these seeds have been identified by Schultes as belonging to the genus Anadenanthera' (ibid. p. 644). Snuffing kits were found in several different graves from different sites, which let the authors suggest that snuffing practice of hallucinogens might have been a well-established practice.

Ogalde et al. (2008) used gas chromatography and mass spectrometry on 32 mummified bodies from the Azapa Valley in Northern Chile which belong to the Tiwanaku age. It aimed to identify which kind of psychoactive substances were consumed. They found the first direct archaeological evidence for the hallucinogenic use although it remains unclear whether the intakes took place in a recreational or shamanic setting (medical, psychotherapeutic, religious). The results were also surprising in another way because in opposition to the snuff analysis at San Pedro de Atacama (Torres et al., 1991) none of the 32 hair samples in the Azapa Valley contained 5-MeO-DMT, but two contained harmine. One was from a child, probably one-year-old, and a man, probably 39 years old, who was buried also with a snuffing tablet and had a sclerotic process at his perinasal area. It seems unlikely that the buried child had ingested the detected substances through snuffing although it also had a snuffing kit as grave good. All of this lets the authors conclude that the snuffing kits used in Azapa valley were not related to Anadenanthera. Regarding the harmine findings, they suggest that the possible consumption of the Banisteriopsis vine might have coincided with the snuffing practice in that age in a social differencing manner. Possible explanations are that the use of ayahuasca without the DMT-compound could have been used for its medical purging effect (Beyer, 2012). If Banisteriopsis was imported from rain forest regions, it is likely that the other DMT containing compounds or the ready-made ayahuasca mixture would have been imported too, if this composition would yet have existed in that age. May be the sniffing of Anadenanthera was combined with chewing the ayahuasca vine. This practice is reported of today's Guahibo people (Torres & Replo, 2006, p. 73). Or, it was combined in other ways with the Anandenanthera seeds like the Piaroa people do (Rodd, 2002). Beyer (2012) supposes that this might be the root of the modern ayahuasca practice to combine the vine with other DMT-containing plants, even when the DMT is ingested parenterally. By all these suppositions, the harmine could have come from other sources such as tobacco smoke, well-cooked food, hair dye, snuff from some virola species (ibid.).

Further evidence against the ancient origin hypothesis of ayahuasca: The late Inca Empire never seems to have discovered ayahuasca when it reached the territory of today's Ecuador. There seems to be no traditional ayahuasca practice of the southern highland natives of the Peruvian Andes.

The first European chroniclers never mention ed ayahuasca. Authors from the 16th and 17th century wrote about the snuffing practice of the DMT containing Anadenanthera as well as tobacco. The first written descriptions about ayahuasca are given from the Jesuits, Pablo Maroni 1737 and the above quoted Franz Xavier Veigl 1798 (Brabec de Mori, 2011, p. 32).

6.1 Interest in psychoactive substances and research

6.1.1 Narco-analysis

The first known modern attempts to use mind-altering substances in the psychotherapeutic process were carried out in the Europa of the 19th century with substances like ether, alcohol, chloroform, morphine and hashish. A weakening of the control functions of the brain, the conscious intellect and wilfulness during states of fatigue and anaesthesia was considered to be helpful for the responsiveness for suggestions during the hypnotic state. Hypnoses induced from anaesthesia were found to be deeper than if produced only by means of psychological techniques (Goldscheider, 1892, p. 85). Albert von Schrenck-Notzing (*1862 – +1929) tried the above-mentioned substances and found the cannabis intoxication most of all helpful for the suggestibility, as he describes in his monograph 'Die Bedeutung narkotischer Mittel für den Hypnotismus: mit besonderer Berücksichtigung des indischen Hanfes' (von Schrenck-Notzing, 1891).

In the middle of the 20th century some psychotherapists tried to find more effective ways for hypnosis and psychoanalysis. Classical psychoanalysis uses the technique of free association in which the patient is obliged to express everything that appears in his mind as open as possible, no matter how senseless, embarrassing or frightening it might be. The aim of the narko–analysts was to find a right balance for the patient between disinhibiting sleepiness and the ability for verbal expression. Intravenous injection of barbiturates like Pentothal and Sodium amytal were used to induce drowsiness, which reduced resistance, unlocked speech and emotional abreaction. With narco-analysis, battle neurosis was treated in the middle of the 20th century. Under the influence of these substances, patients were seen giving detailed report of battle scenes with strong emotional expression. At that time the narco-analysts saw evidence for relieved anxiety, removed hysterical symptoms and restored memory (Horsley, 1943).

6.1.2 Psilocybin

Great interest in hallucinogenic plant use arose from the discovery of the practices of Mexican Mazatec healers from the state Oaxaca in the late 1950s. They used fungi from genus Psilocybe for shamanic healing purposes, which contained the strongly-psychoactive substance 3-[2-(dimethylamino)ethyl]indol-4-yl dihydrogen phosphate (psilocybin) and others (Guzman et al., 1998). The indigenous ritual use of those mushrooms dates back perhaps 3000 years B.C. as mushroom stones give evidence (Carod-Artal, 2011). This psychedelic ritual use was first brought to the public in 1957 by Gordon Wasson when he published his famous article 'Seeking the Magic Mushroom' in Life magazine (Wasson, 1957). Psilocybin was isolated and synthesised around 1959 by Albert Hoffmann. During the 1960s, psilocybin was used in experiential research and experimental psychotherapy. Soon those mushrooms became popular among the new age movement of the 1960s and recreational drug users. Many of them went down to Mexico to search for the magic mushroom experience. In the year 1970, psilocybin and 3-[2-(dimethylamino)ethyl]indol-4-ol (psilocin) became a worldwide schedule 1 drug, and the research was handicapped. Recently, there has been a new scientific interest in psilocybin as a research tool and therapeutic agent. It is frequently used in both animal and human research and plays a role in modelling psychosis (Tylš et al., 2013). Its chemical structure is very similar to DMT and the neurotransmitter serotonin.

6.1.3 Mescaline

Artists and writers of the 20th century had been interested in the psychedelic effects of Mescaline, e.g. Aldous Huxley, Antonin Artaud, Henri Michaux and Ernst

Jünger. The use of Mescaline became also popular for the Hippy–movement of the 1960s. Mescaline, 2-(3,4,5-trimethoxyphenyl)ethanamine, is one of the main psychoactive substances of the Peyote cactus (Lophophara williamsii). The plant was unknown in Europa until the German scientist, Louis Lewin, might have brought it from his American journey in the late 19th century. This brought up some scientific interest, and others conducted their own experiments, e.g. S. Weir Mitchell and Ellis Havelock (Mitchell, 1896; Havelock, 1897). Alwyn Knauer and William Maloney were probably the first who saw in hallucinogens the possibility to gain insight into the world of psychotic patients (Knauer & Maloney, 1913). Mescaline was first synthesized in the year 1920 by Ernst Späth (Späth, 1920). Beringer and Roushier published about Mescaline, and since then it was subject of psychiatric interest as a modelling agent for endogen psychosis (Beringer, 1927; Rouhier, 1927). Beringer and others also thought about the possibility of revealing aspects of character through the Mescaline intoxication. This approach could never be fully established as a personality test, probably due to the complex relationship between personality and intoxication experiences as well as the setting, but others saw the same advantages of insights (Bensheim, 1929). Dario Baroni might have been the first therapist who used hallucinogenic substances to enhance psychodynamic admissions when he applied a mixture of Mescaline and thornapple seeds (Datura stramonium) to his psychoanalytic patients (Baroni, 1931; Frederking, 1953, pp. 342-364). Mescaline was tested and used in the concentration camps of Dachau and Auschwitz for manipulative use and interrogation purposes during the so-called 3rd Reich. The US showed interest in the experiments because they also were searching for a truth drug. Some of the Nazi–scientists later made careers in the US, e.g. the founder of the space travel medicine Hubertus Strughold (Lee & Shain, 1985; Bower, 1988; Lifton, 1988; Hunt, 1991; Roth, 2000).

6.1.4 LSD

Albert Hofmann (*1906–+2008), a Swiss chemist, synthesized 9,10-didehydro-N,N-diethyl-6-methylergoline-8β-carboxamide (LSD) from lysergic acid in 1938. Lysergic acid is a natural substance, which can be found in the ergot fungus Claviceps purpurea. He himself accidently discovered the psychotropic effect in 1943 (Hofmann, 2001, pp. 13-34; Passie et al., 2008, p. 295). First, it was presented in the 1950s by Sandoz AG Pharmaceutical Company (Basel, Switzerland) as a pharmaceutical for experimental psychosis and ousted mescaline, which was mainly used for this before. Soon, its value for analytical psychotherapy in loosing mental constrains and the release of unconscious material was emphasised (Hoffmann, 2001, pp. 45-60). The Psycholytic therapy of Hanscarl Leuner was invented during the 1950s. He understood the subjective phenomenology of LSD-intoxication as a symbolic projection of the biographically-shaped psychodynamics of his patients (Leuner, 1959, p. 97 and Leuner, 1962).

During the late 1960s, LSD spread out as recreational and spiritual drug and became fashionable among international student protests and a psychedelic movement started (Lee & Shlain, 1985; Boskin & Rosenstone, 1969, pp. 1-219; Hunter, 1971). Almost worldwide prohibition hardened the human research and practically stopped the therapeutic use – after LSD was restricted or forbidden in most countries, beginning in the middle of the 1960s. The Convention on Psychotropic Substances of the United Nations treaty, signed in Vienna on the 21st of February 1971 by 71 States, restricted most psychedelic substances, including LSD, Mescaline, Psilocybin and DMT as Schedule I drugs (International Narcotics Control Board, 1971, 2015). A few researchers were repeatedly excluded from the proscribing control politics, e.g. Milan Hausner from Prague (Czechoslovakia), who treated patients with Psycholytic therapy until the 1970s (Hausner & Segal, 2010), Jan Bastiaans from the University Leiden (Netherlands), who treated traumatized victims of German concentration camps until 1980s (Bastiaans, 1983) and Hanscarl Leuner from the University Göttingen (Germany) who was able to continue his research until he retired in 1986 (Passie, 1996). Some physicians had permission from the Schweizerisches Bundesamt für Gesundheit (BAG) in Switzerland for Psycholytic therapy with LSD and MDMA from 1988 until 1993 (Gasser, 1996, pp. 59-65). Since the early 2000s, modern research has been done. One of the most important fundraising organisations, which supports international research activities about LSD and other psychedelic substances is the Multidisciplinary Association for Psychedelic Studies (MAPS). The international legal situation of such studies is still difficult and inconsistent.

6.1.5 MDMA and other entactogens

3,4-methylenedioxymethamphetamine is better knows under its synonyms MDMA or ecstasy. It was firstly synthetized in 1912 by the German chemist Anton Köllisch (*1888 – +1916) who never knew what a strong impact his discovery later would have (Benzenhöfer & Passie, 2006; Freudenmann et al., 2006, p. 1244). The first scientific paper about MDMA was openly published in 1960 (in Polish), although military animal studies had been conducted in 1953/1954 in the university of Michigan and were not declassified until the early 1970s (Biniecki & Krajewski, 1960; Freudenmann et al., 2006, p. 1244). Psychotomimetic effects of MDMA were introduced to the scientific community the first time in 1978: 'Qualitatively, the drug appears to evoke an easily controlled altered state of consciousness with emotional and sensual overtones. It can be compared in its effects to marijuana, to psilocybin devoid of the hallucinatory component, or to low levels of MDA' (Shulgin & Nichols, 1978). David E. Nichols et al. (1986) proposed the term entactogen for this type of substances, which differ in their main psychopharmacological profile from hallucinogens or psychedelics and stimulants like amphetamine and methamphetamine. The word is a composed from the roots "en" (Greek: within), "tactus" (Latin: touch) and "gen" (Greek: produce). It empathizes experiences of emotional openness, empathic resonance and communion with others (ibid; Metzner, 1993). MDMA has been considered from the WHO Expert Committee on Drug Dependence to be an interesting substance for further research (WHO Expert Committee on Drug Dependence, 1985, p. 25). The advantage for tpsychotherapy may lie in its property to give the patient an anxiolytic access to normally frightening and blocked content of his mind (Saum-Aldehoff & Trebes, 1994, p. 58). It has been used for psychotherapy since the late 1970s (Stolaroff, 1997; Seymour, 1987; Adamson & Metzner, 1988), but then its therapeutic use was also restricted in 1986. MDMA had become a great illegal fashion drug among the rave dance movement of the 1990s. Nowadays, there have been accomplished investigations with good methodological standards about the potential values and safety of MDMA assisted psychotherapy, e.g. for PTSD (Chabrol & Oehen, 2013; Mithoefer et al., 2010 and 2012). Psychedelic therapy and Psycholytic therapy

There have developed two different approaches to the substance-assisted psychotherapy: Psychedelic therapy and Psycholytic therapy.

The psychedelic approach, which had been common in the USA, started with the observation that high dosages of LSD and relatively few applications could have a profound and overwhelming impact on humans. The British-born psychiatrist, Humphry Osmond (*1917 – +2004), tried to cure alcoholism with LSD, first, to produce aversive episodes of delirium tremens. Soon, he discovered that some of his patients had mystical or religious experiences that might have been responsible for the effect of giving up drinking. In 1957, he proposed the neologism psychedelic from the Greek words for mind and manifest (Tanne, 2004). Together, with the Canadian biochemist and psychiatrist Abram Hoffer (*1917 – +2009), he designed the psychedelic therapy (Hoffer, 1967). During the 1960s and the early 1970s, neurotic patients, alcohol and narcotics addicted patients were treated (Yensen & Dreyer, 1994). Also, patients with illness in terminal states were treated with LSD after psychotherapeutic preparation with the aims to reduce tension, depression, pain and fear of death (e.g. Kurland et al., 1973). Psychedelic therapy uses high doses of psychedelic substances, e.g. 300–800 μg LSD, to enable mystical or transcendental peak experiences that go beyond personal psychodynamic or biographical insight (Gasser, 2008, p. 260). Mystical experiences and existential topics within the therapy can have an important impact on life orientation, values and psychotherapeutic processes, as empirically shown (Griffiths et al., 1967; McGlothlin et al., 2006; Bucher, 2007). In contrast to the below portrayed psycholytic therapy, a good résumé of the psychedelic approach has been provided by Masters & Houston:

> 'When one considers the enormously rich and varied range of experience open to the psychedelic subject, as to Dante, it can only seem wasteful if not destructive to limit the drug-state explorations to psychodynamic factors ... This journey may prove to be also therapeutic, including the remission of some symptom or symptoms, but such a result is incidental and not the aim of the guide as distinguished from the therapeutic worker.' (1966, p. 109)

In the psychedelic setting patients mostly lay down during the acute period exploring their introspective world, often listening to specially selected music (Mithoefer, 2008, p. 206; Verres, 2008, pp. 281-298; Grof, 1980) and with closed eyes or with covered eyes. During the acute phase, there is only minimal or no verbal communication with the therapist (Styk, 2008, p. 310) but usually the verbal support increases when the acute phase finishes and if necessary (Mithoefer, 2013). A detailed discussion of the experiences immediately after the acute phase is often not recommended because the experience itself is seen as transformative or curative agent and a process of integration shall not be disturbed through a possible intellectualization. Therapeutic post processing in additional talking sessions has been mentioned to be important for the integration of the insight and emotional changes into everyday life (Mithoefer, 2008, pp. 207-208). Often, there is a suggestive verbal preparation phase before the actual ingestion. Body–psychotherapeutic support can be applied during the session to release muscle tensions if needed (ibid., pp. 206–207). Often, the therapeutic process theory is orientated in the Transpersonal psychology or sometimes considered not to be important because the rather non-predictable existential experiences cause the therapeutic effect, not the interaction with the therapist. He remains as protector of the setting, supporter, attendant and sometimes psychotherapeutic midwife (Passie 1997, Mithoefer, 2013, Gasser, 2008).

The Czech-Slovakian-born psychiatrist, Stanislav Grof, had great influence. He connected psychoanalytic ideas about regressive access to early and repressed material with transpersonal and spiritual ideas about perinatal memories and access to the collective unconscious through the psychedelic method. He developed his own theoretical system of perinatal matrices through which he interprets the symbolic psychedelic material (Grof, 1976). The term transpersonal is often used for psycho-techniques that would enable 'experiences in which the sense of identity or self extends beyond (trans) the individual or personal to encompass wider aspects of humankind, life, psyche or cosmos' (Walsh & Vaughan, 1993). Recent research from Mithoefer et al. about MDMA assisted therapy uses a version of the psychedelic therapy method (Mithoefer, 2013).

The Psycholytic therapy uses smaller dosages of psychoactive substances than Psychedelic therapies – to induce a light dreamlike but conscious state in which the patient can gain introspective access to memories, repressed inner conflicts and emotions. This would enhance the psychodynamic therapy because it would bring the psychic content much faster to the psychotherapeutic elaboration than with conventional techniques like free association and dream analysis. Hanscarl Leuner (*1919 – +1992), the founder of the Psycholytic therapy in Germany, wrote, that 'the overwhelming clinical evidence suggests that psychodynamics, which have been activated through LSD, are better available for the psychotherapeutic influence than without a certain level of hallucinogens in the blood' (Leuner, 1981, p. 92, translated). In the early 1950s, he started to evoke mental images into his patients systematically with a guided daydream technique to enhance the access to preconscious and emotional material. The technique was introduced in Germany mainly under the term Katathymes Bilderleben (Guided Affective Imagery). In the middle of the 1950s, he started to use LSD and other substances to intensify therapeutic processes. The other influence, which led to the Psycholytic therapy was the psychiatrist, Sandison. He found substantial recovery in neurotic patients after single submission of LSD (Sandison, 1954). Psycholytic therapy is routed in the psychoanalytic paradigm and its ego-psychological branch. It focuses on analytical talks about the substance-facilitated experiences under the view of transference and resistance and its meaning and integration into everyday life. The aim is restructuring of the personality through maturing and untying of infantile bindings. Psycholytic therapy uses between 5 and 50 sessions. It claims to treat neurosis, psychopathia, Borderline personality disorders and psychosomatic disorders (Passie, 1997). If transpersonal or mystical content appeared, this was a sign to reduce the dosage to focus only on the personal and biographical content. There have been aspirations to combine both in a Psychedelytic aproach (Yensen, 1994, pp. 191-202; Benz, 1989; Gasser, 1996, pp. 59-65). The Psycholytic approach has also been criticised. The regressed material, which was released during therapy sessions, would have been extremely sensitive to the analytic orientation of the therapist. Positive outcomes and the observed phenomena might have been caused by 'the presence of heightened powers of suggestibility' (Grob, 1994).

7 Phenomenology of psychedelic experiences

7.1 Psychotoxic base-syndrome

The psychotoxic base-syndrom from Hanscarl Leuner describes psychic functions regarding the multiple phenomena of hallucinogenic intoxication.

- Light ontogenetic regression of intellectual functions and emotions
- Qualitative Protophatic change of consciousness (Conrad, 1960)
- No loss of quantitative consciousness
- Activation of imagination with perceptional character
- Enhancement of internal stimulus production with a non-specific affective activation of sensory functions, especially regarding the optical sense.

Protophatic change of consciousness means that Gestalt qualities are dreamlike disconnected and released so that 'not humans and landscapes are experienced but only their Gestalt qualities, from which all imagery of dream results' (Leuner, 1962, p. 40). A slightly reduced consciousness lets Gestalt qualities become more evident.

From the outside, it appears like a syndrome of passiveness: Reduced activity of the Ego, regression from the surrounding, loss of a sense of reality and constriction of the perception into a few but intensively experienced items. Leuner emphasised that on the one hand, there can be found a functional regression and reduction of abstract, purposeful and highly subtle thinking and a decomposition of the field of experience, which results in qualitative protophatic changes. A withdraw from the surrounding reality and a turning inside towards the intensified, vivid and dreamlike qualities. On the other hand, he described an activation of internal sensorial production and affectivity that leads to increased emotionality, banked ideas and delusions (Leuner, 1962. pp. 30-42).

Leuner (1962) found two basic forms of the LSD-process: the continuous-scenic form and the stagnant-fragmentary form.

The first one is characterized by scenic imaginations with closed eyes, which sometimes have a movie-like quality. Those scenes are occupied with emotion and personal sense. They flow continuously with the time. Optical content is seen as

© The Editor(s) (if applicable) and The Author(s), under exclusive license to
Springer Fachmedien Wiesbaden GmbH, part of Springer Nature 2020
T. J. Wolff, *The Touristic Use of Ayahuasca in Peru*, Sozialwissenschaftliche Gesundheitsforschung, https://doi.org/10.1007/978-3-658-29373-4_7

psychic projection related to the personal biography. The internal partition in the experience and the cognitive reflection remains.

The second form emerges normally with higher dosage. Content and emotion are dissociated as well as the continuity or understandable logic of the chronology or sequence of the content. Emotional sprinklings, which seem not to have any connection to the content, can appear. Imaginations are disconnected without understandable relations to each other. The extreme form of defragmentation of the experience can lead to a catatonic-like state. The person has no remaining Ego-residue, which would be able to reflect with a certain distance about the experience.

7.2 Stages of the inebriation syndrome of H. Leuner

Hanscarl Leuner tried to modulate the intensity of the therapeutic LSD-psychosis in order to keep it as far as possible inside a moderate level in which a reflecting residual Ego would be able to communicate with the therapist. He found that the intensity and the progressive form of the inebriation differ strongly even with the same dosage and the same person. It also depends on other factors than simply the dosage: constitutional and functional disposition and the psychological or affective starting position (Leuner, 1962, p. 75-76). He found the following stages:

0. Starting position, ordinary consciousness

1. Explorative stage: This is the transitional stage of the increasing or declining effect of the intoxicant or of a low 'pre-psychotic dosage' (ibid., p.75.). Symptoms are: sustained state of consciousness, up-scaled mood, loos e associations, increased talkativeness, increased emotional fragility, sometimes sensorial hyper sensibility. There is often, but not always, insight into the affective changes.

2. Oneiroide stage (ονειρική κατάσταση, Greek: dreamy state): Syndrome of passivity, increased detachment, hyper sensibility against all senses, turning away from the surrounding, dreamlike illusions or other psychotic experiences demand the attention, reduced purposeful thinking, which can be restored with effort. The state of consciousness is slightly reduced but can be restored with effort, dependent on the depth of the inebriation state. The psychosis can be briefly disrupted by apperceptive focussing on the surrounding. Habituation reduces the slight disorders of consciousness.

3. Extreme psychotic stage: Consists of strong oneiroid, slightly-lowered consciousness under LSD and Psilocybin (less under mescaline), together with

unpleasant psychotic manifestations up to deep confusions and delirium. With middle dosages this stage was seldom and transient.

4. Confusion: In this stage, there are strong psychotic symptoms or a full delirious state with the loss of communication to the outside world. If the consciousness is functional, the person is totally occupied. Without any residual Ego, the person has no understanding of the artificiality of this state. Here, Leuner sees no difference any more to a severe endogen organic psychosis regarding the strength of the symptoms.

7.3 Progressive phases of the inebriation syndrome

Leuner (1962) found five different phases of the LSD intoxication:

1. Start-up phase: It starts around ½ hours after ingestion and has an explorative character. 15–60 min later vegetative symptoms indicate the beginning of phase two.

2. Oneiroid-psychotic main phase: All symptoms of the stages 1, 2 and 3 can be experienced. The highest point is reached around 3 hours after ingestion. Phase two lasts 3–5 hours, dependent on the dosage. Between the second and forth hour the most intense experiences take place. The intensity of the inebriation and outside world attention fluctuates. For LSD, the end of phase two often comes abruptly with disillusionment. The patient seems consciously clearer, exhausted and often wants to report his experiences.

3. Onoiroid after-phase: Then, a less deep dreamlike phase of 4–5 hours follows with the stages two or three. The patient is now able to continuously report his experiences. He also can resist against unpleasant content through deflection and withdrawal of his attention to the outside world. In the end, there is increased talkativeness with loos associations and affective fragility. The talkativeness can conceal the affective fragility and the still present thought disorders.

4. Explorative phase: It can last for 6 up to 10 hours with stages one and two. Sometimes there are some sprinklings of stage 3, but the patients are inconspicuous.

5. Late phase: It can last one or two days; sometimes longer. Aftereffects like isolated oneiroid episodes or fluctuations of the affective state have been reported as well as slight limitations in abstract thinking, but the patient is able to live his

normal life. Sometimes there are isolated effects some weeks after the LSD session (Leuner, 1962, pp. 76-77).

7.4 Depth stages of the psychedelic inebriation of Masters & Houston

In 1966, Masters and Houston published their book 'Varieties of Psychedelic Experiences'. There they describe a model of four levels of the psychedelic experience. The empirical base were observations from 206 drug sessions with LSD and Mescaline and another 214 interviews with experienced persons over more than 15 years (Masters & Houston, 1966, p. 2). Their four-stage-model is marked as explicitly relevant for the therapeutic guidance or assistance of psychedelic experiences (ibid., pp. 108-113). On every stage, the most predominant phenomena are described although others from other stages may also be present. The model likely focuses on experiences of North American recipients and does not take into account ethnological perspectives on different regions and different cultural customs, expectations and experiences of psychedelic drug use.

1. Sensory stage: This level dominates in early stages of the psychedelic experience and sometimes later too, if deeper levels are not reached. It consists of 'altered awareness of body and body image, spatial distortions and a wide range of perceptual changes' (ibid., p. 108). Temporal orientation may be altered, and with closed eyes one may experience 'a succession of vivid eidetic images brilliantly coloured and intricately detailed' (ibid., p. 108). If one tries to preserve the normal categories of orientation or resists against the 'psychedelic flood' (ibid., p. 108), this might lead to unpleasant moments. Here the therapeutic guide has to 'steer the subject along the course of gradual intensification and expansion of consciousness' (ibid., p. 108). E.g., the guide might suggest to discover and explore the colours and dimensions of some simple and familiar objects like see shells, flowers, stones, music. He helps direct the attention to focus on friendly and harmonious relational aspects. 'He may cut a door in a green pepper and direct the subject to open it and look inside at the glorious cathedral now revealed' (ibid., p. 108). The use of carefully selected music has been described as helpful. As an intervention example of this stage, Masters and Houston describe a therapist who created a sense of wonder and revelation by placing simply flowers and vegetables in front of the patients and giving the instruction to 'enter into friendly or harmonious relationship with them' (ibid., p. 108). With positive rapport, she put Beethoven's Pastoral Symphony on the music player, and an 'euphoric intermingling of sight, touch, smell and sound' appeared (ibid., p. 108). When the symphonic climax arrived she slowly peeled back the husks of an ear of corn. By this, patients experienced botanical empathy and witnessed a mystery. The guide can use the

responses to sensory stimuli to lead the subject beyond the trivial activity of sensory observation. For the subject, the sensory experience can be a vehicle for 'meaningful consideration of his place in the world' (ibid., p. 109) and lead to deeper levels of the psychedelic experience.

2. Recollective-analytic stage: After the sensory realm with the emphasis on altered perceptions, the subject normally proceeds with the recollective-analytic stage. This level is characterized through deepened immerged thinking about personal problems, relationship problems and life goals. Past experiences are lived through with accompanying emotions. Sometimes cathartic abreaction takes place. Some material of the psychedelically enforced ideation is not accessible under normal conditions. Associations are loosened which gives space for alternative references, new perspectives and logical connections as well as creative connections of the material. It can be accompanied by eidetic images and memory. Images tend to illustrate and clarify the thought content. The material is sifted, analysed and ordered. In this stage, the subject may be able to get a new clear perspective of his life problems and what is needed to solve them.

For long periods, the guide will remain silent not to interrupt the internal processes. In some cases, the guide will intervene and suggest another direction or help to get a new perspective on persistent (self-)destructive ideas. Sometimes subjects become stuck in circular ruts of insignificant content or no longer useful themes. Then, the guide will interrupt and assist in directing the subject. The therapeutic role is more or less an accompanying one, with few suggestions of new dimensions of experiences and some possible new interpretations. Little unconscious mimic or gesture expressions and moods in the guide may be of great interpretative relevance to the subject in this state. That's why a warm and open awareness should be maintained by the therapeutic companion. Sometimes subjects assume that the accompanier is equally sensitized, and that telepathic communication takes place and that verbal communication is no longer necessary, or they think that longer verbal interactions had taken place were there were no such communication. Masters and Houston believe that great insights are possible on this level, which can be sufficient for the revision of thinking, self-image and behaviour but greater gains would be possible 'when the subject uses tins level to effectively formulate his problems and goals and then "carries" this material "down" with him to the experimental level and stage of descent we have termed the symbolic' (ibid., pp. 109-111).

3. Symbolic stage: According to Masters and Houston around 40 % of their participants reached this stage. Here the subject participates in historical, mythic, ritualistic and archetypal scenes. He may process his personal topics on trans-personal symbolic stages and may experience himself beneficially in continuity with

historical and evolutionary processes. The subject often witnesses this by means of eidetic images. Myths, legends, initiation and rituals often are surprisingly conforming to the most urgent needs of the participant. Strange landscapes, architectures and creatures can be seen. The person may fully experience a particular ritual or identify himself with a legendary figure that has similar aspects to main features of his life as personal allegory. The guide helps him to find his way through 'ever more complex and more personally significant realms of symbolic experience until the subject is able to participate directly and wholly in those dramas that will be most beneficial to him' (ibid., p. 162). All these figures seem not to have any symbolic or psycho-dramatic meaning until they are 'recruited as players in the subject's personal drama' (ibid., p. 162). In this stage, there may be seen main differences between, on the one hand, the psychedelic work (in the narrow sense psychotherapeutic work), which reaches out to the participation and completion of the personal symbolic drama, and, on the other hand, the shamanic work, which would invite or convince such figures from the "other word" to give information, protection or to do healing actions for the client. For the psychedelic or psychotherapeutic use of those substances, the direct participation and emotional response to the mythic re-enactment is seen as the premise for the descending to the deepest level, the integral state (ibid, p. 111).

4. Integral stage: Ideation, images, body sensations and emotions are fused, resulting in a sense of full self-understanding, self-transformation, religious enlightenment and mythical union. Experience of Ground of Being, God, mystery, essence, fundamental reality and noumenon have been reported. The experience is sufficiently self-validating that there is left no doubts to the subject about its authenticity. Only around 5% of the cases observed by Masters and Houston reached this psychedelic level. When experienced it was always regarded as religious by the subjects. According to Masters and Houston, the integral psychedelic state of unity typically last from fifteen minutes to two hours and occasionally up to four hours (ibid., pp. 113). All subjects who reached this peak experience were well prepared, had exceptional self-understanding, usually through hard previous effort, and were fully functional in life. Self-damaging behavioural patterns seemed to have been 'effaced, cut through or overlaid in a kind of imprinting or re-imprinting process' (ibid., p. 113). The intense affect, which accompanies such experience, would lead to 'a lasting positive integration of the restructured psychical organization' (ibid., 113). Masters and Houston lament the lack of scientific language for the description of such phenomena like "transformation," "self-understanding," "illumination", "realization of potentials". After such experience, the subject usually has no desire for any new psychedelic experience in the near future. Masters and Houston report enthusiastically as after-effects: strengthened, energized, made more serene, creative and spontaneous, heightened sense of being in harmonious relation with

other persons and with things, sharpened perceptions with a consequent enhancement of aesthetic response to a wide variety of stimuli, bettering of mirror image and body image, subjective feeling of light and better coordination, generally more fit. The therapeutic advice in such cases is to stop at the sill of the integral stage and let the person experience this unique moment of intensity in private. The therapist does not interrupt or interfere but bears witness to the culmination of this process from outside (ibid., pp. 111-113).

The question about the transferability of this model from LSD and Mescaline to the therapeutic use of ayahuasca has not yet been empirically and systematically answered, but its practical value for psychedelic processes seems obvious for now.

7.5 Basic Perinatal Matrices and depth stages after Stanislav Grof

Stansislav Grof, who is one of the most recognosed representatives of the Transpersonal Psychology, has worked therapeutically with LSD before he developed the Holotropic Breathwork. He proposed a similar classification. But his model has some major additional presumptions, which make it very controversial. According to Grof, only after the overcoming of the sensory barrier, psychodynamic content emerges into the consciousness. This corresponds to the concept of the individual unconsciouness as well as to the recollective-analytic level of Masters and Houston (1966). Grofs transpersonal stage beyond the psychodynamic level corresponds largely to the symbolic and integral level of Masters and Houston. But he leaves the purely descriptive field and lets the experiencing person transcend beyond the boundaries of time and space. The connecting door to this transpersonal area would be, according to Grof, four perinatal memory matrices, which correspond to the process of childbirth. In verbal and artistic material from LSD inebriations Grof identified and distinguished those matrices of birth phases as well as corresponding basic traumatic experiences:

- Basic Perinatal Matrix: BPM I (amniotic universe and primal union with mother organism)
- Second Perinatal Matrix: BPM II (cosmic engulfment and no exit or hell)
- Third Perinatal Matrix: BPM III (the death-rebirth struggle)
- Fourth Perinatal Matrix: BPM IV (the death-rebirth experience)
(Grof, 1976)

The model is widely not accepted by the academic psychology and medicine but has influence among the alternative psychotherapy scene and protagonists of the Transpersonal psychology.

7.6 Transphenomenal dynamic control systems

The content of psychedelic and psycholytic experiences vary highly. Attempts have been made to give sense and order to the emerging material. For this purpose, Hanscarl Leuner created his Transphenomenal Dynamic Control Systems (German: Transphänomenale Dynamische Steuerungssysteme – tdySt), which are partly rooted in the psychodynamic paradigm and the school of Gestalt-psychology. He refers to Herbert Silberer (1909, 1912) when he understands the characteristics of the scenic experience and symbolism under the hallucinatory state and to Julius Varendonck (1922) when he connects the altered state of consciousness with the pre-conscious delirious thinking. He also refers to Ludwig Frank (1927) who found a connection of spontaneously arising imaginations in processes of emotional abreaction. Another source of Leuners ideas is the psychology of Kurt Lewin (1926). Lewin postulated 'a great number of relatively separate strained systems stand side by side but are only rarely and usually imperfectly able to relax. They are energy reservoirs of action and without their relative degree of separation an ordered action would be impossible' (Lewin, 1926, p. 25). This system of parallel strained arcs of suspense would not push necessarily for resolution and completion, as Sigmund Freud believed, but form the basic matrix of attention and consciousness (Lewin, 1911). Leuner saw the function of symbolization as a basic mental ability for all spontaneous mental imaging operations. This ability would shape the environment pictorial-physiognomically and retroactively form itself. In opposition to Freud he believed that symbolic imaging would not automatically point towards pathology, regression and the defence mechanism of repression. The emerging content of thoughts, emotions and sensations can be seen as results of a continuing process of projective auto-symbolic self-portraying. They are symbols which illustrate the inner soul state in a rather pictorially and physiognomically way (Leuner 1962, p. 111). During crisis this ability of the normal would lack control and override. There the symbolic expression can calm down pathologic arousal or hinder quick depletion which might take place from biological regressive saturation processes (ibid., p. 111). The psycholytic therapy enhances and uses this ability: 'We gain the phenomenological access from mental imaging processes (Kretschmer) and their experimental steering (Leuner), which are placed at the service of psychodynamic processes' (ibid., p. 2).

The postulated mental strain systems are the basis of auto-symbolic processing. Inner-psychic states do not express themselves directly but are represented vicariously through the changing flow of pictures and scenes (ibid., p.119). The inner state, which expresses itself symbolically, has a transphenomenal property, that means it directs the experience from beyond the emerging and disappearing pictures. This model separates the persisting unconscious transphenomenal systems from its conscious symbolic expressions. Their biographically formed cores are emotional and tensional, and they drive and colour the flow of the experiences. Through the enforced stimulus production under the psychedelic or psycholytic inebriation a transphenomenal dynamic control system activates and determines the corresponding symbolic expressions, biographical and emotional material and transference phenomena. This process of expression would – according to Leuner – lead to an energetic discharge of the determining control system so that it loses its power and another control system can take its place. This principle of operation of the psycholytic therapy works the best under a medium dosage so that the patient is still able to experience and realize the relaxation of the control systems after its discharge.

7.7 Systems of condensed experience

Another but similar system has been developed by Stanislav Grof: A system of condensed experience is a constellation or network of experiences from different ages but with similar topic and emotions. As connecting factors, he sees the quality of the emotion and sometimes the accompanying body feelings. The associated memories would be organized around a root or nodal experience. Depending on the strength or imprint of the root experience and the number and strength of subsequent reinforcing experiences such a system could influence the attention, perception and further processing of new stimuli and information. By this they influence thinking, feeling, expression and communication and affect motivational and decision-making processes of attraction and avoidance, emotional responses, opinion, physical reactions and behaviour. Under normal conditions COEX-systems would be well organized or supressed in a way that enables the person to function in every day life. There is an infinite variety of possible trigger stimuli for the activation of a COEX-system. Most of them would be idiosyncratic and would emerge when the organism focuses on particular aspects of the experience. Every person has a greater number of COEX-systems with pleasant or unpleasant touch. The psychedelic therapy or other ASC techniques would weaken the supressing organisation of COEX-systems so that corresponding elements such as associations, scenes, symbols, episodic memories of the activated COEX-system would appear and accessible to processing and integration. If not disturbed, this process would continue until the core of the COEX-system is reactivated, experienced with its corresponding emotions and body reactions and until it is integrated. After that, the COEX-system loses its leading function and another system would dominate the experience field (Grof, 1976).

8 Ritual elements that influence psychedelic experiences

Ritual and ceremony are used synonymously in this research for practical reasons. They can be defined ‚as a formalised symbolic procedure, which has subjective and cultural meaning and transcendental aspects.' (Presser-Velder, 2012, p. 13), although other definitions exist. The traditional use of ayahuasca has been socially embedded into rituals and their corresponding belief systems.

8.1 Set, setting and substance

Different persons can experience very different effects in strength and content, regarding to the same dosage of a hallucinogen. The same person under different conditions or from session to session can experience a great content variety (Leuner, 1987, pp. 151-161). Set and setting are non-pharmacological factors (Zinberg, 1983, pp. 256-266). Set, setting and substance have varied throughout different cultures and times. Depending on the social and historical context and the psychological state the same psychoactive substance might have different effects (Zinberg, 1986).

The setting variable has been described in general as the situation in which the treatment takes place (Hess, 2008). The following elements can be considered as parts of the setting.

Table 1: Synopsis of setting elements in substance supported psychotherapy from different authors (adapteded and modified from Abegleen, 1996; Leuner, 1987; Metzner, 1994; Hess, 2008)

Setting elements	Examples
Social context and surrounding context	Perceived social roles
	Perceived mutual expectations
	Communicated taboos or no-go
	Economical arrangements (Who has paid whom and how much?)
	Number of participants and their perceived mutual behaviour
	Perceived social and economical relations between participants and the provider
	Language and cultural differences between the persons involved
	Private and individual care or mass session
	Level of privacy
	Level of strangeness of the surrounding environment, nature and sounds
Atmospheric elements	The location (healing centre in the nature, clinical study in a hospital, private trial in a hotel room or at home)
	Room arrangements
	Light design
	Qualities of the personal place
	Distances and height differences between participants and therapists
	The use of music
	The use of fragrance
	The use of atmospheric objects like flowers, etc.
Provider	Behaviour and appearance of the therapist, staff and communication with the therapist
Treatment and ritual	The action and sequence of the treatment

Another possible classification of setting elements was adapted from Hess (2008, pp. 265-280). His perspective comes from the European psycholytic therapy branch of substance supported psychotherapy. He does not only provide a list of setting aspects but also discusses advises for their handling. The following table has been complemented with some considerations about ayahuasca therapy:

Table 2: Classification and considerations of setting elements in substance supported psychotherapy and ayahuasca ceremonies (adapted and extended from Hess, 2008)

Setting elements	Examples and considerations
Receptive or active	In the quiet introspective experience of a MDMA-supported laying down therapy setting it is likely that emotionalized biographical material emerges. But ecstatic dancing under the same substance (here called Ecstasy) to loud rhythmical monotone music in a disco mass event (Rave-party) will bring up resource orientated material and interpersonal material like e.g. sense of community or isolation feeling.
Single, group or pair setting	In beginning of the psychedelic and psycholytic therapy, sessions took place in single settings with one therapist and one patient, similar to the classic psychoanalytic therapy. Sometimes problematic were the strenuous long periods of time and the intense intimacy that enforced transference processes. In South America, local ayahuasca therapy often takes place in the community or relative public of a group. In the Northwest-European influenced culture, the participation of the public in psychotherapy, healing or psychedelic experience is socially not accepted, because psychotherapy is often considered an individual matter, not infrequently associated with a private blemish or at least a personal optimising process. In Peru, ayahuasca sessions for non-local clients provide a compromise between the publicity of a group setting and the individual privacy of the psychedelic process within the participant. In Peru, this compromise is fostered by ayahuasca group ceremonies typically conducted in complete darkness.

	The setting of H. Leuner's *Psycholytic therapy* solved the problems of the single setting through a combination of a group phase in the beginning, a single setting phase with an accompanying "sitter" and another closing group phase. This helped reducing the problematic transference and made it more economic. The Group setting of the SÄPT (Swiss Association for Psycholytic Therapy) also tries to provide a relative individual privacy for the internal processes within a beneficial group setting.
Time frame, bio-rhythm	The time frame for a therapy session depends strongly on substance and its intoxication time as well as the "afterglow" and recuperation time. LSD needs at least one day and MDMA half a day. In terms of side effects, the MDMA use in the morning seems better for so called "morning persons" and its use in the afternoon better for "night persons". The therapeutic use of LSD, and MDMA is mostly done during daytime but Psilocybin, Mescaline and ayahuasca have been consumed traditionally at night in the South Americas. An advantage might be that there is less disturbance and distraction at night time. Also, the release of melatonin during night time may support the visionary work. Colourfull lucent as well as soft and blurred visions with open eyes contrast better in the darkness and are better perceived. The night is associated with ghosts and spirits and the fear of the unknown.
Location	According to Hess, traditional rituals with psychedelic substances often taken place at special locations, e.g. holy or distinctive places in the nature. Such settings can provide a frame to the individual, which helps relativizing, transcending and integrating personal problems into a wider context, opens up the view for alternative perspectives and reconnect with the holy and beauty of the existence.

	In Peru, many of the ayahuasca healing centres, focussed on North American and European and urban clients, are situated in lodges close to nature and emphasise an aesthetic traditional or semi-traditional architecture, which is associated with native cultures.
	For the psychedelic and psycholytic therapies, it is essential to provide a quiet and safe location without any disturbances from the outside since clients might be very sensible and irritable in this particular state.
	Single settings with a biographic focus often would not make it necessary to seek such exclusivity of the location. Psychedelic terminal care for patients with incurable illness is best situated in a single setting at home of the patient, if medically possible.
Conducting guide	Intense processes in big therapy groups need more than one therapist. A male and a female therapist are an ideal combination. The task sharing between the guides should be clear.
	Strongly disordered patients need very formal or ritualized sequences for their participation. This has to be discussed with them before.
	Ayahuasca ceremonies often follow a ritualized sequence.
	South American mestizo ayahuasca therapists often wear special ritual costumes when working with western clientele. Systematic research about the costume habits of ayahuasca healers, working with local or foreign clients, have not been conducted yet.
Music and silence	Psychedelic and psycholytic therapists often use music to prepare and support the inner processes. The use of music should follow the stages of the substance effect as well as the individual process of the client. It should not try to evoke particular emotions or memories but support the autonomous process of experience.

	In order to work focussed on special topics the use of particular music pieces is better done in a single setting. An example is the LSD-therapy for victims of Nazi-concentrations camps that has been conducted in Holland (Bastiaans, 2000). Hess suggests not using a fixed musical preset or discography but prefers a flexible use of music. If available, he chooses life music, that he adapted from the receptive music therapy with various instruments like monochord, overtone singing, tanpura, drum, digeridoo, gong and silence. With 7 process stages the suggested music and instruments are oriented in Stanislav Grof's birth stages. Unlike Grof, he does not reject entirely the use of songs and vocal music. Only in the most intense stages or at high dosages words would confuse. In the syncretic *Santo Daime* Church, participants sing religious vocal hymns during the entire ayahuasca ceremony. They also perform synchronised dance movements in the group. As mentioned, ayahuasqueros frequently sing or whistle special songs called *ícaros* (Quechua) during their healing rituals. They are often used purposefully for protection, to guide the psychedelic process of the client (attune and finalise the ceremony, intensify or diminish visions, enforce purging, etc.), exorcism, summon healing spirits, conduct "healing energy" to the patient.
Further arrangements	Aroma, fragrance oil or incense have been used in different ritual cultures to mark a sacred space. The sense of smell can be subjectively intensified under psychoactive substances.

	Fragances can be helpful to modify persistent unpleasant psychedelic items. They can change the emotional atmosphere of the perceived psychedelic visual world. They frequently used in traditional ayahuasca ceremonies.

Substance supported psychotherapy could encourage the use of special clothing to mark the importance of rituals of transition or special phases. In western cultures, which emphasize individualization and individual development a uniform dress for the ritual group does not seem to be useful. Brazilian ayahuasca churches use uniforms.

A very sensible topic is the use of symbols. Due to the intensified symbolic mental production every detail of the perceived location can become of special importance or meaning for the participant. That is why many psychedelic and psycholytic therapists abstain from any religious symbolism.

In contrast to the ayahuasca therapy, which often claims to be related to the ancestral past of the native Amazonian heritage, modern substance-supported therapy does not have a continuous tradition from which it could take its symbols and arrangements. Here the artistic dimension replaces the traditional. |
| Substance specific arrangements | LSD, psilocybin, mescaline and other hallucinogens intensify the perception and imagination. Intensive body-psychotherapeutic work like holding, pressing, giving resistance, etc. can enrich the process as well as the perception of the nature. |

	MDMA and its analogs enable the intense contact with the self and biographic topics, if the setting is appropriate. Music and photos from the biography, partners and family members can be used for this work. These substances reduce the differentiated perception of music and reduce the perception of pain. The skin contact is intensified, and a gentle touch might be more efficient than intense bodywork. After the most intensive phase it is useful to contact the person and encourage the reflection on the experiences of the session in order to avoid an unpleasant or unproductive drifting-into-the-nothing-experience.

Practitioners of psycholytic and psychedelic therapy give a lot importance to setting variables, as Benz (1989) has shown in an interview study. The common ground of their therapies is characterized through a continuous care in a group therapy setting with alternating meditative silence, music and interaction with therapists and other group members. In the naturalistic environments of touristic and local ayahuasca sessions the setting is also often carefully designed because the social and suggestive setting compounds seem to be a most important and integrated part of the ayahuasca phenomenon. An isolated intake of ayahuasca without the shamanic social context would be unusual and not common in South America. The contemporary traditional and semi-traditional ayahuasca use is accompanied by a number of specific setting elements. They vary from centre to centre, from shaman to shaman and from the supply for locals or foreigners but often have substantial mutuality:

- The use of íkaros (personal vocal healing songs, sung by shamans throughout the Amazonas basin) or other forms of music during the session
- The use of accompanying actions of the conducting healer, e.g. blowing tobacco smoke over potion and clients, waggling or hitting with special plant bunches, laying on of hands
- Special scenery design, e.g. sometimes special clothes, round arrangement of seats or round room architecture, fireplace, altar-like table of ritual objects (Spanish: la mesa)
- Time frame for the session: mostly held at night time

The influence of the setting was missed out in early studies of psychedelics when research was often conducted in a sterile hospital environment or psychiatrist's offices with poorly trained staff. Good results could often not be replicated and a contradictory picture of the therapeutic benefits from LSD therapy arose in the

1950s and 1960s (Abramson, 1967; MacLean et al., 1961, pp. 34-45; Smart et al., 1966, pp. 469-482; Ludwig et al., 1969, pp. 59-69.; Johnson, 1969, pp. 481-487; Grof, 1980; Grob & Bravo, 1996). There have been found adverse effects of the use of psychoactive substances mainly through the inappropriate and unstructured use (Frecska, 2007; Hermle, 2008).

One of the early North American pioneers who recognized the importance of the setting variable for the success and benefit of LSD therapy was M. A. Hubbard. He introduced music, pictures, evocative symbols and flowers in order to create a relaxing atmosphere for the patients (Hoffer & Osmond, 1967). The expression "set and setting" was made popular by Timothy Leary during the 1960s (as an example see Leary, 1966) and later discussed by the above quoted Norman Zinberg (Zinberg, 1986).

The psychological preconditions in general have been defined as the set variable. This can be the psychic conflict dynamics of the patient, motivations, mood and emotional state, personality and resources, stability, structure or ego strength, expectations and pre-knowledge and subjective working model, etc. The preparation of the patient has been recognized as influencing factor for the set as well (Grof, 1980; Leuner, 1987, pp. 151-161; Hess, 2008, p. 265).

8.1.1 Interaction between set, setting and substance

Setting variables have an interactive influence on the psychic set, even without the influence of any mind-altering substance and the perception of the setting is selectively influenced by the set. For Leuner the psychoactive substance is a more or less unspecific enhancer for setting and set influences. It enhances the psychodynamics and the psychotherapeutic effect factors. Expert interviews with therapists of substance-supported psychotherapy with so called empathogenetic substances such as MDMA have revealed that they consider the setting of intention or purpose ‚the single most important foundation for a beneficial experience' (Adamson & Metzner, 1988, p. 64). Although there are differences between emphathogens and more hallucinogenic substances such as LSD, psilocybin, mescaline and probably DMT/ayahuasca, these authors consider all those substance as 'catalysts' for a ‚transformation of consciousness' (ibid., p. 65). Those substances would not directly cause specific insights or revelations but rather enable them. The interactions between the elements set, setting, substance and experience can be considered highly complex. I did not find any study that would provide a model, how exactly those interactions work. A neuroimaging study points towards the interaction of brain areas during the ayahuasca state that are less connected under normal circumstances (see de Araujo et al., 2012).

The working mechanism can be considered a feedback circle. Not only the set and setting, the altered perceptions and interpretation activity shape the experience significantly under the influence of psychedelic substances, but the altered experience also influences the future sets and settings of the individual, which might change over time depending on previous experiences.

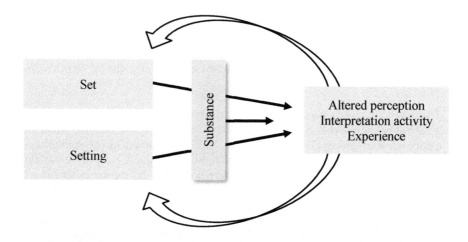

Figure 1: Schematic presentation of the complex interaction between set, setting, substance and experience

8.2 Elements of ayahuasca rituals

8.2.1 Prepatation and dieta

The local diet regulations before and after the rituals vary from tradition to tradition and from shaman to shaman. Most of them have in common certain regulations for bland food like the abstinence from salt, sugar and spice (Luna & Amaringo, 1999) as well as restrictions of red meat, alcohol, drugs and sex. Some emphasise the importance of a long diet before the ritual, some give emphasise to the post-ceremonial diet (Frecska, 2011, p. 163). Spiritual or health reasons are stressed out from the providers. From a medical point of view long diets are not necessary mainly to prevent MAOI-problems – here it would be enough to follow the diet some hours before and during the ceremony – but a tryptophan-rich diet with complex carbohydrates (starch) that does not provide at the same time rivalling other amino acids (with multiple chain, not ring-type) and no concentrated simple sugars is wanted in order to prevent serotonin-depletion. This can be done through fish, poultry, papaya, banana, avocado, spinach, cottage cheese, milk, seeds, and nuts (ibid., p. 163). Diverse variants of fasting is traditionally part of the Amazon medicine and education of vegetalistas. So even longer periods of isolation and fasting are the rule in the training of shamanic healers, even without targeting primarily the refined consume of ayahuasca by that. The goal of traditional shamanic dieting is mostly to get in touch with the world of nature spirits during retreat periods, not particularly to have rich psychedelic visions. The ayahuasca focus of the Western public often obfuscates this. Thus, all possible variations of diet recommendations and corresponding theories about its necessity for rich and safe visions are transported in the international Neo-shamanic or touristic ayahuasca scene. It should also be noted that the food pallets in poor rural areas of the Amazon, are mostly limited to what is now often promoted as a special ayahuasca diet to the Western ayahuasca pilgrims. But regardless of possible physiological effects on the ayahuasca experience, fasting in the retreat setting may well have its value: an introspective and sensitizing influence.

8.2.2 Vomiting

Vomiting is a common physiological effect of ayahuasca. It takes place mainly in the beginning of the intoxication. Therapists and curanderos at the Takiwasi therapy centre in Tarapoto (Peru) consider the beginning of the ayahuasca ritual as a confrontation between the psycho-physiological effects of ayahuasca and the resistance forces of the patient. Thus, vomiting would be a sign of surrender to the process and the person would not only vomit the brew but also the corresponding blockage. In this case spontaneous vomiting during the ritual is seen as energetic purification on a physical, psychological, emotional and spiritual level. To indigenous people vomiting is often a sign of healing. Also, in the Santo Daime church vomiting is seen as a ritual of purification (Labate & Pacheco, 2011, p. 78). Experienced curanderos rarely vomit. This could be a sign of adaption but more often this is seen as progress in the personal process of purification of that person. If a patient never vomits this might be seen as a sign of resistance and a non-satisfactory therapy progress. (Labate et al., 2011, pp. 228-229).

8.2.3 Sopladas (Spanish: blowing)

Amazonian curanderos often work with this intervention of the traditional Amazonian medicine. The curanderos blow tobacco smoke over central parts of the client. For this purpose, they also use vapours from liquids like aqua florida

(Spanish: blossom water – alcoholic blossom extract), camphor, citric or cinnamon extract, other fragrances, essential oils or alcohol. Each of these substances has its particular effect. Camphor and citric scent would reduce the intensity of the vision and other scents would enhance it, protect, strengthen or tranquilize. The fragrance is not always blown over the patient but sometimes the curandero lets the client simply smell it. Sopladas are performed also on objects, medicine and the surrounding. They would change their energetic qualities. The blowing would establish an energetic relationship between the curandero and the client and allow him 'to absorb and assimilate the energetic pertuberances of the patient', as Jacques Mabit, the founder and director of the Takiwasi centre in Tarapoto (Peru) says (Labate et al., 2011, p. 227).

8.2.4 Chupadas (Spanish: sucking)

The curandero sucks out disorders from body parts of the patient where he locates the witchery, disease or blockage. This is done either directly at the skin or with some distance. The curandero takes supportive and protective liquids into his mouth or swallows tobacco smoke. Than he produces special mucus that he regurgitates, in Peru sometimes called yachay or mariri. This phlegm would serve as reservoir or magnet for whatever bad energy he sucks out from the patient. After sucking out the problem of the patient he spits out the mucus. The sucking intervention is frequently performed on the head, the solar plexus or the abdomen. The intervention is considered risky for the curandero and would need a proper formation since he might contaminate himself with what he extracts from the patient. (Labate et al., 2011, p. 227-228). I personally have never attended any ceremonies in which chupadas were performed. The vegetalistas Santiago Enrrique Paredes Melendez and his brother Hegner Paredes Melendez, who I had collaborated with never used this and they did not know any one who would perform chupadas. They considered it a dangerous and ancient technique.

8.2.5 Íkaro and sound

Bernd Brabec de Mori believes that the magical use of music is far older than the use of ayahuasca, and that ayahuasca was embedded into its pre-existing practice (Brabec de Mori, 2013, p. 103). In the native understanding, the songs themselves would be the key to communicate with non-human entities, but in the new-age context the songs would have the role of suggestive elements or psychological leading ropes during the psychedelic experience (ibid., 98). For the traditional healing songs of the Shipibo-Conibo tribe, called Ícaro, Brabec de Mori documented that the lyrics often give detailed descriptions of what happens in the visions and that they even change the perspectives to non-human beings (ibid. 109). The singing is the way to communicate with the shamanic world and its inhabitants, even without any psychoactive substance use. The singing is also the way to report back and communicate the information that the indigenous healer or witchdoctor has gathered. He is the one who must describe and translate his visions and experiences. For the ayahuascsa tourism, a fundamental change took place. Nowadays, the client expects to drink the ayahuasca during a ceremony, not exclusively the healer. The tourist tries to have a look at the spiritual wonderland and wants to describe what he experiences. He can only do this with his own metaphors and symbols. The focus of the interest of western recipients and researchers often lies on the visual imagery or synesthetic hallucination and its dramatic processes. The singing of the healer becomes a supportive tool, similar to the use of music in the western psychedelic therapies. Brabec de Mori argues that this common standart appeared, when the natives realized the western curiosity in the psychedelic aspects of ayahuasca. At least for the Shipibo people this was mostly uncommon until scientists and tourists indicated their interest in those experiences. Before, only in heavy cases – e.g. of a witchcraft wars – the patient also had to drink the brew. Normally, people tried to stay away from such dangerous matters. Economical reasons also might have played a substantial role for this profound change in the ayahuasca usage. Most of the research about the ayahuasca songs was done during this transformative process. (ibid., pp. 110-112). The work of Susanna Bustos (2008) about the ícaro singing bases on the new-way shamanism which focus lies on the psychedelic and visual experience of the ayahuasca potion. She investigated the Peruvian spiritual and healing singing in the eclectic Takiwasi centre for addiction therapy and in the Mayantuyacu centre for western visitors. There, she documented that during ceremonies 15 to 20 songs were performed, interrupted by pauses of silence.

Demange (2002) mentions that indigenous healers emphasise the spiritual origin of the songs and their direct connection to the plants from which they were received in a dieting process. Healers from foreign origin would show a disperse picture when they stress energetic and psychological approaches (ibid., p. 71) like rhythm, vibration, resonance, harmony or the suggestive healing power of words. He continues: "Words call the spirits, and the spirits cure, whether or not those words are understood by the patient" (ibid., p. 74). This would only work if performed by a person who is personally acquainted with the plant and has undergone periods of dieting with the plants or other spirits (ibid., p. 74).

As far as I have witnessed in many ayahuasca ceremonies over a period of 4 years in the Garden of Peace centre near Tarapoto, the Sanctuario Huishtín near the village Honoria and others, the singing was frequently accompanied by simple rhythms on a maraca (seed filled gourd shaker) or chacapa (leave-bundle rattle made from Parina bush or others). Sometimes special gestures were performed while singing. During ceremonies, the vegetalista Hegner Paredes Melendez also had a little mesa on his side (Spanish: table), usually a cloth brocaded with Shipibo patterns with various esoteric objects like stones, figures, crystals and agua de florida (sweet smelling perfume).

The musical repertoire showed a variety from repetitive melodic phrases and little pentatonic melodies towards more abstract sounds, repetitive staccato or long notes. The melodies were sung, whistled or sometimes whispered. Often lyrical phrases or words in Spanish were used, sometimes mixed with other native or unintelligible languages.

9 Research about DMT and ayahuasca

The first synthesizing of DMT took place in 1931 by the Canadian chemist Richard Helmuth Fredrick Manske (Manske, 1931, Ott, 1998, McKenna and Riba, 2015). Before, DMT was found in natural sources in 1946 by the Brazilian microbiologist Oswaldo Gonçalves de Lima. He called it nigerine, when he isolated 0.51% of the alcaloid from a root-bark of Mimosa tenuiflora, which he had collected at the town Arcoverde in the state Pernambuco. De Melo isolated 0.98% of nigerine in 1955 from Jurema preta (De Melo, 1955, mentioned in Ott, 1998, p.10). Then in 1959, when Gonçalves de Lima provided a sample of Jurema preta to a US pharmaceutical company, 0,57% of DMT was isolated (Pachter et al., 1959). Nigerine might have been an impure form of DMT. In between DMT was isolated unequivocally the first time from the seeds of Anadenanthera peregrina by M.S. Fish (Fish et al., 1955). The first investigations on the administration of DMT in humans, which were conducted by Hungarian chemist and psychiatrist Stephen Szára in 1956, found strong effects such as mood changes, thought changes, visual effects, increased blood pressure and heart rate, tremor, mydriasis, tingling interoceptive sensation.

Over 50 different plant species have been found to contain DMT since 1955 (Ott, 1994).

An article from 1961 in the Science magazine from Julius Axelrod started the still on-going discussion about endogenous DMT production in mammals and other animals. He found an enzyme in rabbit lung 'that N-methylates serotonin and tryptamine to psychotomimetic metabolites, bufotenine and N,N-dimethyltryptamine ... and also N-methylates phenylethylamine derivatives such as tyramine, phenylethylamine , mescaline, and dopamine' (Axelrod, 1961). Gillin showed that unlike other hallucinogens DMT does not evoke tolerance in cats (Gillin et. al., 1973). The next decade the research concentrated either on the localization and description of N-methyltransferase or on the search for DMT in body liquids and tissues (Rosengarten & Friedhoff, 1976). Many of the methods before 2001 have been criticised due to a lack of sensitivity and selectivity (Barker et al., 2001). The minimum of required measurement method is the gas chromatography, which is combined the best with mass spectrometry. The best method is a liquid chromatography-tandem mass spectrometry with electrospray ionization (LC-ESI-MS/MS) (Shen et al., 2009). This most sensitive and selective detection method on DMT in body fluids and tissues was used in 2005: 'Endogenous levels of bufotenine and DMT in blood and a number of animal and human tissues were determined' (Kärkkäinen et al., 2005). Within the last years DMT was found in pineal gland microdialysate of rats (Barker, et al. 2013). It was also found to be bio-synthesized in the human melanoma cell line SK-Mel-147. The biological effects of DMT and its metabolites on the cell functions and proliferation are yet not understood (Gomes, 2014).

In 2014 it was shown for the first time an immune-modulatory role of NN-DMT and 5-MeO-DMT. The study points out that DMT 'may act as systemic endogenous regulators of inflammation and immune homeostasis through the sigma-1 receptor' (Szabo et al., 2014).

9.1 Pharmacological and botanical research on ayahuasca

The main ingredient of the ayahuasca brews in the Amazonas valley is the vine Banisteriopsis caapi to which the Quechua name ayahuasca refers to. B. caapi is part of the family Malpighiaceae which belongs to the order Malpighiales. There are 92 species of Banisteriopsis, which are distributed mainly in Peru, Ecuador, Brasil, Bolivia, Colombia (Mabberley, 1997).

Richard Spruce (*1817 – +1893) was the first western scientist who identified B. caapi as the source of a native soutwest american hallucinogenic drink, although he failed to discover the rich ethnopharmacological lore of South Americas tropical region besides the ayahuasca (Schultes, 1983, pp. 140-141). Firstly, its harmala alkaloids (Rivier & Lindgren, 1972), mostly harmine, harmaline and tetrahydroharmine (THH) were wrongly identified as the main cause for the hallucinogenic or visionary effect (Hochstein & Paradies, 1957). Louis Lewin (*1850 – +1929), the founder of modern psychopharmacology, discovered harmine in a sample of B. caapi. He called it Telepathine, due to the psychoactive property of the B. caapi brew and also Banisterine. But it proved to be identical to harmine. Banisterine was seen as the "magic drug" for the treatment of postencephalitic parkinsonism for some years, before it was replaced later in the 1930s by L-Dopa (Lewin, 1929; Sanchez-Ramos, 1991; Wang et al., 2010).

ayahuasca did not find much the attention of western science again until the ethno-botanical fieldwork of the North American biologist Richard Evans Schultes (*1915–+2001) in the middle of the 20th century. It was him who scientifically discovered the commonly used second compounds of the ayahuasca brew: leafs of Psychotria viridis (Quechua: chacruna or chacrona) and Diplopterys cabrerana (Quechua: chaliponga or chagropanga).

1957 Francis Hochstein and Anita Paradies – both chemists from the US – found DMT in aqueous extracts from a plant they called Prestonia amazonicum (Haemadyction amazonicum), which was reported to be commonly mixed with the plant Banisteriopis caapi from Amazonian natives for hallucination purposes. They used paper chromatography besides other investigational techniques and found harmine and the alkaloids, harmaline and d-tetrahydroharmine in B. caapi and N,N-dimetyptryptamine in P. amazonicum (Hochstein & Paradies, 1957). But other scientists had doubts about the correct botanical identification of the plant (Schultes & Raffauf, 1960). Than in 1965 the French pharmacologist Jaques Poisson isolated DMT from leafs of Diplopterys cabrerana (Banisteriopsis rusbyana), which is a common ingredient of ayahuasca, as mentioned, used by the Peruvian Aguaruna (Awajún) people (Poisson, 1965). They resisted against the incorporation into the Peruvian society until the late 1950s. This was one of the first strong scientific evidences for the cultural hallucinogenic use of DMT in South America. In the year 1970 DMT was found in the other commonly used ingredient of the potion: Psychotria viridis (Marderosian et al., 1970). The same researcher also found DMT in another unidentified species of Psychotria, which the Kaxinawá (Cashinahua) people, who live in Peru and Brazil, call nai kawa (Ott, 1996). Other unidentified species of Psychotria, which were part of ayahuasca brews of the Peruvian Sharanahua and Culina people, probably contained DMT as the analysis of the brews showed. They called these admixtures pishikawa and batsikawa or matsi or kawakui. (Rivier & Lindgren, 1972).

Luna (1984) reported Virola surinamensis as an admixture, which 'must be considered to be a potential source of tryptamines' (Ott, 1996).

Depending on the region, people and purpose of use their ayahuasca brew has different ingredients. Ott (1996, p. 221) counted nearly 100 different plant species from 38 different families as admixtures. About a forth of them are known to have so called entheogenic effects and are often used without the ayahuasca-plant as well. Some of the additives may have no psychoactive effect and may be considered medicinal.

Based on the scientific literature Ott (ibid, pp. 212-221) provides six categories for the great number of additives, each with some examples:

1. Tobacco: Nicotiana tabacum and N. rustica (Lewin, 1924, p. 141; Luna & Amaringo, 1991; Schultes & Hofmann, 1979) are commonly used together with the ayahuasca: tobacco juice drunk alternately (Shuar people, Barasana people) or after B. caapi intake (Piro people shamanes) or with the ayahuasca when inducting young shamans (Cocama people), ambíl (an edible preparation) licked by the Campa people after the ingestion of ayahuasca, mixed intake (Shipibo ayahuasqueros) (Wilbert, 1987), clysters or enemas with tobacco syrup mixed with ayahuasca (Aguaruna people) (Schultes & Raffauf, 1990), blowing tobacco smoke over patients and ritual items prior to ayahuasca (Tecuana people) (Ott, 1996b, pp. 212-213) and during the ayahuasca session (Siona and Secoya people from Ecuador) (Vickers & Plowmann, 1984). Tobacco is considered to be one of the most

important shaman drugs of South America for 'magico-religious, medicinal and recreational purposes' (Wilbert, 1991).

2. Guayusa: Some Amazonian tribes add the leafs of the holly Ilex guayusa to their ayahuasca brew. They do this against the soporific effect of B. caapi as several scientists report (Furst, 1976; Russo, 1992; Kohn, 1992; Ott, 1996; Patiño, 1968; Shemluck, 1979; Schultes, 1972D; Schultes & Raffauf, 1990). As Schultes & Raffauf (1990) also mention guayusa is taken in Ecuador against the bitter taste, hangover and for strength to deal with ayahuasca. Paullinia yoco, which is a relative of guaraná (Paullinina cupana var. sorbilis), has been used as additive to ayahuasca among the Siona people for its stimulating caffeine effect (Langdon, 1986).

3. Chiriguayusa or chiric-sananho (Brunfelsia grandiflora, B. grandiflora subs. schultesii): Some native people of Colombia and Ecuador add roots, barks or leafs of B. grandiflora and/or leafs of B. chiricaspi to their ayahuasca (Kofán, Siona, Ingano, Runa, Shuar people) (Kohn, 1992; Langdon, 1986; Plowmann, 1977; Schultes & Raffauf, 1990; Schultes & Raffauf 1992). The Brazilian manacá (Brunfelsia uniflora) is also known as additive. The last one contains the coumarin scopoletin (Mors & Ribeiro, 1957; Plowmann 1977; Schultes & Hofmann, 1980).

4. Huanto (huantuc or huanduj): Species of solanaceous Brugmansia have been reported to serve as admixtures to ayahuasca. An early mention of "tree Datura" as admixture can be found in Reichel-Dolmatoff (1975). B. suaveolens was reported to be added from the Sharanahua, Ingano and Siona people and B. insignis was also reported from Peru as admixture (Langdon, 1986; Schultes & Raffauf, 1990; Schultes & Raffauf, 1992). Ecuadorian Siona and Secoya peope use Brugmansia x insignis species alone and in combination with ayahuasca as enterogens (Vickers & Plowman, 1984, p.29). The Peruvian Mascho are also known to use B. insignis as very important shamanic plant to help find lost objects, healing, and divine the future (Califano & Fernandez, Distel, 1982). Some non scientific web sites provide additional selections of common names for Brugmansia inside of Peru: Floripondio, Maricahua, Campana, Choco pana, Borrachero, Toa or Toe, Maikoa (Líbaro people); Chuchupanda (Amahuaca people), Aiiapa (Amarakaeri people), Haiiapa (Huachipaeri people); Saaro (Matsiguenga people); Gayapa y Kanachijero (Piro-yine people); Kanachiari (Shipibo-Conibo people) (deperu, 2016; peruecologico, 2016).

5. Miscellaneous admixtures: A variety of plants have been reported as admixtures. Ott (1996, pp. 215-218) collected scientific reports of those known additives. It seems not to be uncommon that many other plants and ingredients have been added and tried out together with the ayahuasca plant.

6. Chacruna and Chagropanga: Plants that contain tryptamines like N,N-Dimethyltryptamine are most common admixtures to ayahuasca (McKenna & Towers, 1984; Ott, 1994).

Widely used in Peru, Ecuador and Brasil are the leafs of Psychotria viridis. In Peru it can be found under the name Chacruna, and in Ecuador under the names Sami ruca and Amirucapanga (Kohn, 1992; Miller, 1993). Sometimes Psychotria carthaginensis or two other uncharacterized species of Psychotria were used in Peru instead of P. viridis by the Sharanahua people under the names Batsikawa and Pishikawa (Rivier & Lindgren, 1972; Schultes & Raffauf, 1990).

Another main additive can be Diplopterys cabrerana, previously known under the old scientific name Banisteriopsis rusbyana. In the northern Amazonian region of the Putumayo in Colombia Klug and Cuatrecasas collected this additive plant. It is sometimes locally called Chagropanga, Chalipanga, Oco-yagé or Yagé-úco. Schultes reported its use by native people in this region (Cuatrecasas, 1965; Schultes, 1957). And also, the Siona and Secoya people have been seen adding D. cabrerana leafs to their ayahuasca brews (Vickers & Plowman, 1984). But unlike to Colombia and Ecuador, the use of D. cabrerana was not very common in Peru (Ott 1996, p. 219).

Although the traditional and modern use is well established, the pharmacology of the diverse known combinations is almost unknown to modern medicine (Callaway et al., 1999, p. 244).

Since the 1990s the modern clinical research of ayahuasca started.

9.2 Interaction theory

In 1968 a scientific group discovered DMT in Diplopterys cabrerana (Banisteriopsis rusbyana) (leafs and stems), which is another Colombian admixture to ayahuasca as mentioned before. The DMT of the plant seemed inactive if taken separately oral. They supposed that only in combination with the monoamine oxidase inhibiting harmala alkaloids, which were found in ayahuasca (Yagé) brew, the pharmacological effect of N,N-dimethyltryptamine could take place (Agurell et al., 1968). The working model was that MAO-inhibiting beta-carbolines protect the DMT from being deaminated before it reaches the central nervous system (McKenna et al., 1984). Harmine and harmaline act as specific reverse inhibitors of type-A monoamine oxidase (MAO-A) (Udenfriend et al., 1958). The molecule structure of N,N-DMT is related to the neurotransmitter serotonin. It binds to HT2A receptor sides of the central nervous system (CNS), like other better-characterized substances (LSD and mescaline) and plays an agonistic role in the mechanism of exogenic hallucinations (Smith et al., 1998). Tetrahydroharmine (THH), which is not a strong MAO-inhibitor, may act as a weak neuroactive inhibitor of the presynaptic serotonin uptake (5-hydroxytryptamine, 5-HT), like other 1-methyl-tetrahydro-beta-carbolines (Airaksinen et al., 1980). Therefore 5-HT concentrations increase when the presynaptic uptake is blocked as well as its MAO-A metabolism.

In newer research, it was shown that 'MAO-A inhibitors alter the locomotor profile of 5-MeO-DMT in rats, and enhance its interaction with 5-HT2A receptors' and 'that 5-MeO-DMT can disrupt PPI by activating 5-HT2A, [...] and that MAOIs alter 5-MeO-DMT pharmacodynamics by increasing its accumulation in the central nervous system' (Halberstadt, 2016). The pre-pulse inhibition (PPI) corresponds physiologically to the filter function of the healthy brain for external stimuli.

The interaction theory as the main mechanism for the psychedelic effects of the ayahuasca brew is widely accepted.

9.3 Physiological effects

Ayahuasca has a low toxicity (Domínguez-Clavé, 2016, p. 10) but yet a literature analysis from 2006 did not find any animal model that exactly tested the acute toxicity of the ayahuasca brew and its abuse potential (Gable, 2006). The median lethal dose of DMT and several harmala alkaloids, tested in animal studies, is 20 times greater than the dosage of the typical ayahuasca ceremony (ibid., p. 27). The risk of overdoses seems to be minimized, due to the serotonergic stimulation of the nervus vagus, which induces emesis near the effective dose (ibid, p. 29).

Mello et al. (2018) did not find any significant alteration in alanine aminotransferase, aspartate aminotransferase, bilirubin, creatinine, urea, lactate dehydrogenase, alkaline phosphatase, and gamma glutamyl transferase in the serum of 22 healthy volunteers who had been drinking ayahuasca twice a month for at least one year. Regular ingestion of ayahuasca in a religious context does not seem to alter hepatic function.

As far as Gable (2006) investigated there have been no deaths reported, caused directly from an intoxication of DMT/beta-carboline ayahuasca brews (ibid, p. 29). The safety margin would be comparable to codeine, mescaline and methadone. The dependence potential as well as the risk for sustained psychological disturbances were considered to be minimal (ibid., p. 1). But combinations of the synergic actions of harmine with atropine and scopolamine have been reported severe for some individuals, which Gable finds an additional evidence for the potential danger of creative non-traditional combinations (ibid., p. 29). In contrast to studies which show strong cardiovascular effects of pure DMT (intravenously administrated), the increase of systolic (SBP) and diastolic (DBP) blood pressure seems to be rather moderate with almost no changes in heart rate for the orally administrated common ayahuasca combination B. caapi and P. viridis (Riba et al., 2001; Riba, 2003; Dos Santos et al., 2012). Therefore, the admission of the ayahuasca to healthy individuals seems to be safe in terms of cardiovascular impact (Domínguez-Clavé et al., 2016, pp. 9-10).

One of the most common side effects are vomiting and nausea (Riba et al., 2001). This is often seen as a positive cleaning property of ayahuasca (Domínguez-Clavé, 2016, p. 10), due to the fact that substance induced purging is widely practised as a traditional healing and cleaning method in the Amazonian medicine. Combining ayahuasca with further MAO inhibitors and serotonergic drugs like antidepressants should be avoided as well as the application to individuals with abnormal metabolism or compromised health status (Gable 2006, p. 29).

Like with al psychedelics there is a risk of anxiety reactions and transient dissociative episodes. The risk seems to increase with high dosage use (Riba et al., 2001). The role of dubious or uncontrolled admixtures as well as the combination with hedonic drugs should always be considered. Infrequent longer-lasting psychotic symptoms have been reported (Dos Santos & Strassman, 2011). But the incidence of ransomed psychotic episodes seems to be rather low with 0.1% (0,052-0,096%). Over a period of 5 years the medical section of the Brazilian Unidão do Vegetal church (UDV) documented 13-24 cases out of 25000 ayahuasca users (Joint Appendix, 2002). This rate is seen comparable to those about LSD (Dos Santos & Strassman, 2011; Gable, 2006). The general 12-month prevalence rate of psychosis or schizophrenia lays approximately around 1,1% for the USA (National Institute of Mental Health, 2016). Compared to the low incidence rate of under 1% of the UDV data Gable (2006) finds evidence that the use of ayahuasca serves not as a triggering event for prolonged psychotic episodes. He further quotes the Joint Appendix document of the UDV (2002, p. 623) that reports that many or most of the psychotic episodes were transient in nature and resolved spontaneously (Gable, 2006, p. 30). The responsible therapeutic use of ayahuasca should consider a contraindication for individuals with a risk for psychosis like previous episodes or a known family risk.

9.4 Psychological effects

9.4.1 Subjective experiences

After the oral admission acute subjective effects start after 45–60 minutes. They reach their maximum between 90-120 minutes and are fully decreased after 4–6 hours (Riba, 2003). Effects follow a classical dose-response pattern and their intensity curve correspond with the amount of DMT in the blood plasma (Riba et al., 2001; 2003; 2005; 2006). The ayahuasca ingestion changes the quality of the state of consciousness. Visual, auditory and tactile perception, sensations as well as thought content and emotions are affected (Riba et al., 2001). For the traditional users in South America the ayahuasca brews are considered to produce visionary effects, which are used for deeper insight and healing. For this purposes curanderos (healers) and shamans would be able to communicate with different spirits such as plant spirits and animal spirits. Spirits like ayahuasca itself are considered to be teachers.

As neuroimaging of ayahuasca experiences shows, areas in the brain get activated, which are related to episodic memories, emotional arousal and introspective awareness. It enhances the intensity of recalled images up to a level of natural images and lets users see complex visual pattern with closed eyes. Certain areas that are responsible for receiving visual stimuli are normally without activity, when eyes are closed. But under ayahuasca and closed eyes, these areas are activated along with those regions responsible for imagination. This explains the realistic and vivid visions (de Araujo et al., 2012). ayahuasca experiences are frequently accompanied by visual imagery (Riba et al., 2006). Synesthetic experiences are common. Visions are simultaneously seen, heard and smelled (Luna & Amaringo, 1999, p. 38).

The before mentioned study of Barbosa et al. (2005) investigated dimensions of the altered states of consciousness in first time users in the ritual setting of the urban Brazilian ayahuasca-churches Santo Daime and Unidão do Vegetal. Visual phenomena like 'extraordinary visual experiences, kaleidoscopic lights, geometrical forms, tunnels, animals, humans and supernatural beings' (ibid. p. 198) were experienced by 64,3 % of the 28 participants of the study. 53,6% mentioned a sensation of peace, silence, harmony and inner calm. 'A mixture of terror and fascination, which results from the sense of superior and powerful presence' (ibid. p. 198) was reported from 42,9%. Alleged insights, such as 'elucidating thoughts about biographic, existential and behavioural aspects', which sometimes were 'attached to great fascination and profundity and to a deep meaning of ritual events' and 'frequently were perceived as received from outside' (ibid. p. 198) were experienced from 39,3%. 32,1% reported alterations in self-body image, like fusions with the environment and separations between consciousness and body. One person (3,6%) experienced a reaction of spiritual crisis. After 7-14 days after the ayahuasca ritual 28,6% of the participants reported more serenity towards previous stressor psychosocial aspects. 17,9% experienced more assertiveness towards previous psychosocial aspects. 14,3% more happiness and energy in daily life and the one person who had the distress experience reported a lot of preoccupation.

Shanon (2002, p. 431) found that items such as animals, phantasmagoric creatures, royalty and religious figures, magic and art objects and divine beings are frequently seen. Autobiographical content appears less frequent in experienced drinkers (ibid. p 432) but can reveal patterns of personality to the drinker (ibid., p. 114). Benny Shanon provides a typology of visions that include two-dimensional pop art or comic style, complex geometry and architecture with fluorescent-coloured lines, expanse panoramic view on landscapes and worlds, enchanting paining style of Henri Rousseau and finally visions of baroque flair and fairy tales (ibid., pp. 96-97). Also mentioned are several communications with phantasmagoric beings (ibid. p 97). Some individuals would have no or sparsely visions (ibid., pp. 96-98).

The appearance of supportive entities (de Rios, 1972; Luna, 1986; Beyer, 2009, pp. 239-244) as well as receiving teachings from the personified ayahuasca are reported from traditional ayahuasca-ingestion and the immediate subjective evidence of such personal "teachings from entities" plays an impressive role in traditional Upper-Amazon vegetalism (Luna, 1986; Beyer, 2009, pp. 110-111; Shanon, 2014, pp. 65-67). But it also has been reported from the ibogaine-induced state of consciousness (Schenberg et al., 2017) as well as occasionally from western substance-supported psychotherapy, e.g. guiding spirits from family members during psilocybin ingestion (Belser et al., 2017, pp. 365-366). Psilocybin and (a little less) Ketamine are also known to produce complex and elementary imagery (Studerus et al., 2010). This may point towards the high influence of personal set and ingestion setting, which even may be able to affect the perceptional content from different substances in a similar manner.

I suggest distinguishing visions from hallucinations. Hallucinations, in contrast to ayahuasca vision, give the subjective impression that the perceived content would be part of ordinary reality - in such a way that the person can hardly distinguish between deemed 'reality' of the surrounding and the hallucinatory phenomena.

Emotional release is known not only to be a typical phenomenon of the ayahuasca inebriation (Shanon, 2014, p. 64) but also of other psychedelics such as LSD and psilocybin in psychotherapeutic settings (Gasser et al., 2014b; Belser et al., 2017). It points towards typical process-elements that have been previously described from therapies with entactogens and are typically accompanied by emotional activation: 'acceleration of psychological processes', 'regression', 'rescripting of past behaviours', 'problem actualization and corrective new experience' as well as 'transpersonal experiences' (Passie, 2012). Emotional release is seen as closely related to meaningful experiences, especially those described as 'alternative simulations of formative situations from the past, encapsulated in an inner realm' (ibid., 2012).

Gaining diagnostic insight into other peoples' social and psychosomatic issues may be of particular interest in medical antropology because ethnographic literature documents that local vegetalistas of the Amazon claim to gain insight into the causes of the diseases through ayahuasca (Luna, 1986) - diseases are often attributed as being physical symptoms of social causes (Beyer, 2009, pp. 178-180).

A typical narrative of members of the Brazilian religious ayahuasca movements seems to be the central insight of the necessity to return from a self-destructive path in life as Grob et al. (1996) have reported. All of the 15 interviewed participants of the ayahuasca church UDV had this profound impact on their course of life. Most important seems to be the first experience of the psychedelic ritual. Many had drastic visions how their life would become worse if they would not change radically their personal conduct and orientation. They reported pervasive dysfunctional behaviours prior to their membership and gave insight how their life had changed since they entered. They saw ayahuasca as an enhancer or catalyst for the psychological and moral evolution within the UDV (Grob et al., 1996).

9.4.2 Mental health

In 2009 Barbosa et al. published another study about first time users in an urban religious Brazilian context. They investigated 23 individuals in a naturalistic pre-post1-post2 design within a 6-month period and surveyed minor psychopathological symptoms, subjective general health status and personality variables. A reduction of somatic pain complains could be shown for some of the participants as well as a partly reduction of minor psychiatric symptoms and some improvements of mental health, a change towards more confidence and optimism, attitude change towards more independence and no adverse effects were reported. The two big ayahuasca churches Santo Daime and Unidão do Vegetal were statistically compared. Unfortunately, the study lacks a control groups with ritual participation without ayahuasca, a waiting group with no treatment at al. and larger sample size.

Bouso et al. (2012) published a better-controlled large study about religious Brazilian long-term users of ayahuasca (min. 15 years of active membership in a religious ayahuasca church). The participants as well as the control group were recruited from different regions and different religious groups. A personality questionnaire (Temperament and Character Inventory: TCI), mental health questionnaire (Symptom-Check-List-90-Revised: SCL-90-R), purpose of life questionnaire (The Purpose in Life Test: PLT), well-being questionnaire (The Psychosocial Well-Being: BIEPS) and spirituality questionnaire (The Spiritual Orientation Inventory: SOI) were applied twice (the second time after one year). This retrospective study setting could compare between the samples from different religious ayahuasca groups and samples from other religious groups (control group) and it could make statements about the stability of found differences. But it could not analyse directly the influence of ayahuasca onto the wanted variables. The study cannot show directly if the found changes between the groups are caused in the ayahuasca use or if the ayahuasca use is caused in the observed differences between the populations. The selection of the individuals out of the same population into the different analyse groups was not controlled before the systematic variation of the independent variable started. For such a direct analyse a prospective study would be needed.

Regarding the personality differences the ayahuasca users showed significantly lower Harm Avoidance and higher Reward Dependence. The lower harm avoidance came from significantly lower scores in the subscales anticipatory worry, shyness, fatigability and asthenia. The higher reward dependence came from significantly higher scores in the subscales attachment and dependence. The sample groups from the jungle showed higher attachment and dependence and a trend to higher persistence but no higher scores on the sub-dimension sentimentality, compared to the urban sample groups. The authors explain this finding with the possible adaption to the life in a small community in a hostile ecological environment in the tropical rainforest, which needs the ability to persist as a group despite isolation. The lower scores of the ayahuasca groups on the harm avoidance scale might indicate a need for this personality feature for people who undergo such regular ayahuasca use for such a long time (ibid, p. 10).

Significantly lower scores of the ayahuasca group were shown for the character dimension self-directedness and higher scores in self-transcendence. The lower scores on the dimension self-directedness came from significantly lower scores in responsibility, purposefulness, resourcefulness and self-acceptance. The higher scores on the dimension self-transcendence came from the facets self-forgetfulness, transpersonal identification and spiritual acceptance. In the dimension cooperativeness were no differences shown but on the subscale helpfulness they had higher scores and on the subscale compassion lower scores. The higher self-transcendence in the ayahuasca groups was seen as a direct effect of the ayahuasca, since the character dimensions of the TCI – other than the temperament dimensions – can be modified through life experiences but the religion as secondary variance was controlled (control groups were chosen also from religious settings). The lower self-directedness in the ayahuasca groups could also be a result of the strong psychedelic substance, which might enhance the adherence to religious indoctrinations of community values over individuality. At the same time as the self-transcendence and spirituality was greater in participants of ayahuasca churches, the willingness to cooperate was equal to that seen in conventional churches.

The second assessment after one year showed again lower scores in Harm Avoidance but no higher Reward Dependence. Again, ayahuasca users had lower scores on self-directedness and higher scores on self-transcendence.

Grob et al. (1996) found no differences in reward dependence in 15 long-term ayahuasca users compared to 15 non-users, but also found significantly lower scores in novelty seeking and harm avoidance.

In the study of Bouso et al. (2012) the examination of the psychopathological status reported that all 9 dimensions of the SCL-90-R showed lower scores for the ayahuasca group: somatization, obsessive-compulsive, interpersonal sensitivity, depression, anxiety, hostility, phobic anxiety, paranoid ideation, psychoticism. In the second assessment 7 from 9 scales showed lower scores for the ayahuasca group: obsessive-compulsive, interpersonal sensitivity, anxiety, hostility, phobic anxiety, paranoid ideation and psychoticism. The general symptom index was lower for the ayahuasca group on both assessment times. Also, the number of positively marked symptoms. The intensity of the marked symptoms was the same as in the control group.

According to this and other investigations ayahuasca seems to have a low potential to induce psychopathological symptoms.

Similar findings from Santo Daime long term users (min. 10 years) in a double-blind, placebo-controlled study have been presented from Santos et al. (2007) who found significantly reduced scores of panic and hopelessness under the acute effects of ayahuasca in the long-term users. There was no reaction on state or trait anxiety. The variables were measured with the Beck hopelessness scale (BHS), the anxiety sensitivity index (ASI-R) for panic-like related states and the state–trait–anxiety inventory (STAI) for anxiety. The authors conclude, 'the brew, as solely a pharmacological agent, can produce beneficial effects on mood and anxiety' (Santos et al., 2007, p. 512). Also, a study in which 32 long-term Santo Daime ayahuasca users from the US were investigated found reduced scores on 7 out of 9 dimensions of the SCL-90-R (Halpern et al., 2008).

In the study of Bouso et al. 2012 the spiritual orientation was measured with the Spirituality Orientation Inventory (SOI: Elkins et al., 1988). It has 9 major domains: transcendent dimension, meaning and purpose in life, mission in life, sacredness of life, material values, altruism, idealism, awareness of the tragic, and fruits of spirituality. The first assessment showed significant differences towards higher scores of the ayahuasca sample on all 9 domains of the SOI. The results remained stable after one year.

Also, higher scores of "purpose in life", measured with the Purpose in Life Test (PLT) were found. These results were not stable. There were no group differences in the second assessment after one year. The test bases on the therapist

Victor Frankl and measures 'meaning in life' vs. 'existential vacuum' (Crumbaugh & Maholick, 1976).

The psychosocial wellbeing was measured with a translated version of the Psychosocial Well-Being (BIEPS: Casullo & Castro, 2000). The analysis showed stable significant group differences towards higher values in ayahuasca group. Urban sub group comparison showed stronger differences between ayahuasca and non-ayahuasca groups (Bouso et al., 2012, p. 10).

As Franquesa et al., 2018 point out, documented improvements in different pathologies have been attributed to the introspective qualities of ayahuasca, although the possible underlying psychotherapeutic processes are yet not well understood. Anecdotic benefits are usually related to processes of ego dissolution, higher consciousness of important things, contact with oneself, improved ability to understand others, acceptance of oneself and life events and and personal growth (Bresnick & Levin, 2006).

Mystical experiences such as oneness, ego-dissolution and connectedness predict the long-term increase of well-being as well as clinical improvements after psychedelic therapies (Griffiths et al., 2006, Carhart-Harris & Goodwin, 2017). Carhart-Harris et al. (2018) believe that a feeling of connectedness is a key factor of mental health because evidence was found that it mediates psychological wellbeing (Cervinka et al., 2012) and the sense of disconnectedness is seen as a feature of depression (Karp, 2017). Experiences of connectedness have previously been attributed to ayahuasca. (Shanon, 2002, p. 205).

Franquesa et al. (2018) found evidence of therapeutic processes in ayahuasca inebriations, which are also known from other psychotherapies: decentred introspection, attribution of meaning (which was also proposed by Shanon, 2003) as well as alterations in meaningful, guiding values in life (which are also pointed out by Kavenská & Simonová, 2015; Liester & Pricket, 2012 and others). Some psychedelic therapies aim towards 'meaningful visual phenomena' as well as changes in the personal narratives of patients (Belser et al., 2017, p. 372). Concepts of generating and altering meaning are common in psychotherapy and were described under various terms (see Yalom, 1980; Frankl, 1986; Cade, 1992; Mattila, 2001, Roediger, 2011; Ruf & Schauer, 2012; Batthyany & Russo-Netzer, 2014; Lichtenberg et al., 2016; Mittelmark et al., 2017) and have also been generalized as a psychotherapeutic effect factor: 'new narrative about the Self' in a broader sense is defined as the development of a coherent rewording of the patient's life history as well as a new assessment of his identity and his relationship to the environment (Jørgensen, 2004).

9.4.3 Neuroimaging

Ayahuasca activates brain systems, which are connected to emotional processing and introspection. Frontal and paralimbic areas in the brain are significantly affected. Under the acute influence of ayahuasca the anterior insula shows bilateraly an increased blood perfusion, but its activity is stronger in the right hemisphere. Also, the cingulate/frontomedial cortex of the right hemisphere shows increased activity. These regions have previously been identified as central for somatic awareness, emotional arousal and subjective feeling states. Also, the left amygdala/parahippocampal gyrus was affected. This structure plays a role in the emotional arousal. To obtain these findings 15 participants received ayahuasca, equivalent to 1.0 mg DMT/kg body weight, in a randomized double-blind placebo controlled clinical trial and their blood flow in the brain was measured by means of single photon emission tomography (SPECT) (Riba et al., 2006).

As mentioned, the altered states of consciousness (ASC), which are induced by ayahuasca, relate to changes in perception and cognition. They increase the self-orientated mental activity. 'A remarkable increase in introspection is at the core of these altered states of consciousness' (Palhano-Fontes et al., 2015, p. 1). Self-oriented mental behaviour co-varies with particular physiological brain activity pattern. It has been linked to a network of brain regions which is known as Default Mode Network (DMN). The DMN is more active during rest and is less active during goal-oriented tasks and meditation. As its central parts it includes the Posterior Cingulate Cortex (PCC)/Precuneus and the medial Prefrontal Cortex (mPFC). Palhano-Fontes et al. observed the brains of 10 experienced ayahuasca users under the substance induced altered state of consciousness with the functional magnetic resonance imaging method (fMRI). The results show that during the ayahuasca induced altered state of consciousness the functional connectivity with core DMN structures such as the PCC/Precuneus decreases and the relationship of the DMN and the TPN (task-positive-network) remains with no changes. This could be explained through the increased internal mental activity, awareness and the mind effort demanded during the ASC. Previously the decrease of the DMN activity during meditative states had been linked to the decrease in mind-wandering (Brewer et al., 2011). This should not be the case in psychedelic states of consciousness. Experienced users of psychedelics like psilocybin have reported increased experiences of mind-wandering (Carhart-Harris et al., 2012). The comparison with meditation shows a similar (but not identical) brain activity pattern (decrease of DMN activity), introspective awareness and self-perception are increased, and the awareness of mind-wandering is altered in both states (Palhano-Fontes et al. 2015, p. 8).

Regular ayahuasca users seem to show changes in the brain structure compared to a control group. Bouso et al. (2015) compared magnetic resonance imaging images of a group of 22 individuals with those of a control group (matched in age, sex, years of education and intelligence). They found significant differences in midline structures of the brain, with thinning in the posterior cingulate cortex (PCC). Based on that the authors suggest that regular use of ayahuasca might lead to changes in brain structures, which support attention processes, self-referential thought, and internal mentation. They suppose that the previously reported changes in personality structure could be related to their founding (Bouso et al., 2015).

In another neuroimaging study from De Araujo et al. (2012) the authors conclude that the brains of the participants interpret their inner ayahuasca experiences with a status of reality. Thus, they explain how ayahuasca facilitates mystical revelations of visual nature to shamans of the rain forest. The visual effects stem from an extensive network, which is involved in the experience of vision, memory and intention: The researchers investigated the vivid seeing of potent imagery with eyes closed, which users commonly report about their acute ayahuasca experiences. Under the acute state of altered consciousness participants had to fulfil a closed eye imagery task, which produced a distinct activity increase in several occipital, temporal, and frontal areas. The activation effect of visual imagination was such strong that its activation in the primary visual area is comparable to that of natural visual content with open eyes. The activation effect in the visual field was correlated with the occurrence of subjective changes in perception. Areas which are involved in episodic memory and contextual associations like the BA30 and BA37 were also potentiated during imagery as well as the frontal area BA10, which is known to be associated with episodic memory and the processing of contextual associations (de Araujo et al., 2012).

9.4.4 Executive functions and working memory

The acute intake of ayahuasca seems to impair the working memory as measured through the computerised Sternberg memory working memory task (Sternberg, 1966). Participants had to recognise before presented letters. Reaction time and performance (errors) were measured. The test recruits the ventrolateral and the dorsolateral prefrontal cortex and the inferior frontal and anterior cingulate regions, among others (Bouso et al., 2013). At the same time the acute intake of ayahuasca seems to increase the ability to deal with stimulus-response interference. This was measured through a modified computerised Stroop colour and word test, in which the colour of the ink of the presented words interfere with the written content of the words, e.g. the word "green" was written in a blue colour (Golden, 1978). Participants had to react to the ink colour of the word but not to the colours to which the content of the words referred. Reaction time and performance (number of errors) were measured. The test activates the anterior cingulate cortex and the dorsolateral prefrontal cortex (DLPC) (Bouso et al., 2013). The Speed in the Stroop test was increased, without an increase of impulsiveness or inaccuracy. 'Mean values of incorrectly answered incompatible stimuli were lower after ayahuasca ...' (ibid., p. 7). Experienced ayahuasca users showed less incapacities in executive function than occasional users. The higher cognitions of executive functions like planning, inhibition of impulsivity and working memory, were measured in the complex task 'The Tower of London' from Shallice (1982). Participants had to arrange coloured beads in pegs using the least number of movements and the least time possible. During this task a network is activated that includes the DLPC, the anterior cingulate cortex, and parietal regions (Bouso et al., 2013). The performance in this task correlated negatively with the lifetime ayahuasca use. This indicates compensatory or neuromodulatory effects related to long-term use of ayahuasca (ibid, pp 1-2).

The larger investigation of Bouso et al. (2012) with 127 long-term ayahuasca users (minimum 15 years) investigated also neuropsychological functions. There was no evidence at al of neuropsychological or frontal impairment found. The results maintained after a second measuring time after one year and are in line with others who did not find working memory deficits in ayahuasca users (Grob et al. 1996a) nor Stroop effect impairments in adult ayahuasca users (Da Silveira et al., 2005) nor neuropsychological impairments in long term Peyote users from the Native American Church (Halpern et al. 2005). Bouso applied the following neuropsychological instruments: the Stroop colour word test, the Wisconsin card sorting test (WCST), the Letter-number-sequencing (LNS) from the Wechsler Adult Intelligence Scale (WAIS-III) and the Frontal Behaviour Scales (FrSBe).

These tests have been used previously to identify damages of the prefrontal cortex and neuropsychological deficits in various groups of drug abusers.

9.4.5 Dependency risk

Another important concern is that of a potential dependency risk. The tolerance development of the body has to be seen differentiated. Early studies demonstrated no tolerance development of DMT (Cole & Piper, 1973; Gillin, 1973). Later, one study had found no tolerance in subjective effects of intravenous applied DMT in humans, but the study did find tolerance in some physiological measures like the change in body temperature (Strassman et al., 1996).

Dos Santos et al. (2012) did not find a tolerance or sensitization development in EEG variables but 'ayahuasca increased relative power in the higher end of the beta EEG frequency band' which is an objective measure for the effects of ayahuasca on the CNS.

All together until now there seems to be some evidence that there is no tolerance to subjective effects of DMT but to cardiovascular and other peripheral effects of DMT (Carbonaro et al., 2016).

Does the first time use of ayahuasca trigger a chronic use? Negative evidence comes from the UDV-church. The UDV reported that 15-20% of their first-time participants of their ayahuasca ceremony later become a regular member of the church (Joint Appendix, 2002, p. 700). As Gable (2006) mentions, this equates to the number of first-time visitors of US-American Christian churches who later become one of their members (Miller, 1987).

Another important finding of the before described study of Bouso et al. (2012) is that the scores on the personality dimension Novelty Seeking did not show differences in the long term ayahuasca users group and control group. No subscale of Novelty Seeking, including Impulsiveness, showed any higher values for the ayahuasca users group. High scores of those have been previously associated with drug abuse (Verdejo-Garcia et al., 2008; Pedrero-Pérez, 2006). Other researchers also found no change in Novelty Seeking in ayahuasca users (Barbosa et al., 2009). They administered the personality questionnaire TCI shortly before and 6 months after the first ayahuasca use of 23 naive participants in a religious setting. A positive correlation between the decrease in Reward Dependence and the intensity of ayahuasca use was found. Halpern et al. (2008) investigated 32 members of Santo Daime church. Out of 24 subjects who reported drug or alcohol abuse or dependence in their history 22 were already in full remission. Al 5 participants who had prior alcohol dependency reported that their participation in the church was their turning point (Halpern et al., 2008).

In 2005 a qualitative study was published, which conducted interviews with 28 adolescent members of the ayahuasca-consuming União do Vegetal church (UDV). No psychosocial destruction was observed on the youth who usually participates in the ayahuasca rituals together with their parents and other relatives. It was shown that the teens 'appear to be healthy, thoughtful, considerate and bonded to their families and religious peers' (de Rios et al., 2005).

The scientific data up to the present give some evidence that the non-hedonic use of ayahuasca in a well-controlled structured setting seems relatively save. The addiction potential seems to be low.

9.5 Psychological scales

Pharmacological studies from 1994 until the present, which took a quantitative look onto subjective effects of DMT or ayahuasca, have preferred for that purpose the Hallucinogen Rating Scale HRS (Strassman, 1992). It measures substance-induced subjective psychedelic effects on six scales. 1. Somesthesia: somatic experiences. 2. Affect: emotional and affective responses. 3. Volition: capacity to wilfully interact intra-individual and with the environment. 4. Cognition: modifications in thought processes and thought content. 5. Perception: visual, auditory, gustatory and olfactory experiences. 6. Intensity: strength of the overall experience. The range of scores for all HRS scales is 0 to 4. The scale was constructed from interviews from the rather small sample of experienced DMT users through factor analysis (Strassman et al. 1994).

Another very common scale for the quantitative report of drug effects is the Addiction Research Centre Inventory (ARCI), which was developed in 1958 on detoxified opiate addicted prisoners (Martin et al., 1971). They were exposed to different psychoactive drug experiences, including a non-drug and placebo group (Strassman 1992). It consists of five scales or groups, which describe the measured experiences as, e.g. more or les "LSD-like" or "morphine-like". 1. MBG scale: morphine–benzedrine group, measuring euphoria and positive mood. 2. PCAG scale, pentobarbital– chlorpromazine–alcohol group, measuring sedation. 3. LSD, lysergic acid diethylamide scale: measuring somatic– dysphoric effects like anxiety, tension, depersonalization, changes in perception and sensation. 4. BG, the benzedrine group scale: measuring intellectual energy and efficiency. 5. Amphetamine-like effects scale.

The Abnormal Mental States questionnaire (APZ) from Dittrich (1975, 1998) and its revisions Altered States of Consciousness Rating Scale (OAV with 66 items) and the newest 5D-ABZ version with 94 items (also called 5D-ASC), are often-used instruments to differentiate subjective effects of different induction methods of altered states of consciousness (ASC). They are also used for the investigation of dose-response relationships and to relate subjective effects of ASC to various neuronal, psychophysiological and behavioural variables. Unfortunately, there is some confusion about the different versions and names of the questionnaire, e.g. 5D-ASC, 5D-ABZ, OAV, OAVAV. In 2010 approximately 70 international experimental studies were counted, in which a version of this questionnaire was used for retrospective analysis of ASC. Dittrich wanted to observe inter-experience features of those experiences, which are invariant for all ASC, regardless of their induction method. He tried to differentiate them from normal waking consciousness, in order to establish empirical indicators for his underlying ASC construct and to find a taxonomy of ASC. For that psilocybin, ketamine and MDMA was administrated to healthy volunteers. Dittrich postulated three primary dimensions and one etiology-independent dimension (G-ASC): 1. 'Oceanic boundlessness' (OBN) measures positively experienced depersonalization and derealisation, positive mood and experiences of unity. High scores would indicate states similar to mystical experiences. 2. 'Dread of ego dissolution' (DED) measures unpleasantly experienced derealisation and depersonalization, cognitive disturbances, catatonic symptoms, paranoia, loss of thought control and loss of body control. High scores would indicate so called "bad trips". 3. 'Visionary restructuralization' (VRS) measures visual (pseudo)-hallucinations and illusions, auditory-visual synaesthesia, changes in the meaning of percepts. The secondary dimension describes the general consciousness alteration.

In 2010 an evaluation of the OAV version scale with a large sample from 43 experimental studies was published (Studerus et al., 2010). The original 3 factors did not fit to the data and could not be confirmed.

The following 11 factors were necessary to achieve model fit:

1. Experience of unity (e.g. item 21: 'It seemed to me that my environment and I were one.')
2. Spiritual experience (e.g. item 56: 'I experienced a kind of awe.')
3. Blissful state (e.g. item 7: 'I enjoyed boundless pleasure.')
4. Insightfulness (e.g. item 52: 'I had very original thoughts.'; item 34: 'I felt very profound.')
5. Disembodiment (e.g. item 43: 'It felt as though I was floating.')
6. Impaired control and cognition (e.g. item 45: 'I was not able to complete a thought; my thought repeatedly became disconnected')
7. Anxiety (e.g. item 32: 'I experienced my surroundings as strange and weird."; item 38: "I felt threatened.')
8. Complex imagery (e.g. item 25: 'I saw scenes rolling by in total darkness or with my eyes closed.'; item 49: 'I could see pictures from my past or fantasy extremely clear.')
9. Elementary imagery (e.g. item 8: 'I saw regular patterns in complete darkness or with eyes closed.')
10. Audio-visual synaesthesia (e.g. item 11: 'Noises seemed to influence what I saw.')
11. Changed meaning of perception (e.g. item 37: 'Objects around me engaged me emotionally much more than usual.').

10 Health and health theories

In the study, subjective health theories of western ayahuasca users in South America were examined. Some general scientific western perspectives about health are presented here.

> 'Health is a state of complete physical, mental and social well-being and not merely the absence of disease or infirmity' (WHO 1948).

This general definition of the World Health Organization has remained since 1948 until today. With the central criterion "well-being" the subjective perception and interpretation of the health status is strongly emphasised. The WHO actively prevents the negative definition of health from the possible criterion of the absence of disease with this social-psycho-somatic view. A bio-medical view from a western perspective defines health much tighter as the undisturbed functionality and concurrence of the organs to ensure their contribution to life.

The health status can be interpreted subjectively from the concerned person but also from an outside view onto the objective process events. The objective appraisal comes from a consensus of experts on the basis of recognized criteria of health. Such criteria take in account medical diagnostic findings, risk factors, physiological, psychological and social operativeness related to certain areas of life and their requirements (Schröder, 2008, p. 178).

Health is defined from different instances. Firstly, there are subjective health theories of layman. Secondly, there are medical definitions from culturally recognized experts, which apply as official theories. Thirdly, there are holistic theories, e.g. the bio-psycho-social models (Udris et al., 1992) or bio-psycho-social-spiritual models. A transactional bio-psycho-social definition is provided by Schröder (2008, p. 117): Health is a transactional state between the potentials of the individual to organize itself autonomously, to develop itself and its social-economic surrounding. Health is a quality of the psychophysiological regulation and expresses a stabilized system and a dynamical balance within the contradictory relation between human and environment. Levels of health can be experienced subjectively and described through signs of health. Disease is seen as an expression of the disturbed interdependency between the organism and its surrounding.

One-dimensional considerations see health and disease as opposite poles on the health continuum and the individual point on this continuum as a result of

© The Editor(s) (if applicable) and The Author(s), under exclusive license to
Springer Fachmedien Wiesbaden GmbH, part of Springer Nature 2020
T. J. Wolff, *The Touristic Use of Ayahuasca in Peru*, Sozialwissenschaftliche Gesundheitsforschung, https://doi.org/10.1007/978-3-658-29373-4_10

longer efforts to stabilize the system. The two-dimensional concept sees health factors and risk factors independently. A person can subjectively feel ill if the balance between protective and pathogenetic influences is shifted towards the last (ibid.).

Integrative bio-psycho-social views of the human see the health regulation activity in three areas: External regulation competences for the control and coping of environmental and situational demands, self regulative competences for the internal stabilization, self control and self development and finally the meaningfulness of experiences under the individual attitude towards the world and life values.

10.1 Loads, demands and consequences

Influences or stimuli on the organismic system, which make it necessary to perform regulating activity, can be called loads (German: Belastungen). Complex self-regulating systems like organisms try to measure and interpret those loads. They establish and obtain their states of optimum or homoeostasis within the proportion between the surroundings and their body-functions. They follow aims and satisfy needs.

Subjective impacts of loads on the physiological, psychological and behavioural level can be called demands or strains (German: Beanspruchungen). The proportion between loads and demands is interactive and contains feedback loops. Load experiences and the quality and quantity of demanded reactions are influenced by prior conditions like personality, habitual and situational factors (Scheuch & Schröder, 1990). Loads and individual conditions constitute the demands and demanded reactions can be within a psychophysiological range of homeostasis or beyond. On example of a typical demand reaction is learning. If those necessary regulative reactions are outside the homeostatic range far distant or for a longer period of time demand consequences follow. They are changes in function or physiology, which arise directly from the overstraining load or from the attempts to cope. Positive examples of demand consequences are better adaption, emotional stability and improved competence of action. Negative examples are fatigue through the excessive demand, monotony through low demand, stress through threat and saturation through frustration. Fatigue through excessive demand and chronic stress lead to exhaustion of the system and symptoms appear (Schröder, 1996, p.13).

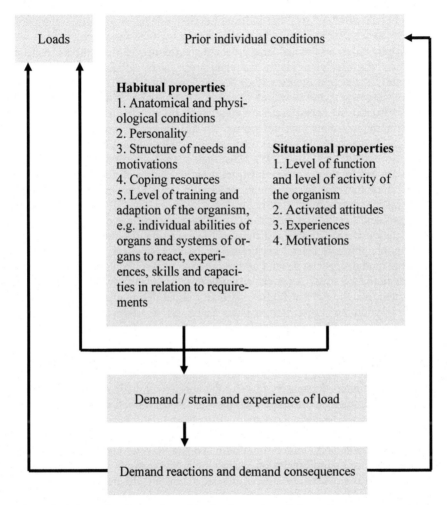

Figure 2: Schematic presentation of loads, demands and demand consequences from a health psychological perspective (adapted from Schröder, 1996)

10.2 Stress

As far as I found out in the literature research, the use and effects of ayahuasca have never been examined under a stress theoretical view, but previous investigations have found psychological benefits, like e.g. improvements in the well-being

(Bouso et al., 2012, p. 10), that indicate possible relevance for stress regulation. That is why a closer look onto the theory of stress will be done here.

In general, stress is considered a demand consequence. Many theoretical concepts from the research of loads, strain and stress can be categorized as a) theories of stimuli, b) reaction theories or c) transactional theories. The connections between loads, strains and health on one side and long-term and short-term consequences from badly coped stress are varicoloured (Udris & Frese, 1999).

Stimulus concepts interpret stimuli as situations, which produce stress. The research of stressful life events is difficult because individuals react very different in the same situations (Filip, 1995). Nevertheless, there are certain types of stimuli, which are experienced as stressful from a large number of persons showing the typical stress reactions in such situations (ibid., p. 430). Reactional concepts define stress independently from it's trigger through the reactions of the organism. The main problem here is that the same physiological reaction can be triggered from completely different stimuli, which even can have opposite psychological meaning (e.g. happiness or fear). Measurements of stress parameter do not necessarily correlate, and results can depend on the criterion chosen for the measurement. In the beginning of stress research, reaction-orientated and physiological models dominated, like the fight or flight syndrome from W. Cannon or the General-Adaptation-Syndrome (G-A-S) from Hans Selye (Selye, 1946, 1976). He defined stress as an unspecific reaction of all organisms to any demand (Filip, 1995; Selye, 1951). Three steps are passed through: 1. Tensional state of the alarm reaction, 2. Resistance state against the load, 3. Exhaustion and Disease of Adaption (Selye, 1951).

Transactional concepts try to solve the conceptual difficulties. Because they include psychological considerations they can separate better between positive states of arousal, euphoria, challenge, eustress and unpleasant stress. Individual variables like perception, interpretation of stimuli and anticipation of success or no-success, needs and aims, estimation of coping abilities and resources have a strong influence on the generation process of stress reactions. Greif (1991, p. 13) defines stress as an intensive unpleasant state of tension within a strongly aversive, threatening and long-lasting situation, which leads to the subjective interpretation that avoidance is important. Lazarus's transactional stress concept cannot predict exactly which reactions follows out of which circumstances or combinations of circumstances. The model will be described later in detail. Other ideas also focus on similarities between concepts of loads and stress. Stress arises if aim-oriented action is hindered through obstacles of regulation or excessive demands (Leitner, et al., 1993). Or stress arises through additional regulation activity, uncertainty of regulation or aim (Richter & Hacker, 1998; Semmer, 1984). Another important idea is the concepts of cumulated micro-stressors (Schönpflug, 1987) or "daily hassles" (Kanner, Coyne, Schaefer, Lazarus, 1981). In a typical work surrounding regular small occasions are mostly seen as more relevant for health-related stress reactions than rare big incidents. Their accumulation leads to multiple load and chronic cognitive and emotional strain (Dunckel, 1991).

Transactional concepts can locate the stress-generating process and the stress-reduction process on different processing levels.

Table 3: List of process levels of the stress reaction in humans in transactional stress models

Process level	Examples
Physiological level	Alarm reaction ability Vulnerability of the organs for disease General-Adaptation-Syndrome Psychosomatic diseases (e.g. gastric ulcer) Coronary heart disease Prostration Death
Behavioural level	Escalated level of attention Problem solving Interruption or inhibition of action Rigid or stereotype behaviour Self-aggression Social behaviour (social avoiding behaviour, help seeking behaviour, abrasiveness/aggression)
Emotional level	Primary and secondary emotions Defence mechanisms (renouncement of the threat, rationalisation, etc.) Alexithymia Depression Burnout
Cognitive level	Creativity Reframing, cognitive validation Perceptual limitations Self validation

10.2.1 Transactional model of stress

Besides from the physiological and immunological mechanisms stress reactions in human organisms depend from different factors: The cognitive validation of a situation has a substantial influence on the triggering and the development of stress reactions. Interpretations of difficult situations can differ from threat to challenge and facilitate, prevent or moderate stress reactions. The general load from multiple sources in life may decrease the threshold for stress reactions. The availability of resources like pre-experience, coping skills and coping style, access to society resources, social support, social network, physical constitution and personality presuppose and moderate the process as well as the cognitive appraisal of the resources in relation to the stressor.

Table 4: List of influential factors on stress reactions, according to transactional stress models

Factors	Examples
Cognitive appraisal	Threat or challenge or neutral
Load from multiple other sources	Quality of sleep Social problems Financial problems Environment of arbitrariness Time pressure Noise pollution Overcrowding Many overlapping and unfinished actions
Availability of resources	Pre-experience Coping skills and coping style Access to society resources Social support, social network Physical constitution Personality
Cognitive appraisal of resources	

Transactional models empathize the importance of interpretation and appraisal of load factors one hand and on the other hand the appraisal of the personal ability to accomplish or cope. Psychic stress generates from the individual interpretation between demands (which can be contradictory) and personal resources, which subjectively puts the resources to the test or overstrains them (Lazarus, 1990, p. 213). The interpretation of loads as being un-solvable or the appraisal of the coping actions as unsuccessful can lead to stress reactions on the different process levels.

The mostly known stress coping model is the transactional process model from Lazarus and Folkman (1984). It puts first the objective situation, which provides the load or potential stressor. But more important is the way in which the person subjectively processes the load from the objective situation. A primary appraisal takes place. This is said to be a phylogenetic old processing step on a subcortical level. The situation is basically evaluated as relevant or irrelevant to one's well being regarding its interpretation either as a threat or a challenge. A secondary appraisal of the stressor takes place, which evaluates the relation between the demand and the coping competences and the estimated extent of endeavour which will be necessary to solve the challenging situation. If the result is positive, coping activity will be performed. After the subjective detection of success, the additional activation of the organism will decrease. Both appraisal steps contain feedback loops. The stress cirquit continues until the load/strain is subjectively solved or faded out (e.g. through distraction, alcohol).

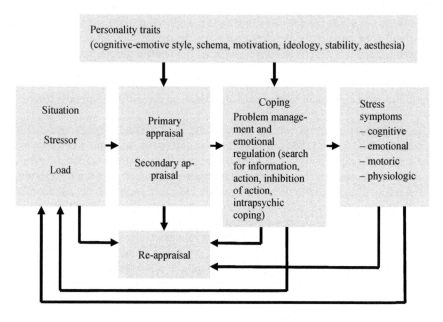

Figure 3: Schematic presentation of the transactional stress model of Lazarus (Lazarus & Folkman 1984; Lazarus, 1999; Yong Wah Goh et al. 2010)

Both appraisal steps can be accompanied by different emotions, e.g. interest, hope and reliance if the situation is interpreted as challenge and chance. These emotions stimulate both activity and perseverance. Anger, grief, despondence and helplessness can appear if the situation is interpreted as harm or loss; anxiety, worry and excitement if the load is experienced as threat, and the personal coping competences are appraised as insufficient.

There are different coping categories: Direct action, inhibition of action, search for information and intra-psychic coping processes (Lazarus, 1974).

Table 5: List of different coping styles in the transactional stress model of Lazarus

Types of coping	Explanation and examples
Direct action	Direct change of environmental loads, external emotional coping (e.g. violence, intrigue, relaxation exercises)
Inhibition of action	Omission of ineffective or threatening behaviour
Search for information	Analyse of the loads and search for alternative or additional coping possibilities
Intra-psychic coping	Cognitive emotive coping (e.g. through the inner monologue, trivialization, self encouragement, denegation, phantasy, daydream, dissociation, distraction, etc.)

On the basis of these coping types, Lazarus has created a taxonomy of two big domains of coping strategies: problem centred external coping and emotion centred internal coping.

Table 6: Taxonomy of coping strategies on the basis of differnet coping styles in the transactional stress model of Lazarus (adapted from Lazarus, 1975; Schröder, 1996)

Coping domains	Examples
Problem centred external coping Actions with the aim to influence the stressor directly or to make changes in the relationship between person and stressor Modification of stress inducing circumstances	Fight or flight Search for alternatives to fight or flight, e.g. negotiation and compromise Prevention of anticipated stressors Activities that reduce the anticipated intensity of stressors Activities that reduce the anticipated impact of stressors (self preparation for the improvement of resistance, activation of resources)
Emotion centred internal coping	Modification of physical circumstances, e.g. relaxation techniques, biofeedback, medicines, drugs

Regulation of inner conditions without direct affection on the stressor	Modification of cognitive emotive circumstances, e.g. distraction, phantasy, daydream, reframing, increase of the cognitive distance through inner logical arguing, acceptance of logical errors to maintain cognitive consonance, relativization through reducing the identification with the problem, meta-level view, mindfulness meditation, dissociation, lowering of the pretensions
Optimizing the reaction of psycho-energetic appropriation to prevent overstimulation or understimulation	
	Unconscious/preconscious and automatic biased processes, which affect and deform the perception and appraisal of the reality, e.g. defence mechanisms

Different authors extended the transactional stress model. For this study the extension from Folkman and Greer (2000, pp. 11-19) seems especially relevant. They added the meaning-based coping in addition to the problem-related and emotion-regulation coping, in order to increase the predictive power of the model for patients with life threatening diseases (Taubert & Förster, 2005, pp. 147-157). When recent coping attempts fail or are ineffective in reducing the stressful activation of the organism, meaning-making is often used to reassess the situation. In the light of meanin- based coping, elements of magical thinking in subjective health and disease concepts can be understood (fait, guilt and punishment, Karma, higher will, lesson to learn, pain as teacher, etc.). The search for meaning regards as a predictor for the development of a pleasant emotional state (Knoll et al., 2005). A longitudinal pilot study on 27 adults supports this: A negative correlative connection of perceived stress and spiritual well-being had been found (Tuck et al., 2006). A one-year follow-up study with 99 patients of depression identified higher spirituality and harm avoidance as predictors for the recovery from depression after one year. The authors distinguish between spirituality and religiousness. Mostly Catholic religiousness was not a predictor for the recovery (Mihaljevic et al., 2016). Meaning-making may serve as a mediator between stress and emotional well-being.

Amazonian shamanism is substantially based on magical thinking and invisible meaning behind situations, surroundings, health and disease. But, when reflecting about Amazonian shamanism, the use of the expression might be inaccurate because of its connotation to the word belief. The term does not distinguish enough between a belief that lacks its empirical basis and a conviction that is not doubted because of its subjective evidence in the personal experience. For mestizo or even for native American ayahuasqueros, intelligent and communicating spirit-beings and their actions behind our visible world might be as real as a taxi driver talking about his opinion on football. For them, there is no magic (in the sense of ‚unusual' or ‚miracle') in matters that we would easily call ‚magical thinking'. In opposition to them, we mostly do not have any subjective empirical base for such stories. Carlos Tanner, the owner of an ayahuasca centre near Iquitos, once talked about the convincing power of ayahuasca experiences in this particular setting. Often, one night-ceremony would have been enough to change the subjective theoretical system of participants substantially (Carlos Tanner in a personal talk on the 3rd of October 2014 in Lima). Regardless of the reality or illusion of the perceived psychedelic items under the influence of ayahuasca in a shamanic setting, it often produces strong subjective evidence of meaning. This itself would have therapeutic relevance, Carlos Tanner emphasised. Elements of magical thinking as part of the meaning-making and subjective theories about disease, healing and the working processes of ayahuasca will be analysed in the investigation about expectations, subjective effects and evaluations (Tarapoto sample of Garden of Peace centre in Peru).

10.2.2 Self regulation and environment-focussed regulation

As seen above in the taxonomy of coping activities one can separate two substantial regulatory circuits. One is focussed on the fit with the environment through changes in the problem or object of concerns. In general, this seems to be the so-called alloplastic and autoplastic regulations (Pawlowsky, 2009), which are known from different psychodynamic authors (Ferenczi, 1919, Freud, 1924, Laplanche, 1972, Stern, 1992). The other focuses on the self-regulation to secure and stabilizes the person as premise for the successful interaction with the environment. It contains internal processes of homeostatic exchange on the emotional, cognitive and physiological levels.

One-sided regulation attempts can be dysfunctional. If in an objectively problematic situation, which requires additional regulation activity, the preferred strategies are exclusively self regulation, a current quick reduction of the acute stress reaction might be possible, but it does not lead to the change of the circumstances in which the stress reaction occur. If this is a habitual reaction pattern, adequate competences of environment focussed regulation activity can not sufficiently be purchased and a real lack of these (e.g. social) competences fix the limited, rigid, dysfunctional reaction pattern with a feeling of insufficiency or ideological justification.

The stress coping should be adapted to the quality, length and intensity of the stressors.

External regulation strategies can be insufficient, if the unregulated emotional involvement and activation increase more and more and avert prospective and unerring action.

Both regulative systems are mostly necessary for successful regulation activity but can also be conflictive, e.g. if the autoplastic adaptation activity demands actions which do not harmonize with narcissic self prospects or if alloplastic regulation activities clash with internal moral or religious convictions. Such conflicts of the regulatory systems can be themselves potent stressors and pathogenetic causes for overstrain, chronic stress, diseases and death.

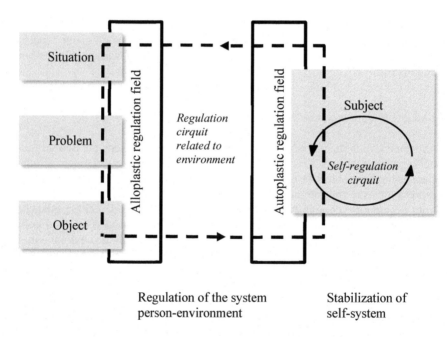

Figure 4: Schematic presentation of aspects of human regulation activity (adapted from Schröder, 1997)

Schröder (1996) defines stress as useful additional or alarm regulation. It always appears in critical strain situations if basic physiological or psychological needs are threatened. In the model of Schröder acute and chronic stress operate on the continuum of health and disease within a process of destabilization. This process of additional regulation and destabilization under strain pressure (ibid.) works over four steps:

1. Adjustment and behavioural routines: Demands within a homeostatic range and without threatened basic needs will be adjusted automatically. If any additional adjustment is needed, e.g. if contradictions within the process of adaptation of the person to the dynamical environmental system appear, regulative operations like emotion-based regulation and cognitive controlled actions) will be performed under the central cognitive control, in order to maintain the homeostatic balance.

2. Activation of action: If the discrepancy between person and environment can not be regulated and is appraised as a threat in terms of strain and coping abilities, an action activation program will be initiated. The individual has to perform a self-controlled and organized adaption due to the changed conditions. The acute stress reaction is functional because it provides the necessary additional energy for the adaption effort. The outcome depends from the appropriateness of the coping effort.

Pleasant emotions and the interpretation of the situation as challenge, which can accompany such repeated acute stress reactions will lead to a higher self esteem and improved competences. This can have a preventive and protective effect. If the additional activation of acute stress reactions and the problem solving or adaptation activity fail over a longer period of time, the situation leads to the 3rd step.

3. Permanent activation (chronic stress): The permanent activation through imbalance of the person-environment-system leads to a depletion of psychophysiological reserves. The situation can be accompanied by impairments of well-being like lowered self-esteem, anxiety, helplessness, depression, agitation, high sensitivity and breakdown of defence mechanisms. The organisation of actions lacks effectiveness. Flexibility and ability to adapt are limited and coping strategies are dysfunctional (e.g. abuse of alcohol). The person is tired but unable to relax or sleep. Psychosomatic symptoms appear as pathogenic precursors.

4. Psycho-vegetative reactions: Psychopathological disorders, vegetative disorders or physiological organ-damages are seen as consequence of chronic overstimulation. Chronic disease follows. The disease often changes into a dynamic process, which is independent from the original conditions of its emergence.

Stress is seen as an adjustor between health and disease. Models of stress in general try to show psychophysiological and psycho-endocrinological mechanisms that adjust between suboptimal environmental conditions and impairments of the organism (Schonecke & Hermann, 1986).

10.2.3 Elements of pathogenic transformation

Schröder (1996) identifies tree pathogenic domains: Inappropriate appraisal, emotional transformation elements, psycho-physiological elements. These domains contain specific elements of stress, which have been proved to co-determinate the harming effect.

1. Inappropriate appraisal: Psychological defence mechanisms for the fading-out of threads may have a helpful stress reducing short term effect but the long term effects of excessive cognitive defence is unfavourable; hostile defence with strongly unpleasant emotions; the experience of helplessness and loss of control while a connection between actions and results can not be established, desperateness ("My actions just make it worse.")

2. Emotional transformation elements: unpleasant emotions like depression, anger, fear and anxiety; fluctuations between hope and disappointment.

3. Psycho-physiological elements: psychophysiological over-reactivity in stress situations and according to that limitations of endocrinological, immunological and autonomous answers of the organism; reduced times of relaxation and recuperation; higher vulnerability of the overloaded regulation systems (endocrinological, immunological and physiological systems – cardio-vascular diseases) and lowered resistance against infections; reactivation of cured former diseases, dysfunctions (e.g. gastric irritation or ulcer) and pathological behaviour (e.g. addiction behaviour, social aggression).

10.2.4 Strain consequences and stress reactions

Negative consequences and stress reactions go from short-term reactions to chronic symptoms. They affect physiological, psychological, behavioural and communicational levels.

Table 7: List of examples for strain consequences and stress reactions (Greif 1991; Kaufmann, Pornschlegel & Udris, 1982; Kaluza, 1996)

	Short term, acute reactions	*Middle and long term, chronic reactions*
Physiological	Increase heart beat frequency Increase blood pressure Release of cortisole and adrenaline	Psychosomatic problems and diseases Dissatisfaction Resignation Depression Burnout
Psychological, cognitive, emotional	Tension, nervousness Agitation Frustration Anger Monotony, fatigue, saturation	
Individual behaviour	Fluctuation of performance Decrease of concentration Spurious action Poor sensorimotor coordination Eagerness and hastiness	Increased consume of nicotine, alcohol and medicine Absence from work Inner resignation
Social behaviour	Increase of testiness Social conflicts Mobbing Quarrel Aggression against others Social withdrawal and isolation	

10.2.5 Possible connection of ayahuasca motivation and internal stress coping activity

Previous investigations have shown evidence that the greatest part of the motivation to consume ayahuasca may be a wish for general improvement of well-being related to psychotherapeutic and spiritual matters. Only a minority comes explicitly to heal specific physiological diseases. Hedonistic motivations, which might typically be a strong factor in drug users seem to be of subordinate interest. This study aims to explore the evidence for the possible motivations to the ayahuasca experience to minimize effects of psychic strain and stress.

Emphasising the individual interpretation of stimuli situations and loads as important part of the stress generating and coping process, transactional models of the complex regulation activity between individual and environment could serve for the understanding of some of the often-claimed positive subjective effects of ayahuasca to the well-being and coping.

If seen under such a stress theoretical view, for the substance assisted psychotherapy and possible effects of ayahuasca ritual therapy the influence on the self regulation and emotion centred coping domain might seems relevant. It is likely that categories which relate to this will be found in the interviews of ayahuasca tourists.

10.3 Salutogesis und SOC

Pathogenesis was the viewpoint of traditional health research and health education. Questions which arise from this are: What is disease? How does it develop? Which are the risk factors and how can it be dissolved. Additional to this perspective the Israeli American sociologist Aaron Antonovsky (1987) asked about the predictions of health and its protective factors: How and why can individuals stay healthy, in spite of their loads and how is it possible to re-establish health (Lindstrom & Eriksson, 2007, pp. 938-944). Both views presuppose and complement each other.

The salutogenic model describes determinants, which help to maintain health and how health can be obtained. Health is not seen as static or categorical state other than illness but as a bi-directional dimensional continuum between illness and health. Antonovsky describes three general factors for the determination of health:

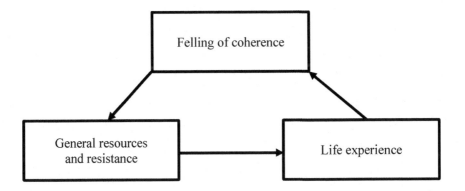

Figure 5: General components of the model of Salutogenesis

General resources for resistance are seen within the individual, within the closer social space and within the environment of life and work. Individual resources refer to the physical and psychic status, which is determined from constitution, immunological system, intelligence, self-esteem and ego identity. Social space refers to the social relations and their quality, social affiliation, embedding, support, participation and material resources. The environment of life and work refers to the cultural and social status and its stability, individual transparency and the involvement in socially recognised processes of decision.

Stressors lead to the generation of tensional states in order to provide energy and prepare the system for regulating actions. The coping behaviour, it's quality and appropriateness can lead to a decrease of the tensional state in the case of successful coping actions, but it also can become chronic in case of unsuccessful coping. Successful coping strengthens the general feeling of coherence and the general resources for resistance.

10.3.1 Sense of coherence

The sense of coherence (SOC) is one of the central concepts of the idea of salutogenesis beside life experiences and resources for resistance. It was the answer to the salutogenic question of how some people can stay healthy even despite stressful situations while others do not (Lindstrom & Eriksson, 2007).

The SOC consists of three components:

- Meaningfulness (wanting to cope)

- Comprehensibility (understanding the challenge)
- Manageability (being convinced of the availability of coping resources)
(Antonovsky, 1996, pp. 11-18)

Meaningfulness describes the conviction that it is worth to invest cognitively and emotionally into the demands of life (Antonovsky 1979; 1987). People who are orientated towards meaningfulness find meaning in challenges. The meaning that is found in life provides motivation (Antonovsky, 1987). Another definition describes meaningfulness as "an emotional connection that promotes motivation" (Landsverk & Kane, 1998, p. 422).

Comprehensibility refers to the possibility to find logic and consistency in life events, to create order to experiences and situations, to be able to review life and that the life events make ‚cognitively sense' to the person (Antonovsky, 1979; 1987).

Manageability refers to the conviction that a person has the resources to cope with the loads and demands or adversity in life (Antonovsky, 1979; Sullivan, 1993, pp. 1772-1778). The efficacy of the coping depends in parts on the conviction to have the right coping strategies (Antonovsky, 1979; 1987).
The strenght of the SOC results from the synergic interaction of its three elements. According to Antonovsky it would have "direct physiological consequences and, through such pathways, affect health status" (Antonovsky 1987, p. 154). A strong SOC would lead to succesful coping through a realistic appraisal, a focus on adaptionally relevant aspects of an encounter and appropriate evaluation of coping options in relation to the actual demands and coping ressources (Lazarus & Folkman, 1984, p. 79).

The SOC concept had been subject of much research but has also been criticised. As examples a few of these studies are mentioned here. An evaluation study of the SOC scale found evidence that the SOC positively correlates with psychological well-being and adaptive coping strategies (Pallant & Lae 2002, pp. 39-48). A large number of validity-research across different populations and countries provides evidence for the SOC (Amirkhan & Greavessense 2003, pp. 31-62). This literature review shows that a high SOC correlates with lower level of stress and symptoms. A Swedish study with a large number of participants found a strong relationship between a low SOC and mental and circulatory health problems. The SOC level seems to vary between different social classes and age groups in the investigated population. Men and women did not show any difference. (Lundberg & Nyström, 1994, pp. 252-257). Marais & Stuart (2005, pp. 89-105) found evidence among journalists that a high SOC supports the ability to cope with traumatic experiences.

Also, Feigin & Sapir (2005, pp. 63-74) show that the SOC would be central regarding the ability to cope with stressful stimuli among substance abusers. Data from a large longitudinal study of adults could show that the SOC is related to the adaptivity to adverse life events (Surtees, Wainwright, Khaw 2006, pp. 221-227). Among a population of patients who had previously attempted to commit suicide low SOC seems to be a better predictor of further suicide ideation and attempts than depression, hopelessness and low self-esteem (Petrie & Brook 1992, pp. 293-300; Polewka et al. 2001, pp. 335-9).

The critics on the SOC concept argue that it is psychometrically problematic, emotionally confound, contradictory, deficient in the prediction of the physical health status and lacks evidence for its time stability (Volanen, 2011, p.28). The critics on its validity might be the most serious (ibid.): It had been complained that a negative correlation between the SOC and measures of mental health would indicate that it does not substancially differ from them (Geyer, 1997, pp. 1771-1779). The same suggestion was made in regards of psychopathological factors of depression, anxiety (Kivimäki et al. 2000, pp. 583-597; Konttinen, Haukkala & Uutela, 2008, pp. 2401-2412; Frenz, Carey & Jorgensen, 1993, pp. 145-153) and neuroticism (Feldt et al., 2007, pp. 483-493). How can the SOC be a cause of mental health and at the same time be itself an element of the mental health concept (Volanen, 2011, p. 28)?

The relevance of meaning-based coping (Folkman and Greer 2000, pp. 11-19) for well-being and coping with difficult situations has been discussed above in the chapter about the transactional model of stress. Meaning-making is also a characteristic element of a high SOC, which has relevance for the mental health and might be a protective factor for stress related disorders. The possible influences of shamanic ayahuasca therapy on meaning-making have also been discussed. Different aspects of subjective disease theories, healing theories and health theories, their relevance and the possible impact of ayahuasca therapy shall be discussed in the following chapter.

10.4 Subjective health and disease theories

The subjective health perspective focuses on the well-being and the experienced cooperativeness. Convictions about signs of health and disease and causal process theories as well as procedures for the maintenance and recovery are part of the subjective perspective. Subjective theories are relevant because they determine the processing of health-related information and they influence the health behaviour (Schröder, 2008, p. 178).

Within this study the reflections of participants about their expectations and experiences are examined. This includes their subjective view on health, disease and their subjective working model of the ayahuasca interventions within their subjective models.

Health perspectives focus on the salutogenic way from disease to health and what it needs to perpetuate the subjective defined health status whereas in opposite disease perspectives describe the pathogenic way and the subjective logic of a disease and its symptoms. Faltermaier, Kühnlein & Burda-Viering (1998) define "subjective health concepts" and "subjective health theories" as sub-constructs of the main category "subjective health perspectives". The latter is "the overall of convictions, considerations and ideas of a person or a group of persons about health" (translated from German; ibid. p. 37). Health concepts are the subjective understanding of health and health theories construct connections between the different positive and negative influences on the health (Faltermaier, 2005; Faltermaier & Kühnlein, 2000). The subjective representations show a continuum between health and disease. They are no exclusive categories. "A person can be sick and at the same time far up the continuum of health, a person can be at the bottom of the health continuum and does not have to suffer a disease" (translated from German; Faltermayer, 2005, p. 153).

Flick (1998, p. 8) identified dimensions or elements of which health concepts can consist of:

- Negative demarcation, e.g. to be free from strains
- Positive definition, e.g. to feel good
- Description of the state, e.g. to be in peace with one self
- Health as a premise, e.g. everything else will come by itself if one is healthy
- Health as a result of certain actions, e.g. healthy life style, nutrition, regular health care
- Health as a phenomenon of social functioning, e.g. talking about one self, emotions, and doing activities with friends.

Weis (1998, pp. 13-23) identified two main dimensions of subjective disease theories:

- Conviction about the locus of control
- Causal attribution

The psychological concept of control convictions – also called locus of control – bases on the theory of social learning from Julian B. Rotter (1966, pp. 1-28). Locus of control means the dimension in which on one hand people are convinced that they have control over a situation and the success of their actions in life and on the other hand that external uncontrollable forces, Persons or conditions would determine or dominate. For this theory the objective locus of control of a particular situation is les relevant. The belief of the person about the locus of control will substantially determine its action. There are two main control convictions: 1. Internal locus of control: The outcome of an action or situation can be influenced or controlled by one's own actions. 2. External locus of control: The outcome of an action depends on external circumstances. Today some authors divide the external control conviction into a) social-external locus of control (other people determine the outcome) and b) fatalistic-external control conviction (fait and chance determine the results). Generalized control convictions are based on larger numbers of previous experiences. They are relevant for new and unpredictable situations. They are based on a smaller number of specific experiences and actions. Specific expectations are built in situations in which some experiences or clues about the locus of control already exist (Amelang et al., 2006).

Intrinsic religious orientation seems to correlate positively with intrinsic locus of control and extrinsic religious orientation seems to correlate negatively with intrinsic locus of control. This was measured on 519 college students (Kahoe, 1974, pp. 812-818). Holt et al. (2003) distinguish between an active spiritual locus of control and a passive spiritual locus of control in relation to health beliefs about breast cancer in African American women. The active conviction lets God empower the individuals in their health belief and behaviour and the passive conviction lets them rely on a higher power (e.g. God, etc.) to determine their health outcomes. The active dimension was negatively related to the perceived benefits of mammography and positively to the perceived barriers to mammography. The study was based on 1227 participants.

Becker (1984, p. 318) identified five factors that influence subjective disease theories:

- Type and time frame of the disease
- Biography and personality
- Present scientific model
- Magical thinking
- Reactive need for causal attribution

The development of health concepts depends especially on the context in which ideas about health become relevant for the concerning person (Flick, 1998, p.8). The emotional states, e.g. fears, can be seen as part of this context and must be kept in mind when investigating the development of subjective health theories (ibid., pp. 14-15). But emotional factors were not considered in earlier research about subjective health theories, e.g. by Groeben et al. (1988). Flick quotes Alfred Schütz, who defined theories during the early 1970s in general as knowledge that is organized in the form of constructs. Constructs of the first grade would be the constructs of participants of a social field. Constructs of the second grade would be constructs about constructs of these participants, e.g. of the sociology (Flick, 1998, p. 12). The ideas of subjective theories have evolved also from the idea of personal constructs of George A. Kelly (1955). He believed that ordinary persons form and test hypotheses and construct their knowledge about the world, just as scientists do. They build theories of causes and effects. A mentioned earlier this building process of implicit theoretical models is influenced by the person's attribution style, which was firstly described by Fritz Heider (1958). Heider also saw humans as naive scientists in their everyday life but identified two types of causal attribution that effect the subjective modelling in naive psychology:

- External attribution, which imputes the own behaviour to reasons, which lie outside the person.
- Internal attribution, which assigns behaviour to internal factors like e.g. personality, character convictions.

The causal attribution is done retrospectively but it is subjectively interpreted as a predictor of future actions. Regarding unpredictable and negative situations causal attribution has often the functions of stabilizing the emotional state and the self-esteem and provides understanding in order to reject the feeling of helplessness (Filipp & Ferring, 1998, pp. 25-36; Faller, 1998). Herewith the causal attribution serves the earlier described sense of coherence: The world is comprehensible, meaningful and manageable.

Causal attribution has three dimensions that influence the coping behaviour:

- Localisation
- Control
- Stability

If a person interprets the cause of an unpleasant effect as stable and uncontrollable the probability is high that this person will not put much own effort in active coping behaviour.

Subjective theories sometimes have other functions than scientific theories. They provide orientation in particular situations in life, give later explanations or predict the future, facilitate decisions, control actions and stabilize the self-esteem (Dann,

1983, pp. 82ff). They serve for the emotional coping (Bischoff & Zenz 1989, p. 13) and the current rejection of intolerable emotions (Verres, 1989, p. 18). A person becomes expert about a particular topic in life through the subjective theories about it but due to its dependency from the actual context those theories change (Verres, 1986). The functionality of subjective disease theories has been examined for particular diseases, e.g. cancer (ibid., 1986). The quality of such personal theories is subjectively evaluated either through their practicability for that particular topic and through their empirical confirmation. Social and emotional factors also play a role for keeping a conviction, despite of its evidence of disprove. Subjective theories can be distinguished from scientific theories by their partly logical inconsistency, their instability in time and dependence on the context of experience, their use for the guidance or justification of action and their emotional elements and psychodynamic function, e.g. containing symbols, metaphors, the function of denegation of perception as coping against fear (after Verres, 1986). The so called 'magical thinking' has also been identified as an influencing factor and element of those theories, as mentioned above: E.g. an analysis of subjective disease theories of cancer patients had shown that 1/3 of the sample saw fait or guilt and punishment as substantial pathogenic factor (Becker, 1984, p. 315).

Three general types of subjective health theories were divided in early research (Herzlich, 1973):

- Vacuum theories, which define health as the absence of disease
- Storage basin theories of a quantity of resistibility against harming influences
- Equilibrium theories which define health as a state of perfection which can be characterized by wellbeing, good mood and supporting social surrounding.

- Flick & Niewiarra (1994) added a forth type which they call 'health as life style'.

According to this, Herzlich (1973, p. 104ff.) also found types of subjective disease concepts:

1. Disease as destruction: The loss of the social role, social isolation and dependency from others dominate this type. The person experiences himself as a victim to whom harm or violence was done. It leads to inactivity.

2. Disease as liberation: Here the disease provides the possibility to escape incriminating situations and demands of the society. The disease is experienced as protection and protest. It is seen as dormancy and opens up new possibilities, e.g. more intellectual activities, rediscovery of personal interests and personal growth.

3. Disease as a task: Characteristic is the active fight against disease, the fear of the disease but also the acceptance of the disease. Disease is understood as an opportunity or task to learn from it and healing is the natural outcome of this process. Chronic diseases still offer the possibility of adaptive coping. Patients see possibilities to take part in the healing activities. The relationship to the healing professionals is cooperative and interchanging. This type is complementary to the subjective health concept 'health as life style'.

The dynamic aspect of subjective health models can be grouped as four types (Faltermaier & Kühnlein, 2000):

- Switch model with on-off dynamic: Health and disease are seen as two different states.
- Battery model: a person loses more and more health over the span of life
- Rechargeable accumulator model: The health status can be influenced; health can be regenerated.
- Generator model: Health can be amplified under very propitious circumstances.

Newer research combined dynamic aspects and content aspects and created four general types (Faltermaier, Kühnlein & Burda-Viering, 1998):

- Theories of risk: Health is threatened by external environmental risks, burdens and risky behaviour. To maintain health, these risks have to be minimized.
- Theories of resources: Extern and intern resources have to be built-up, maintained and strengthened in order to maintain and optimize health (such as lifestyle, social network support, predisposition)
- Theories of equilibrium or adjustment: Health can be maintained by equilibrate risks and resources such as physical, psychic and social factors. Risks turn to harming strains only if necessary adjustments are not realized.
- Theories of fate

Subjective theories about health and disease have an influence on the experience and the behaviour. In healthy individuals these believes influence mostly the prevention behaviour and additionally the coping behaviour in ill individuals (Burkert, Knoll, Daig, 2012). Many symptoms and problems never reach the professional medical systems because the amateur and folk medicine knowledge of the affected as well as his social environment have always been used to recognize and treat diseases (Flick, 1998, p.25).

Dörner (1975) emphasises that subjective concepts about health and disease play different roles on every level of the socialization process of patients. At the first stage, where first symptoms are experienced, the individual feels the need to search for explanations and definitions of his state (Dörner, 1974, p. 153). His own ideas, but also the concepts of his social environment, will determine when and how he realizes that the disease has to be treated. In the second stage ("I am ill."), when he comes to the conclusion to be ill, he decides were, how and when he seeks medical help. Before this decision, an amateur diagnosis is made (ibid., p. 157). Medical knowledge and beliefs influence this process. In the third stage ("I have to go to the doctor") and in the forth stage ("I am a patient") the trust, cooperation and compliance are also determined by individual ideas and the ideas of the social field. In the fifth stage ("I am healthy") the perception and interpretation of the person as healthy depends on the subjective concepts about disease and health (Flick, 1998, pp. 25-26).

Cultural theoretical models, which are more or less collectively believed from a social group, are called folk models in the literature of cognitive anthropology (D'Andade 1987, p. 112). They contain elements and relational connections between those elements, e.g. causal sequences. Often, they are used intuitively, without explicit knowing about its existence. One example is the folk model of the mind from D'Andade (1995), which might be valid for a great number of cultural groups. D'Andrale could show that for many people it is subjectively evident that their (as well as other's) minds would work as a processor and a container for knowledge. Someone who believes in this cultural model would always assume that events and perceptions form thoughts and not that thoughts would generate events. Thoughts than would generate feelings and wishes and this would generate intentions, which generate actions. Sometimes feelings also would influence the thoughts.

The individual shape of this cultural model may be more or less simplified, more or less consciously reflected and more or less consistent or interspersed with additional elements.

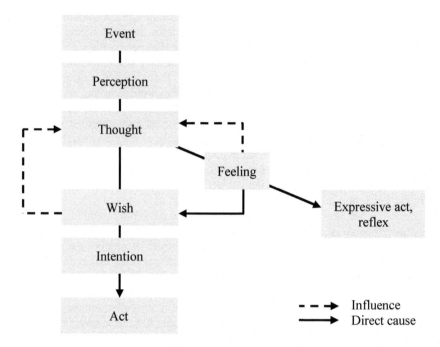

Figure 6: Schematic presentation of the folk model of the mind (adapted from D'Andrade, 1995)

Some exceptions of the general sequence are common, e.g. that actions sometimes can appear as effect of impulses and not from rational thinking or that thoughts occasionally could appear spontaneously without any previous event or that sometimes perceptions are influenced by emotions.

The model provides propositional information and can be used for problem solving and prediction of effects, thoughts, feelings or of the behaviour of others. It guides the person's attention to relevant aspects, e.g. if someone wants to understand the other's behaviour the model leads to focus on the other's intentions, wishes and thoughts. If a person knows what someone else things about a certain topic this person may be able to make predictions about the others behaviour, since the model connects both. If there are information of one part of the model one may be able to suggest about other parts.

Shore (1996, p. 315) emphasised that such shared implicit models help to communicate experiences within the same social group because they all use the almost same cognitive experience filter. The shared model may not only provide shared mental processes to the individual member but also shared content and thus orientation, certainty and easier communication.

The ritualized ayahuasca intake within the South American curandero-settings might be imbedded into its own folk models, belief systems, health theories, supposed expectations of their customers as well as the folk models, belief systems, health theories, expectations and interpretations of the participants themselves. It is likely that the cultural folk models of disease, health and healing of local South Americans from the past differ from the ones of nowadays and from the ones that foreign visitors bring with them from the North Americas and Western Europe. The development and change of the ayahuasca traditions and working models over the time probably take place within the dynamic tension and interaction process of these sides. Within the ayahuasca scene there is a strong tendency of emphasizing the importance of the ritualistic and guided intake as well as the shamanic interactions with e.g. plant spirits that provide hidden diagnostic information and therapeutic actions. The substance intake in another but the curandero set and setting or even a more or less contextless consumption of ayahuasca seems to be seen as unethical, dangerous or inefficient from many insiders (C. Tanner, personal communication, October 3, 2015). Not infrequently this discussion is lead on one hand under the points of preserving the supposed traditional dogmas, authenticity and high therapeutic quality or on the other hand under the idea of adopting and transforming some native or shamanic elements – or what is seen as such – into other neo-shamanic, therapeutic or experimental framework with different theoretical environments.

'Because the conditions of action do not have an exclusively delimiting or even enforcing character but also a facilitating one, they are submitted to continuous interpretation from the protagonists and by this to modifications' (translated from German, Witzel 2010). Different authors have formulated this view: 'self organization' (Heinz, 2000) and 'productive reality processing subject' (Hurrelmann, 1983). Protagonists are seen as manufacturing their own development. Conditions give a certain orientation and suggest actions, but they do not determine them (Elder & O'Rand, 1995). The relation between subject and its environment is interactional. In the case of ayahuasca tourism, very different living environments come together, and different folk models interact and are exchanged. Zacharias (2005) has shown that the personal theory of Mexican curanderos about disease and healing differ, dependent weather their main clientele comes from urban or rural environments. It is likely that the exchange with foreign clients (their expectations, problems and healing theories) will change the subjective disease and health theories (and healing practices) of local healers in the Amazon.

In general, subjective health theories are formed through the interpretation of the interaction process of the person with the (social) surrounding (social interactions, health related situations, experiences and places, media, etc.). But at the same time the health-related theories and convictions influence this interaction process. They are dynamic structures (Flick, 1998, p. 16).

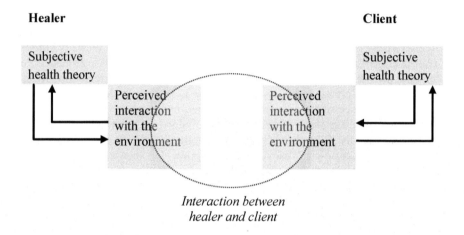

Figure 7: Schematic presentation of the mutual influence of subjective theory, perceived interaction process between individual and environment in healers and clients

In western health sciences the acceptance of professional disease theory and health theories is often seen as important part of the targeted healing process, because it improves the patient's compliance, cooperation and appropriate coping behaviour regarding the disease and its treatment. In psychotherapeutic treatments the shared acceptance of a theory that was commonly developed within the therapeutic work between the therapist and the client and its saturation with the sensation of truth might have a healing effect itself and might often be seen as evidence for the healing progress. Flick (1998, p. 16) and others writes about psychotherapy in general as a process of negotiation about the subjective disease theory.

11 The empirical research

11.1 The research field of the healing centre Garden of Peace

Here comes the story of my first data collection and participant observation. As researcher in a shamanic jungle seminar for western tourists, I believe that I am also a kind of tourist. Or, let's say it the other way around: I treat the tourist participant just like another kind of subjective researcher. My purpose is to find out about their personal research methods, their findings from the experience field of subjective occurrences, their interpretations, theories and backgrounds.

I take my double role as a researcher and tourist participant purposefully. The following report is mostly written from my very subjective perspective as a participant. This chapter is, therefore, not a scientific text but still scientific material. It does not aim to argue for or against any of the esoteric hypotheses or convictions but gives an episodic picture about this type of tourism. I refer to the anthropological research tradition of the going native of participatory observation (Kawulich, 2005).

11.1.1 Opening the field

I contacted the retreat-centre Garden of Peace via Facebook as I had contacted some other centres before. English-speaking closed Facebook groups intensely discuss questions about the use of ayahuasca, shamanic and esoteric aspects, psychedelic experiences, integration, search for suitable shamans and other topics. For some of those groups, this comprises recommendations and advertisement. In one of these groups, a young woman reported her own current ayahuasca-assisted healing diet with medicinal plants in the relative isolation of a 10-day retreat in the jungle. Lara represents a retreat centre near the Peruvian jungle town Tarapoto. I contacted her, and we arranged a Skype appointment. Lara turned out to be the manager of the Garden of Peace centre and is responsible for the marketing as well. She was born in New Zealand but has been living in Peru for several years and runs this small retreat-centre together with her partner, Ashley. After discussing my request with Ashley and their 'master shaman,' Hegner Paredez Melendez, they agreed that I could do my research with them as long as the disturbance of the participants would be kept as low as possible. From the very beginning, I tried

© The Editor(s) (if applicable) and The Author(s), under exclusive license to
Springer Fachmedien Wiesbaden GmbH, part of Springer Nature 2020
T. J. Wolff, *The Touristic Use of Ayahuasca in Peru*, Sozialwissenschaftliche
Gesundheitsforschung, https://doi.org/10.1007/978-3-658-29373-4_11

to be as transparent as possible so that they would feel themselves involved in the research process. On their part, however, no restrictions were imposed on the design of the data collection. They desired that I, myself, would take part in their initial Tobacco purgation ritual and also would drink ayahuasca with them at least once. I agreed to their request. I had planned to deploy the widely-used participant observation methodology in order to develop familiarity with the interviewees and to keep the artefact formation as low as possible in the interpretation and categorization of the interviews.

11.1.2 The beginning of the retreat

The data collection took place in 2017. The participants of the 10-day retreats were informed beforehand by e-mail about my research request and asked to complete the baseline online-questionnaire before their arrival in case they wanted to participate in the research. The manager of the retreat centre met the group of participants and me early on day 1 in a café in the small Peruvian town, Tarapoto. The procedure was roughly explained, and the payment settled. This gave me the opportunity to briefly present my research proposal and to ask for their participation. Also, remaining baseline questionnaires could be filled out. From this point on, the fasting began. The rest of the day, we did not take any more solid food because in the evening the initial purging ritual should take place. We were transported on the loading compartment of an off-road vehicle over country roads. The atmosphere between the participants was warm and sarcastic joking while driving through the impressive landscape of wide jungle valleys. The last part of the trip went over sandy earth roads directly into the jungle nature. The moist smells of the Jungle welcomed us. Rich greenness overwhelmed the view. We continuously had to hide from branches hanging over the path. After some hours of driving over humps and puddles, we suddenly stopped at a crooked metal-door in an overgrown, barbed wire-fence, which I would have otherwise overlooked. The Peruvian driver started to unload backpacks and vegetables. Some hippy-looking young men and some dogs welcomed us at the Garden of Peace. Here, we were quickly distributed individually to small huts, where we set up to wait for the beginning of the late afternoon cleaning ritual. The huts were connected by small natural paths throughout a steep, bushy and moist terrain. Huts were made of coarse wood and covered with palm trees. They were about 4 square meters of space, just enough for a bed with a mattress and a mosquito net, a clothes line, and a stool (which was missing in mine). The huts were open on all sides; always three sides were protected against insects with a close-meshed plastic net while the view-side was left open. The cabin offered a beautiful view over a small jungle valley. Very closely down the hill behind leaves, trees, and bushes, I could hear a constant stream. I spent time ordering my equipment for the night and unsucessfully trying to relax myself.

In the dawn, we were individually guided to the central maloka by a volunteer helper. The maloka was an open, wooden rotunda on stilts, covered with palm fronds. There were mattresses in the circle, and in the middle were some esoteric or aesthetic objects (for example, a large crystal, a candlestick and a bowl with a few palos santos - Peruvian incense wood, etc.). Each was assigned a mattress as a personal place.

Ashley began to explain the retreat rules, the master plant diet and the rules for the post-diet after the retreat. He stressed that contact with each other should be kept low for the duration of the retreat and that there should be no deeper talk than some small talk. Mutual contact should only be brief and easy since individual words, remarks and gestures would inadvertently exert much greater influence than in normal everyday circumstances. Visits to other huts were, therefore, generally forbidden. As a social environment and also for possible Yoga exercises or meditation, the maloka would serve those who wanted it. Contact with the centre would take place twice a day through the helpers who would bring food and tea. Here, it would be possible to have a little talk so that they would know that the participants are doing well. Only in emergencies should it be possible to visit the main and kitchen house in order to get in touch with the retreat management. The food, twice a day, would consist of unsalted rice, platano (plantains) and some vegetables, as well as unsweetened herbal tea. On the day of an ayahuasca ceremony, there would be only one meal in the morning.

The use of fluoride-containing toothpaste and perfumed cosmetics such as soap, detergents and creams were forbidden for participants by the diet, since their strong smells would be particularly penetrating and disturbing in the sensitivity of such a comprehensive master-plant diet. The same applied for masturbation, alcohol and other drugs, as well as coffee and tea. It was recommended to avoid reading novels or other kind of literature or watching movies. Participants were cautioned about the use of electronic devices, because they could be damaged by the damp jungle weather. Since there was no mobile phone reception, the use of the Internet was not possible anyway. Such fasting rules were very familiar to me, because I knew most of them from Buddhist seminaries and from my previous activity in a psychosomatic therapeutic community in Germany.

Ashley explained the schedule to us. Overall, there would be three ayahuasca ceremonies during the retreat. On the two days in between the ceremonies, plant and flower showers would be offered at the riverside, and the shaman would bring each participant a brew from an individually selected master plant. He, however, would choose this master plant only after the first diagnostical ayahuasca ceremony and an initial conversation the day after.

11.1.3 Initial tobacco purge

For the tobacco ceremony, we then went outside and grabbed a plastic bucket. Here we saw the first time Hegner, our shaman. As the website of the centre indicates, Hegner Paredes Melendez is a master ayahuasquero and vegetalista, originally from the Pucallpa region of Peru. He comes from a powerful lineage of healers, and he also brings immense depth of experience and a profound personal connection with the land, plants and spirits. Furthermore, he has a particular affinity with palos fuertes (hardwood trees) and he also has spent many years in solitude and exclusive diet with these master teachers. Hegner, not especially traditionally dressed as a western tourist might have expected did not give any explanation, nor did he celebrate any initiatory/ ritual performance. Everything went on objectively, calmly and quickly. He came out of his stilts-house with a plastic jug, surrounded by his little kittenish daughter. She seemed not especially curious or afraid of western strangers about to perform a collective purging vomit in front of her home. Hegner handed Ashley a cup filled with tobacco juice, one after another, after he had blown tobacco smoke over it. Then, the first one swallowed the tobacco juice, waited a few minutes, and started to drink quickly 4 litres of water out of an old plastic bottle. I saw myself nervously taking care of my dirty yellow bucket when my turn came nearer and nearer. It was not long until everyone threw up into the buckets. The liquids were spouting out almost like from a water hose under pressure. I immediately started to feel dizzy and weak when standing up to empty the bucket onto the ground. This ended the surprisingly unpretentious purging ritual and officially started the diet. Like everyone, I quietly tottered back to my hut, preparing for the night before it got dark.

I spent the night inside my hammock, which I had brought along and wrapped myself into my mosquito net. I did not want to use the bed at all, because it gave me phantasies of insects that would crawl up on me.

During the night, I woke up because I had to pee. I found myself surrounded by complete darkness and the strange noises of the jungle. No one had told me to bring a flashlight. I still felt weak and dizzy inside the unsteady hammock. Because of that, I tried to avoid getting out of my place as long as possible. My worries of insects or snakes on which I could accidentally step brought me into quite a tricky situation. One idea could have been that I would just throw something to the floor before getting down myself to startle the creatures on the floor. After recognising that, I had nothing with me to throw down, I had to give up that idea. When I realised that I would not succeed in figuring out a reasonable elegant solution, I found the whole scene fairly comical. Finally, I had no other choice. After several trials of bringing myself into a position from which I would be able to pee over the edge of my hammock without falling down into the darkness or making myself wet, I finally relieved myself. I listened how it splashed onto the floor through the mosquito net. The same procedure had to be carried out four times more that night. In the morning, the comedy finished when I found out that I had piddled onto my own shoes, which were placed right under the hammock. I mention this episode here because it shows how uneasy, helpless and awkward one can feel and act in such an unknown surrounding, being just an inexperienced tourist. Since we know the significant influence of the set-setting complex onto the psychedelic experience, we can imagine how influential the unknown jungle surrounding can easily become, especially under the condition of altered states of consciousness. A couple of days later, I realised how unfounded my worries of that first night had been. After all, the episode might sound silly, but at that time I was convinced that I had a real problem not being able to go to the toilet.

During that night, I also had a lucid dream about heavy car traffic which frightened me. I left the dream with the feeling that it would have an important message, which I did not understand. When I woke up, I still could taste the tobacco from the night before. Moreover, there were some hardly describable bodily sensations, and I still felt a bit dizzy.

The insight of the morning: I realised that I had underestimated the seriousness of the process and the retreat centre, even though they had told us before.

Eventually, the friendly volunteer came by and brought a plastic plate with rice, plantains and some cabbage, all unsalted and unseasoned. This would be the last food for the day of the first ayahuasca ceremony. Following a sudden inspiration, I wrote the following: "When you give, give only what the other is able to accept - and a little more". During that moment, this seemed to be a very important and personally relevant message.

11.1.4 First ceremony

I spent the day of our first ayahuasca ceremony dozing, dreaming and waiting for the night. When the evening began to dawn, I prepared myself and went to the maloka. Everyone was there already, only our shaman was still missing. Muted conversations were heard. In the middle, there was a candle and a bowl of smoking palo santo (Peruvian incense wood). Many of the participants had dressed in special clothing, many in white. Mapachos were smoked here and there (filterless jungle cigarettes made from pure tobacco of nicotiana rustica). Ashley, the head of the centre, explained the sequence and gave helpful details about the handling of puke buckets, finding the right shoes in the darkness, going to the loo, etc. When it was quite dark, Hegner entered the maloka very silently. He had dressed himself with a long robe but could hardly be seen in the dark. One after another was called to sit in front of Hegner to drink the ayahuasca from a small wooden cup after it was blown upon tobacco smoke. Then again, the waiting began in complete darkness and silence. Between dreaming and drifting thoughts, I repeatedly checked whether my visual perception had already changed. After about 45 minutes, the visions abruptly started. Hegner began singing at the same time. First, I saw neon-coloured lines on the floor in the dark. They moved quickly towards me from all directions like thin, agile snakes that joyfully had noticed that I was there. This raised fright, and I guess I resisted against this so that the snake lines disappeared, and other patterns appeared. This made me think about the degree of one's own influence on the psychedelic ayahuasca experience, which is often reported by somewhat experienced persons and often discovered and tried out by beginners. The initial colourful patterns changed, and biographical and current relational content dominated. It was a mixture of contemplation and emotionally recalled scenes or fantasized relationship episodes from which rational insights emerged. Or, vice versa, biographical scenes and imagined episodes, which arose from rational insights. For example, at the end of an intense, but rational, thinking process about my relationship to my son, I experienced a playful fight with him with toy laser swords. This vivid scene came after I had understood some issues of my relationship on a rational level. I was increasingly touched by our intense encounters and the expression of connectedness and love between father and son. This scene was, at the same time, an emotional summit, quintessence and climatic of this theme. Afterwards, I suspect that the emotionality and episodic reality character of the psychedelic phantasy contribute to a stronger embossing or anchoring of rational insights, just as the combination of experience and cognition within psychotherapy. In retrospect, I can easily access the feeling of being connected with my son about the vivid memory of the encounter in the laser fight game. A retrospective reproduction of rational knowledge about my relationship with my son, however, seems to me more difficult and, therefore, afterwards less relevant than the reproduction of episodic, emotionalized memory. I can just play with him in a similar way to enable this kind of experience for us in reality, and this is possible without understanding it rationally. After this particular episodic conclusion, similar and connected themes emerged.

After a while, the singers exchanged. Ashley and the volunteer helper also sang their songs. This irritated me at first and pulled me out of my current experience back into the world of the maloka.

From time to time during the ceremony, Ashley sprayed various floral perfumes among participants, the scent Agua de Florida and others. On me, this had the pleasant effect of awakening and interrupting dreamlike pondering and phantasies. I remember myself being on a visionary voyage (intense imagination with stronger reality character) in a greenish and reddish-looking forest with strangely constructed vine-like curved, high buildings. I admired this architecture and regretted that I was not able to adequately memorize it in its beauty and complexity. Then, I suddenly saw three or four dark, luminous insect-like creatures hovering on me from about a meter away. They were quite large with a diameter of about 50 cm and did not look particularly friendly. I was frightened and swayed between trying to ignore them or scare them off. In any case, it was hard for me to concentrate on the architecture; I had to keep an eye on them. Somehow, I realized at that moment that they probably had to do with my frequently-occurring, unpleasant pondering-thoughts, which sometimes absorbed me completely. In this frightened, suspicious condition, I suddenly felt a strong, pleasant tingling sensation on the skin and immediately afterwards smelled an intense, but light, floral perfume. I could not explain what that was, but the colours and visionary content changed radically. The forest, the buildings and my thoughts were gone. Instead, I found myself in an orange-yellow world of flowers. I was so surprised that I noticed only after a while that someone was standing in front of me, asking if I would like to have another cup. He had sprayed me with the flower water Agua de Kananga before he spoke to me. Later, when I saw the bottle I was surprised that it was exactly the orange colour of my vision.

The ceremony ended when everyone had to puff a bit on their mapacho that Hegner previously had handed out after he had come to each participant, lighted the cigarette with his own, and had blown its tobacco smoke over the person's head and hands. The music now was performed by Ashley, a pleasant mixture of spiritual peace and love songs with guitar, harmonica and flute. It was up to us to stay and sleep inside the maloka or go back to the cabin. The next morning Lara gave us a basic yoga class.

11.1.5 Informant H.

That morning I had a talk with H., our volunteer. Originally from Asia, he lived and worked as a cook in the US before he came to Peru. He bought property nearby the centre and plans to build his house there. H. followed the shamanic path for a couple of years now. He produced different spiritual fragrances based on jungle healing plants that can be sprayed for enhancing or cleaning the room air.

I asked H. about different topics. We started with the use of tobacco and its high regard as a powerful healing plant of the Amazon. He mentioned that the main reason for smoking is an animistic connection to the spiritual world. Basically, the tobacco smoke takes the prayers and wishes of the smoker to the spiritual world. That's why the intention of the smoker would be highly significant for the development of cancer. He stated, 'If you always send your emotional shit up, over many years, then you finally get shit.' Normal cigarettes, which contain a different type of tobacco, would have additional toxic and addictive ingredients. In contrast, mapachos are pure and healthy because they contain only plain (nicotiana rustica) tobacco. The addiction of so many westerners, which comes from the wrong usage of tobacco, shows how the powerful tobacco plant spirit keeps hold of them.

We also talked about the formation of a shaman. Hikaro stated that a shaman receives his songs (ícaro) directly from the plant spirits when doing strict diets with such master-plants. When singing an ícaro, the healer calls a spirit with whom he has developed a special relationship during his own diets. Some sing, some only whistle the songs. The plant recognises its own melody and the singing person. That is why it is not useful to perform someone else's song without one's own personal introduction to the spirit. The ícaro would not come but just wonder why someone strange is singing his song.

The words are less important; plants listen to melodies. But sometimes the songs contain plant-language, which can appear to us like words of infants or nonsense. There are legends about shamans having allegedly received and learned an indigenous language in just one night. It would have been uploaded into their brain from the spiritual world.

The formation begins usually with diets of reasonably easy to handle spirits like the Ajo Sacha (Mansoa Alliacea). An advanced or master shaman "diets" big trees and other powerful plants. Such dietas would become a very serious matter. Retreat and diet are agreements with the plant spirit that is studied by the shaman. The plant spirit is invited to be inside the person, and there it needs appropriate preconditions. If the diet is broken, a plant spirit can become very upset, which entails sometimes serious medical issues. One would have to restart the plant-diet again and resolve the problem. If a person has already departed to Europe or North America where the specific plant may not be available, the symptoms can hardly be cured because they are neither somatic nor psycho-somatic but spiritual-somatic in nature.

H. explained that the Chacruna based vision would appear more colourful, and the ayahuasca- vine based vision would be more monochromatic. He does not believe that the potential to produce visions is just an exclusive matter of physiologically activated DMT. During the ceremony, the master shaman calls his befriended spirits for help and healing. Through his singing, he can deepen or reduce the visions. Another important part of his work is the protection from evil spirits, which he sends away when he detects them. During the ceremony, Hikaro himself drinks ayahuasca and helps to take care of the participants. He sends good energy to the ones who might have a difficult time, and he also helps them to stand up and walk, if needed. Often during the ceremony, he has the opportunity to sing his own ícaro songs.

11.1.6 Masterplants

During the diet, participants drink their individual master plants only during those days on which no night ceremony is planned. After the first ceremony and an initial talk, Hegner decides which plant matches the participant. Typical master plants for a 10-day retreat are Ajo Sacha (Mansoa alliacea), Mucura (Petiveria alliaceae), Bobinsana (Calliandra angustifolia) and others. Serious issues and medical conditions may require other plants and longer diets.

11.1.7 Interview with a healer

For the characterisation of the conducting ayahuasquero, I asked Hegner Paredez Melendez for an interview. Some of my questions might have been strange for him or irrelevant because they were asked from my point of western curiosity and psychological background. I know him as a friendly and simple man from the jungle area of Pucallpa with no academic education. It should be kept in mind that it is not part of the Peruvian culture to say, "no" or, "I don't know." Sometimes, the impression is given that interview partners offer the answer that they suppose the other wants to hear. They tend to answer, even if the answer does not fit the question just for the sake of politeness or the avoidance of social discomfort. It is sometimes hard to distinguish between social answering and true answers.

The interview took place at the Garden of Peace healing centre on April 4th, 2017. After smashing ayahuasca pieces all morning and cooking them in several large cauldrons under open fire, we sat down on a fallen trunk, and I could ask Hegner my questions. These were recorded with his permission. No other person was present. The following narration is a close translation which includes grammatical distinctives used by the interviewee.

When and in which situation did you drink your first ayahuasca?

'I took ayahuasca the first time when I was 14 years old. I had pain here [he shows where]. My uncle was a healer. Because of that, I took ayahuasca to heal me. Then, I left for years. I was studying. Then, when I was 31-years old, I started to diet until now.'

What was your development and personal history in becoming a healer?

'Well, I started to diet also by means of solitude. I suffered from liver and lung conditions. Then, I went to a doctor, and they did not do anything for me. Because my brother was already a healer, my brother Enrique became my teacher. I go to his centre. He gives me some plants, and I start to diet. That was how the diet begun, diet, diet, diet. From the centre, I went to town for a year. After a year,

I felt the improvement of my lung and my liver. And so, I started to travel little by little. And then, I started to learn how to sing little by little.'

How do you know or determine the diagnosis of the client?
'To diagnose, the diet of at least one month or longer is mandatory. With the diet, you can see the patient…, the illness he has. To make a diagnosis, the diet of more than a month (is required) to observe at the patients, which disease they have. Also, one has to follow a diet of some plants, trees to be able to diagnose the ill friends.'

For example, if someone has a stomach disease, can you see it in the darkness of the ceremony?
'Yes, and I also know which medicine I will give. I do that in the second day.'

I read that some ayahuasqueros can see the network in the patient's body and can discern the problem of the person in this network.
'Yes, exactly. It is the diet that serves for all this. Without the diet, we are worthless.'

What are the reasons for the problems or diseases of your clients?
'The reasons they come to cure their problems that they mostly have inside, more related to emotions issues. And, you have to know what medicine has to be given; what medicine we will employ for each person.'

How do you know the reasons for the problems of your patients?
'How do I know? Well, looking at them, looking [at them] during the ayahuasca ceremony. The problems they have are spiritual. Some tell us what problems they have, and [we know] by means of what they tell us.'

Do you have to know the reasons in order to give medicine?
'One asks the plants to help us. The plants you have taken are asked to support us, whether it is the medicine you are going to use or not.'

Who heals in your treatment? You? The plants? How does one cure?
'The plants are the ones that heal. The healer only shows. With a breath, the healer does not heal. But plants do. A healer does not cure. The healer is the knowledge, no more. Plants are what heals.'

And what does the soplo [particular blowing technique of the shaman] do?
'The breath is just a breath. Sometimes, they are a little down and the blow serves to raise their morale.'

Which types of diseases do you treat?

'Mostly the ones of women. Vaginal problems, uterus. There are many plants. I cure all emotional problems. I also cure cancer. But, here there is no medicine especially for cancer. That one is bought, and about purchasing it, I want to say that this means that it is already manipulated, has another energy that is not good. That's why I work with few plants here, no more. There are not many plants here. Because of that, we obtain them to give them to the patient. The most feasible is to take them yourself from the same stem, one with another energy, from there. There, where my brother Enrique lives in Pucallpa in the Sanctuary (a healing centre), from there is all the medicine. My brother does not buy from the village. There is a lot of medicine there. And there is also a plant, a tree to cure cancer. Someday you'll meet.'

Do you work with concepts like susto [fright], daño [wounds by witchcraft], mal aire [bad air], mal ojo / mala mirada [evil look], brujería [witchcraft]?

'Yes, susto [fright], mal aire [bad air] mostly grip the children. For that, there are medicines, brujería [witchcraft] too, because witchcraft exists.'

Do foreigners or gringos have other problems or diseases or are the reasons for their problems different from those of Peruvian or local clients?

'Different problems, mostly emotional, because they live in a different world, different from ours. Sometimes they are stressed from their jobs, or they, themselves, make problems. And, the other diseases outside are like here.'

Do "gringos" from abroad also have problems like susto, daño, mal aire, mal ojo / mala mirada, brujería?

'Susto, that is the only one they have. Susto is a fear when you get mugged, you know... with pistols or with a knife. That is a fear or fright they have.'

And is witchcraft also a reason of the problems that foreigners have?

'No, less because there, sometimes, they collide with evil spirits from the space,
not with witchdoctors, but they are negative spirits that collide among them, so the foreigners come here with pains, and the healer must know how to remove them.'

Do some healers use other techniques, e.g. how to suck diseases out of the body? Like darts from witchdoctors or other bad objects? Do you work with these techniques if necessary?

'No, I don't work with that. Other healers get some patients who have pain in a certain part of their body, they suck it with the mouth and take it out, but I don't. It seems to me, that they did so earlier, our ancestors. Now, not any more.'

Do healers exist who use that, nowadays?

'Yes, they exist but I don't use that. For me it is dangerous. Suddenly it's a witchcraft and if you are not prepared…'

How is it for you to work in a centre for foreigners?

'For me, it's very nice to work here because I worked with the friend since I was 29 years old, and that's why I know how to work with foreign friends.'

Would you work differently with local customers out here?

'Yes different, because foreign friends are more sensitive. We, Peruvians, are more rustic. That is why I have learned to heal everyone, all the persons who trust me.'

Do you have to change something in the treatment to work here in the centre? With Ashley (the owner) and the foreign clients?

'Well, my work is only to heal, no more. Now, I am cooking this ayahuasca, it is my will to teach how to cook. That's normal.'

Tell me the history of working together with the owner of the centre?

'When I was working – since 2001, I worked with my brother – I helped him, I worked in the field, in the ceremony, so I am his student. My brother is my teacher. Many foreign friends go to the centre, and at that time in the sanctuary Ashley and Lara (the owners of the Garden of Peace) were going to diet there in the Sanctuary and there they met me. And at that time, I was the person who brought the food to the dieters, just like here from the kitchen to the fields, to take the medicine to the fields (…?). That's how I met Ashley and Lara. And he said: Don't you want to work with me? I would like to, I said, I want to get out of here. Get an email account, he said. Then I took his advice. It took 2 or 3 months because I had nothing, no mail, no Wi-Fi, no cell phone, nothing. I created an email, sent a message to Ashley. At that moment, he was sending me an invitation, through a Chinese friend, Daniel. Daniel asked if I did not want to work for Ashley, a better option than working in the Sanctuary, so that I would develop more. That was my story with Ashley.'

What do the "gringo" clients expect from you?

'They expect me to heal them, to give them love, patience more than anything. They expect healing.'

Is it different to what local clients expect?

'Some foreign friends come to experimenting, come to test the strength of each healer, they do not only come to a healer, but also want to go to another one and know what the strength and energy of each healer is.'

Some years ago, a congress of ayahuasqueros in Iquitos took place to which many healers attended. Some of them had their indigenous, traditional clothing with feathers, etc. And more gringos wanted to participate in the ceremonies of the ones who were dressed more indigenous. Is this something that you experience here, something that they look for?
'Yes, they are looking for that too. Because in the way I dressed there, when I was in the Sanctuary, I had a crown of feathers and necklaces, well. But not here.'

And for the Peruvian clients? Is the traditional clothing and the indigenous symbols less important?
'It seems to me they do not give it so much importance. It is difficult for me to cure the people of the town here. It depends in which places, in Lima I can heal. But here, people who are from here, from the land, I don't heal them because they do not diet when they are given a medicine. They are told how long they have to diet, that they don't eat this, and they do not. And what do they say? That healer knows nothing. But how can they know, if they do not believe and do not diet either? The plant is what heals and not the healer. And if you do not diet, and have a disease. And if you have a disease, the disease will attack you even more when you break your diet. That is the reason that I do not want to cure people here from the village, because they are not responsible. Instead, the friends that come from another place, the foreigners, they follow their diet, because they come from far, spending their money and time.'

What do you think of the ayahuasca tourism of the foreigners to Peru? There is a lot of money in this business. And a person can earn a lot while the neighbour cannot even afford to buy a taxi.
'Yes, there is a lot of money. For me, it is profitable because it serves us to diet, to learn. Because the diet is a sacrifice. Through this sacrifice I get to know many friends and can earn a little to take care of my family. Although it is not much. The one who earns more is the owner. The owner of the centre earns more, which is fair, since he buys all.'

Are the owners of many centres gringos and not Peruvians?
'I don't know that, I only know Ashley.'

Do the owners earn most part of the money?

'Because of that I am thinking about getting my own centre. Where I am not just a worker.'

Do you do the majority of the work?
'Of course, in the ceremony it's me who sacrifices myself. And if your body is not prepared another spirit might come and pull you down. Healers are everywhere, all over the world, good and bad.'

Is the tourism of ayahuasca a sale-out of the Peruvian culture?
'No, but it's happening nowadays. And many people, foreigners, take it from here to other places.'

Sometimes the foreigners have only little information but serve ayahuasca to people in Europe and some do diet and others not, but they call themselves ayahuasca shamans, they rob the culture...
'Anyone can invite (give), and when the patient gets sick, how do they lower it without knowing? And that is happening nowadays with the foreigners and they do not sing ícaros (healing songs, obtained during formation), no more, they record, and they play it there, so that the patients listen.'

And what do you think about this?
'For me, it is not good but they all do it for money. For me, the money is good. It is for food, for the family. But they want more.'

Does the tourism of the gringo centres change the curanderism in Peru?
'Yes, they change it because they do not carry the same tradition, habits. They want to have the same tradition, but they don't know.'

And what exactly changes?
'Because they don't know which medicine. That is why some friends ask. They ask me which medicine for which disease. I tell them because I am not an egoist. But other healers don't tell the truth. They tell other things, the opposite. I tell the truth; I don't like egoism. If it is for them to learn, they should learn. That is how I have learned with love.'

And do the foreigners have more interest in the visions of ayahuasca than in other medical plants?
'Yes, there is more interest there. That is what they come for, to look, to experiment.'

And how is it in the tradition, normally only the healer takes ayahuasca and the patients not?
'Both things, in the beginning when they come I give ayahuasca to diagnose what medicine I will use, what disease they have. Second, I take care of them spiritually so that they do not get sick, I take care of them, and so on.'

Is there a tradition in which only the healer takes ayahuasca?
'I have never seen that. I give it always to the patients and myself.'

Is there something else you want to say, something I didn't ask you?
'To learn, I ingested many plants. It starts from the smallest plants, and it goes to the trees, trunks. I have made many diets. Now, I diet little to strengthen my body, my spirit, my soul. Because if you do not diet, you are spiritually weak. I used to diet a lot, but now I diet little.'

Is it a dangerous way, the way of being a healer?
'No, it's not dangerous. Better if you diet. I feel better when I diet. I do not eat other food, nor do I have sex. This way, one has more strength for the ícaros.'

Nowadays there are more Peruvians who get interested in becoming a healer?
'There is more interest because of the tourism. In Pucallpa, there are many.'

Do you have Peruvian students?
'No, at the moment I don't. I have just left my masters house. But, once when I have my own centre, I will have students.'

Thank you very much!
'Yes, friend, very good. Whatever, I am here for you.'

12 Main questions and general research ideas

For the beginning Helfferich (2011, p. 28) suggests presenting an overview about the research interest, questions, research objects, material and methods so that the reader can have a quick idea about the project. Below this brief overview the appropriateness between the object of research and the proposed methods will be developed in more detail.

Research interest:

A mixed methods research shall be done on the increasingly growing ethno-tourism in Peru related to the psychoactive jungle tee ayahuasca.

Research questions:

1a. Which meaning has ayahuasca in the life of western ayahuasca tourists and what do they expect?
1b. Is there evidence for a relationship between the motivation to consume ayahuasca and the mental health status?
2. How do they experience ayahuasca.
3. How do they interpret and integrate their experiences?

Object of research:

1a. Subjective localization of the ayahuasca experience within motivational patterns of subjective sense, influences of expectations, personal health theory and working models of ayahuasca.
1b. Mental health status.
2. Process experiences.
3. Interpretation, sense and meaning of the experiences.

Material / data:

1a. Biographical narratives subjectively related to ayahuasca by the narrators and explications about expectations, subjective health theory and subjective working theory, demographic questionnaire.

© The Editor(s) (if applicable) and The Author(s), under exclusive license to
Springer Fachmedien Wiesbaden GmbH, part of Springer Nature 2020
T. J. Wolff, *The Touristic Use of Ayahuasca in Peru*, Sozialwissenschaftliche
Gesundheitsforschung, https://doi.org/10.1007/978-3-658-29373-4_12

1b. Selected quantitative mental health variables and interview data.
2. Quantitative information from questionnaires and participating observation about the use and narratives about the experiences.
3. Narratives on subjective meaning and sense of the ayahuasca experience.

Methods of analysis:

- Semi-structured interviews during and after retreats and qualitative content analysis.
- Participating observation with field protocols.
- Demographic questionnaire.
- Quasi-experimental investigation with psychometric questionnaires and pre-post statistics within a concurrent nested mixed method design.

12.1 Why qualitative methods?

The examination of subjective concepts and theories is done the best through mainly qualitative investigation methods. Quantitative methods such as questionnaires can map only preselected specific aspects of subjective theories without focusing on the individual development of a theory (Faller, Schilling & Lang, 1991). Within more or less structured interviews the relationship of subjective content and dynamic aspects and biographical context of meaning has to be compiled (Faltermaier & Kühnlein, 2000). This explorative work examines not exclusively subjective theory but also subjective experiences and effects. It asks about both, the 'what and which' and the 'how'. That is one of the reasons why both paradigms, quantitative and qualitative, are used in this study. Highly structured data collection, such as a psychological test or a rating scale, is used to collect information and is best analysed with quantitative methods. This paradigm asks questions like: To what extend did you recognise a symptom reduction? What is your precondition? What type of personality are you? A less structured data collection method, such as a semi-structured or even narrative interview, is used best to ask questions like: How did you experience it? How do you give sense and meaning to it? Although there are always more or less conscious expectations and assumptions of the researcher the qualitative main part of the study is heuristically conceived without explicitly testing hypothesis. The quantitative part does not provide a full hypothesis testing design but merely serves as a flanking or descriptive support for the qualitative part.

Primarily, this heuristic, mainly qualitative study is interested in the variety of phenomena in the field, including what significance individuals attribute to them. It is not yet a question of quantifying them, or, in other words, of assessing their statistical significance and representativeness. Therefore, it is less important whether a phenomenon is reported often or only by one person. If something is reported by one person, it does not automatically mean that it is less relevant. In the interpretation of the qualitative results, hypotheses are formed, about particularly interesting phenomena, which seem more relevant than others. Those could then be tested in later investigations.

13 General design

The investigation is divided into three empirical studies:

- Study 1: Motivational structure for the ayahuasca ingestion in members of social networks in the Internet
- Study 2: A phenomenological analysis of some subjective experiences of ayahuasca in Upper Amazon vegetalismo tourism
- Study 3: Expectations, motivation, experiences, meaning and subjective effects effects of subjects participating in ayahuasca retreats in Upper Amazon ayahuasca tourism in Peru.

The first study had the purposes to establish the first contact through the Internet, collect demographic data, test the openness of potential participants for research and to verify the motivational distribution of ayahuasca users which was found in previous studies.

A phenomenological analysis of subjective ayahuasca experiences in the Amazon region followed. In this study I used narrative interviews during ayahuasca-retreats in a Peruvian jungle retreat centre near the town of Iquitos. On the one hand, the interviews were used to extract relevant categories of the ayahuasca experience in foreign clients participating in traditional mestizo-vegetalismo rituals in the Upper Amazon region. And on the other hand, to develop interesting questions for the following study. A radical data-driven strategy was used for the extraction of relevant categories to build the coding frame.

The third study was conducted in a Peruvian retreat centre near the town Tarapoto. Here ayahuasca-tourists were followed from before the retreats, during the retreats, untill 6 weeks after the retreats. This investigation consisted of three parts:

a) Quantitative questionnaire investigation (pre-post and peri)
b) Process investigation during the retreat by participating observation
c) Qualitative investigation of motivations, biographic narratives and subjective healing theories.

© The Editor(s) (if applicable) and The Author(s), under exclusive license to
Springer Fachmedien Wiesbaden GmbH, part of Springer Nature 2020
T. J. Wolff, *The Touristic Use of Ayahuasca in Peru*, Sozialwissenschaftliche Gesundheitsforschung, https://doi.org/10.1007/978-3-658-29373-4_13

13.1 Ethics and confidentiality

An informed consent form about participation in the study was signed prior to al data collections and full information was given about the study purposes, scope and kind of data collection, exclusion criteria, data protection, involved researchers and institutions as well as possible risks and safety instruction. For the Internet data collection, participants agreed by clicking on a "yes, understood, proceed" button after reading the informed consent form and information sheet.

Regarding the field studies, only individuals who had already booked the retreat independently of the study were invited to participate. Participants were not invited to ingest ayahuasca specifically for this study. The independency of the study from the ayahuasca facility was made clear to participants verbally as well as in the information package.

Confidentiality and the voluntary nature of participation was assured and reiterated throughout the research and publishing procedure. The procedure was aligned with the Declaration of Helsinki – Ethical Principles for Medical Research Involving Human Subjects (WMA, 2013). Guidelines of the British Psychological Society have been followed throughout the study design. The protocol has been reviewed by PD Dr. Torsten Passie (MD) and Prof. Dr. Henning Schmidt-Semisch. Further advice was obtained from professionals at the International ayahuasca conference 2016 (Rio Branco, Brazil).

In line with BPS guidelines, the following practical measures were taken:

- Informed consent obtained via briefing document.
- Participant data are anonymous. Codes assigned to each participant.
- Participants have the right to withdraw at any point.
- Participants were debriefed prior to testing and interviewing.
- Information packs were provided that contain some resources on helping to integrate psychedelic experiences. They were given alongside the retreat centres typical material.
- Contact information of the researchers were provided to participants for any queries.

The studies contain no areas of deception or anything that could be considered harmful to the participants. The researcher had no conflict of interests.

As there are documented cases of negative outcomes as a result of participation in ayahuasca ceremonies, this study included only those who would be participating in the ceremonies regardless of the research project, there are no extra measures the researcher could take to minimise potential harm. Furthermore - the legal status of DMT and ayahuasca is not an issue as the study is conducted in Peru - where traditional practices are accepted.

13.2 Quality criteria for qualitative research

In qualitative research common criteria of quantitative research that have been developed and defined for highly standardised methods (such as experiments) are problematic to apply. They are often replaced by other criteria that are considered more appropriate to the method and content of the rather less standardised, low formalised and often inductive qualitative research. Steinke (2003) offers a list of criteria that can be modified and adapted to the individual research project. A study should be evaluated by using a variety of these criteria.

Inter-subjective comprehensibility:
- Through a broad documentation of the research process that contains the pre-assumptions, data collection process and its context, sources, transcription rules, data, methods of analysis, history of decision-making and problems during the research process as well as the actual aims of the study.
- Through the interpretation discourse within a group process.
- Through the application of a codified algorithmic research methods.

Indication of the research process:
- Explanation of the choice of methods, transcription rules, sampling strategy and further decisions.

Empirical grounding:
- Theory making should be done as close as possible to the empirical data and on the base of systematic analysis. For this, codified methods should be used as scrupulous as possible.

Limitation:
- The range and the conditions of the theory have to be explored during the research. Contrasting, cases and the analysis of divergent or negative cases are methods that can be useful to find limitations.

Coherence:
- The developed theory should be consistent and divergent data and interpretations must be discussed.

Relevance:
- How useful are the findings and to what extend does the study contribute to science?

Reflective subjectivity:
- The role and influence of the researcher has to be critically discussed. That includes self reflexion and reflexion of the relationship between researcher and informants during the research process.

The common quality criteria objectivity, validity and reliability are often operationalized differently for qualitative research.

A high degree of objectivity means that other researchers that apply the same methods on the same matter will come to similar result. Objectivity can be increased by the extensive description of the applied methods.

The validity of an instrument describes the extent to which it captures what it is supposed to capture. A coding frame that adequately represents the concepts of the study through its categories can be called valid. There are two contentious areas in the field of validity. One is the validity of the assessment of manifest and latent content. The other is the extent to which valid conclusions can be drawn from the content analysis. Four types of validity have been distinguished (Neuendorf, 2002, pp. 114ff.):

- Face validity refers to the impression of an instrument to really measure what it claims to measure. This type of validity is especially important for the inductive description of material.
- Content validity means the extent to which an instrument covers all dimensions of the measured concept. This type of validity challenges deductive coding frames.
- Criterion validity means the extent to which the measurement of the instrument is related to another already established valid indicator.
- Construct validity relates the concept of the study to other concepts and tests the relationship between these different concepts.
  The last two types of validity go beyond the description of the material if inferences have to be validated.

Analysing the relationship between the categories and residual categories is a method to assess face validity of data-driven coding frames. If the categories are not able to cover the meaning of the material the face validity of the coding frame is low, and this is represented in a higher number of assignments to residual categories. Finding common details and creating additional subcategories increases the validity.

A high number of assignments to only one subcategory compared to other subcategories of the same main category can indicate that the material is not represented in sufficient detail, but several aspects are covered under the subcategory that shows the high coding frequency. Dividing the subcategory into relevant aspects increases the validity of the coding frame. The abstraction level also has direct influence of the face validity. A highly abstract coding frame with few general categories loses a lot of the distinct information of the material. Discussing concept-driven coding frames with experts can increase content validity because they analyse to what extent the coding frame adequately represents the measured concepts (Schreier, 2012, pp. 186-190).

The criterion of reliability is discussed in detail in the chapter 2.4 A phenomenological analysis of some subjective experiences of ayahuasca in Upper Amazon vegetalismo tourism.

14 Motivational structure for the ingestion of ayahuasca in the Internet

The accessibility of the research field of western ayahuasca-tourists was investigated by means of a quantitative internet survey. Its purpose was to explore the motivation as well as demographic data. It provided a first orientation for the following qualitative investigations.

Psychedelic tourism and the international spreading of ayahuasca strongly benefits from the Internet. Social networks play a significant role in the re-invention of ayahuasca culture and it's spreading into new contexts (Conrad, 2018). According to Facebook, the biggest closed Facebook-group named 'ayahuasca' had 74100 members (Dec. 15th 2017).

Motives and characteristics of ayahuasca-interested individuals need more attention in order to further investigate which role they play for the experience and integration process, how they are linked together and how they may influence ayahuasca practitioners and their corresponding working theories.

This part aimed to explore characteristics of active members of the international Facebook community of ayahuasca by an online questionnaire. Motivational aspects and their distribution within western ayahuasca drinkers that have been previously identified as relevant by heuristic qualitative methods were examined in this study by quantitative methods.

14.1 Research questions of the first study

Motivational structure for the ingestion of ayahuasca in the Internet:
1. Is the worldwide ayahuasca scene accessible to psychological research?
2. Which demographical data characterise activists of the Internet scene?
3. How are known categories of ayahuasca motivation distributed in the sample of members of ayahuasca Facebook groups?

14.2 Location and associated institutions of the first study

The main location of the international ayahuasca-scene is the Internet. Facebook provides the possibility to create private groups that cannot be entered without

© The Editor(s) (if applicable) and The Author(s), under exclusive license to
Springer Fachmedien Wiesbaden GmbH, part of Springer Nature 2020
T. J. Wolff, *The Touristic Use of Ayahuasca in Peru*, Sozialwissenschaftliche Gesundheitsforschung, https://doi.org/10.1007/978-3-658-29373-4_14

being accepted from the moderator. This gives a certain feeling of pseudo-privacy although some of those groups are very large with thousands of members all over the world. The biggest groups have many very active participants. Others serve as advertising platform for retreat centres and roving healers. Because the western ayahuasca scene is a global phenomenon the online data collection is the only economic way to gain access to this scene and reach a reasonable number of potential participants.

14.3 Ethics and confidentiality regarding the first study

No approval of the Ethical Committee was required because no experimental or other intervention was performed on the human sample in this investigation. Although risks from answering anonym questionnaires in the Internet are very low, high ethical standards were applied: Strict anonymity was guaranteed through the whole process by the online procedure. Participants agreed to proceed by clicking 'OK' after having read an informed consent form and information sheet. Confidentiality and voluntary participation were explicitly assured and would be kept throughout the research and publishing procedure. Full transparency about aims and content of the study as well as the contact details of the researcher and affiliated institutions had been provided previously participation. Participants were not encouraged to ingest ayahuasca or any kind of substances for this study.

14.4 Data collection of the first study

The self-selected sample consisted of 40 participants from ayahuasca-specific online-forums. All given responses were included in the analysis.

An online-questionnaire about demographic data, pre-experience and motivation for ayahuasca was developed in three languages (English, German, Spanish). It was placed online through a German Internet-based provider: www.umfrageonline.com. As many as possible Facebook groups about ayahuasca were identified and entered. Most of those groups are closed. One has to ask for admission. The research request was posted together with an explanation and the related Internet-link of the informed consent form and the questionnaire. The questionnaire was accessible for one month. After that the data was downloaded and deleted from the server. Members of the following Facebook groups were asked to participate:

- European ayahuasca Forum
- Ayahuasca

Data collection of the first study   139

- Ayahuasca Spain / España
- Ayahuasca Yage Austria
- Ayahuasca Madre Tierra Berlin
- Ayahuasca Germany
- Ayahuasca & Sjamanisme Nederland, België
- Ayahuasca & Shamanism
- Familia Yage "ayahuasca" Barcelona (España)
- Psychoactive Experience Group DMT, Iboga, ayahuasca, Salvia, Mushroom, Weed
- Chaman ayahuasca; Centro Botanico Naturalista
- Ayahuasca – Yage Patrimonio Cultural para la Nacion y la Humanidad Colombia
- Ayahuasca (Yage) Colombia

14.4.1 The questionnaire

Participants were asked to provide demographical data, pre-experience with ayahuasca and other mind-altering substances. We asked about the general interest in ayahuasca: 'What are your main interests in having the ayahuasca/yagé experience?' Motivational elements of modern ayahuasca-drinkers that were proposed by previous studies were collected, analysed and merged into four general categories. Each of these motivational categories was represented by only one item that had to be rated on a 6-step rating scale (from 'not true' to 'absolutely true'):

- Self-awareness and/or self-exploration
- Solve some physical health issues
- Spiritual purposes
- Interesting or exciting experience

Several of the proposed items could be selected. For compliance and validation purposes, semi-structured answer fields were added.

The desire for 'self-awareness and/or self-exploration' was described as personal development, understand and integrate psychological childhood trauma, heal depression, overcome social fears, confrontation with struggles in life, find meaning and purpose in life, find identity, decrease confusion and indecision about desires and preferences.

The motivation regarding 'spiritual purposes' was described as to feel one with something greater, awake the own spirituality, overcome reductionist and atheistic education, follow a 'call' from ayahuasca, be part of the spiritual development of mankind, understand everything with mind and soul, reflect the development of the soul and 'to connect with the source of understanding of the game of the matrix' (participant 36).

Only two motivations to treat physical issues were qualitatively described: fibromyalgia and Alzheimer's disease.

No participant reflected qualitatively about the desire for ‚interesting or exciting experiences'.

14.5 Analysis methods

The data were statistically analysed through descriptive and inference statistical procedures:

1. Test of normal curve distribution by Kolmogorov-Smirnov test and Shapiro-Wilk test, nonparametric comparison of central tendencies through the Kruskal-Wallis H-Test.
2. Mann-Whitney U-Test for each possible paired combination of motivational categories (Bonferoni-corrected).
3. Correlation coefficient from Kendall (Bootstrap with 1000 samples).

14.6 Demographic summary

An average participant of this study is a member of a closed ayahuasca Facebook group, approximately between 22 and 67 years old, holds a rather high education degree and might be pre-experienced in psychedelics such as psilocybin ('magic mushrooms'), MDMA ('ecstasy'), cannabis and LSD. It is likely that the participant has experience with psychotherapy or counselling and has tried ayahuasca once or a few times before. The person would probably be willing to drink ayahuasca again within the next 6 months.

15 Phenomenological analysis of experiences of ayahuasca

15.1 Research question and methodical considerations

How do foreign tourists experience acute ayahuasca effects in the setting of a shamanic jungle retreat in the Amazon rainforest?

The heuristic study wants to contribute to the investigation of subjective relevance of ayahuasca for western clients as well as possible implications for psychedelic assisted psychotherapy. For this, the study aims to explore more comprehensively, the common structure of acute subjective experiences and emotions elicited by ayahuasca in the context of ceremonial western ayahuasca tourism in the Amazon.

It is known in general, that there is a high inter-individual and intra-individual variability of subjective phenomena of hallucinogen intakes. The research interest is about the diversity of different subjective phenomena and asks about the subjective importance of perceived phenomena.

For this purpose, a radically inductive or data-driven strategy is appropriate. It does not test explicit hypotheses, e.g. about the appearance of certain pre-selected categories and their frequencies or probabilities but generates categories directly from the material. The appropriate method to generate the research material is the narrative interview. This strategy avoids the interference with the generation process of material as much as possible. Participants are not forced into fixed answer alternatives, pre-selected categories or any directions. The idea is to generate categories from unbiased material, as far as possible. If a phenomenon is mentioned during the narrative interview without explicitly having asked for it, the probability is high that it has subjective relevance for the participant. If is mentioned often during the interview process it has even more subjective relevance. During the process of generating material, the narrative interview strategy leaves the decision about important and unimportant content in the hands of the participant. In general, the phenomena and details that were spontaneously reported by the interviewees, without having asked for it explicitly, are considered to be subjectively more relevant than what remains unremembered or unmentioned. If content is reported more often it might be even more relevant to the interviewee. That is why the

© The Editor(s) (if applicable) and The Author(s), under exclusive license to
Springer Fachmedien Wiesbaden GmbH, part of Springer Nature 2020
T. J. Wolff, *The Touristic Use of Ayahuasca in Peru*, Sozialwissenschaftliche
Gesundheitsforschung, https://doi.org/10.1007/978-3-658-29373-4_15

responsibility to choose between relevant and irrelevant content remained on the side of the participant during the stage of material production.

One can hardly discriminate whether the interviewee is reporting an aspect because it is of high importance to him or to what extend he does so because he believes that the aspect is of particular interest to the interviewer or the later audience of the investigation. This might be a restriction of the method especially when searching for subjective importance by counting numbers of appearances of relevant topics in narrative interviews. Consequently, this uncontrollable secondary variance has to be considered, when interpreting results of subjective importance.

15.2 Case Selection

Gläser & Laudel (2010) recommend the selection of typical cases and later an enrichment with contrasting cases. Literature from previous studies and discussions with field informants helped to gain initial knowledge about typical cases. Such informants were ayahuasca therapists, owners of retreat centres, medical doctors and psychologists who are engaged in the field of post-retreat integration counselling, professional researchers as well as scientifically naïve informants from Internet groups that had been entered previously. The pilot study had served to get an impression of the demographic and motivational situation of the international ayahuasca scene from the Internet. Many Internet activists who participated in the pilot study either had already been at an ayahuasca retreat or were about to do so.

Due to these sources, typical cases were considered having the following properties:

- Rather well educated
- Middle class income
- White native English speaker
- Pre-experienced with mind altering substances
- Pre-experienced with other self optimizing techniques (e.g. yoga, counselling, meditation, or others)
- Between the age of 25 and 45
- Spiritual motives, self-exploration and personal growth as main motives.

Cases were chosen in the beginning of the retreat after a first acquaintance and initial talks. A mixture of similar and contrasting cases was already present, regarding relevant variables like age distribution, pre-experience, psychiatric conditions, pre-experience in counselling, education level, as presented below.

Upon signing an informed consent form a demographic questionnaire was completed. 6 ayahuasca ceremonies were conducted in group-settings, at night. Interviews took place in the morning immediately after the second ayahuasca night ceremony had finished.

15.3 Reliability

15.3.1 Methods to increase coding consistency

Tests of the reliability are always statistical estimations on the true reliability (Raupp & Vogelsang, 2009, pp. XX-XXI). 'An instrument is called reliable to the extent that it yields data that is free of error' (Schreier, 2012, 167). Content analysis conceptualises reliability through consistency. Consistency is operationalized through the level of inter-subjective agreement or stability over time. The concept is related to the plausibility of the interpretation. The last is a very common criterion in qualitative research.

A reference list of exact definitions of the categories was written during the construction of the coding frame (see appendix). It contains the names of the categories, the definitions, excluding rules where it was necessary and typical examples of coding units. This insured a maximum of consistency during the actual coding process.

15.3.2 Strategy to measure the reliability

In the assessment of coding frames, two main strategies have previously been devised in order to estimate the extent of reliability of such instruments. One strategy compares the coding results of different coders. The other strategy compares the coding results of the same coder across different time points. The first strategy refers to the concept of inter-subjectivity and the other strategy to the concept of stability over time. Comparisons across points in time are typically used if no more than one coder is available (Schreier, 2012, p. 167).

For the re-test reliability strategy of this study, a period of 3 weeks between the first and second coding was chosen. Two coefficients of agreement were calculated across subcategories belonging to the same main categories as well as for main categories themselves.

Percentage of agreement:

$$\%_A = \frac{\text{numbers of coding units on which coders agree}}{\text{total number of coding units}} \times 100$$

Cohen's kappa for inter-rater agreement for category items. Cohen's kappa excludes the random of agreement by chance:

$$\kappa = \frac{(\text{observed agreement} - \text{agreement by chance})}{(1 - \text{agreement by chance})}$$

The results of the two procedures for determining consistency are presented in the table below.

Table 8: Reliability coefficients for the study categories about the phenomenology of the ayahuasca experience (Iquitos, Peru) generated by content analysis: Cohen's kappa, percentage of agreement

Category	No. of included (sub-)categories	$\%_A$	Cohen's *kappa*	Approx. sig.
Preparation	2	98,8700565	0,805	0
Visions or hallucinations	2	98,30508475	0,939	0
Properties of visions or hallucinations	5	96,04519774	0,873	0
Aesthetic or negative visions or hallucinations	2	98,02259887	0,526	0
Own phantasies, imaginations, thoughts	1	96,61016949	0,486	0
Voice inside the head or hallucinated voice	1	98,30508475	0,791	0
Who talks	4	98,02259887	0,743	0
How it talks	4	97,74011299	0,681	0
Content interpretation	3	94,91525424	0,553	0
Personal meaning	1	95,76271186	0,554	0
Personal meaning	5	95,19774011	0,435	0
Relational meaning	1	96,32768362	0,692	0
Relational meaning	7	95,76271186	0,677	0

Another person's issues	1	99,43502825	0,644	0
General wisdom	1	98,58757062	0,73	0
General wisdom	6	97,74011299	0,572	0
Mystical content	1	97,74011299	0,738	0
Mystical content	5	97,74011299	0,709	0
Acting inside the vision	1	100	1	0
Acting outside the vision	1	96,61016949	0,71	0
Acting outside the vision	7	96,32768362	0,728	0
Pleasant target emotion	1	95,76271186	0,765	0
Unpleasant emotion	1	98,02259887	0,819	0
Hedonistic emotions	1	97,45762712	0,514	0
No emotional response	1	99,43502825	0,797	0
Cognitive reaction	1	95,48022599	0,759	0
Cognitive reaction	7	95,19774011	0,755	0
Process character	1	98,30508475	0,563	0
Difficulties	1	98,02259887	0,623	0
Difficulties	1	98,02259887	0,605	0
Helpful	1	99.71751412	0,908	0
Appreciation	1	94,91525424	0,43	0
Role of the Ícaro	1	98,8700565	0,729	0
Role of the shaman	1	99,43502825	0,748	0

As presented in table 8, all measured categories have been found reasonable reliable. After the second coding, the places of disagreement were analysed again under the perspective of the dedfinitions of categories in the category reference list. Than the final coding frame was appointed.

15.4 Data collection

15.4.1 The retreat at the Ayahuasca Foundation (Iquitos, Peru)

Shamanic retreat centres that offer ayahuasca-ceremonies were identified through their Web pages and Facebook entries. A number of centres that offered their service in English were contacted and asked for collaboration.

This part of the investigation took place at the Ayahuasca Foundation facility, located in the Amazon rain forest near the Peruvian town Iquitos: www.ayahuascafoundation.org. It is a typical "healing centre", run by an US-American apprentice of a local vegetalista, offering shorter and longer ayahuasca retreats for western clients as many other centres in the region do. Contact was established through Internet search and personal contact. Upon commencement of a 13-day retreat, all 10 participants agreed to be interviewed during the retreat. A Portuguese woman who previously had gone through a longer shaman formation course that is offered by the ayahuasca Foundation and now works at the facility conducted the seminar.

Table 9: Schedule of the retreat structure at the Ayahuasca Foundation (Iquitos, Peru): study about the phenomenology of the ayahuasca experience

Day	Retreat	Investigation
1	Initial ice-braking round talk in Iquitos	Demographic data collection
2	Journey to the jungle facility First ayahuasca night ceremony	
3	- Purgative plant medicine intake - Counselling with the shaman: feedback from the initial diagnostic ayahuasca ceremony and treatment plan	
4	Ayahuasca night ceremony	
5	Purgative plant medicine intake	Interview
6	Ayahuasca night ceremony	
7	Indicative plant medicine intake	
8	Ayahuasca night ceremony	
9	Indicative plant medicine intake Research interview	
10	Ayahuasca night ceremony	
11	Indicative plant medicine intake	
12	Ayahuasca night ceremony	
13	Journey back to Iquitos	

The interviews took place during the seminar, the morning after the second ayahuasca ceremony.

15.5 Methodological considerations about narrative interviews

A narrative interview strategy was chosen (Helfferich, 2011, p.114; Küsters, 2009) to minimize any potential bias from my own interests, which would possibly manipulate the reports through all too specific leading questions (Patton, 2002, p. 39). I wanted to map the elements that were subjectively most relevant to participants. This would eventually reflect in the decision of the interviewee to report such elements.

As mentioned above a maximum of openness seems to be helpful for the facilitation of the narrative space, which allows the enrolment of systems of subjective relevance and interpretation patterns (Helfferich, 2011; pp. 114). These systems within the interviewer have to be deferred so that the interviewed person can enrol hers, as freely as possible. The limitation of this freedom lies in the research question, the capability of the interviewer to understand, the interview situation and its interpretation from the interviewed person. That is why interview technics of paraphrasing, interpretation and confrontation were put in abeyance for the narrative parts. Only few interventions were allowed and only if really necessary. 'The spontaneously-made report had priority' (Helfferich, 2012; p. 180) Allowed interventions:

- Narration generating open question.
- Nonverbal signals of understanding.
- Keep-up questions for retention of the narrative process.
- Mirroring without verbalization of additional or supposed subconscious content.
- Steerage questions – only to insure the thematic limitation of the interview question or the intelligibility.

Optional questions for the inquire part:

- Attitude questions
- Meaning questions
- Sometimes it can be necessary to serve the participant with a psychological analysis when he requires this. Such interpretations can be done explicitly labelled but should be kept only a few.

The decision for a deeper or confrontational questioning had to be done consciously. Impulses for confrontation of un-verbalized sense were protocolled after the interview in order to reflect them.

15.6 Preparation of the narrative interviews

Narrative interviews were conducted. For this purpose, an interview guideline was developed which defined the questions and interview strategy as well as allowed interventions. The initial question was this:

- 'Tell me as open as possible about your experiences last night.'
  Unspecific conducting and leading questions were allowed:
- 'Tell me more about this.'
- 'What does it mean to you?'
- 'Did it have any significance to you?'
- 'How do you mean this?'
- 'Can you explain this?'

An open question about involved emotions and about the most significant parts were added subsequently to the narrative interview, since, in contrast to traditional local ayahuasca use in the Upper Amazon region (Luna, 2004; de Rios, 1972), the focus of the providers of ayahuasca for western clients rather lies upon psychotherapeutic processes of 'emotional purging' and 'emotional healing' (Beyer, 2009, p. 348). Interviews were sound-recorded.

- 'Were there any particular emotions involved?'
- 'What was the most significant part?'

After asking these additional questions, sometimes participants remembered another episode of the psychedelic experience, which they had not mentioned in the first place. Here, apart from that, interviewees mostly gave overall evaluations of the process.

15.7 Constructing the coding frame

A strictly data-driven strategy was used to describe the material in detail and filter relevant categories out of the analysis units (interviews) during the pilot phase of the pre-investigation. This inductive strategy has been said to be appropriate for the rather naturalistic depicting of the material without producing bias from pre-knowledge or theoretical assumptions of the researcher in which the material otherwise may be pressed into (see Mayring, 2015, p.86). The first interview was analysed progressively summarising the material (see Mayring, 2015, pp. 69-90; Schreier, 2012, pp. 107-110) after splitting it into coding units by using a thematic segmentation criterion:

- Paraphrasing.
- Streamlining.
- Paraphrasing paraphrases that have something in common to their shared content.
- Generating category names and definitions taken from paraphrased paraphrases

For the rest of the analysis units the so formed main categories were used to perform a subsuming strategy. It takes advantage of already existing main categories under which appropriate coding units will be either subsumed into already existing subcategories or into new appropriate categories in order to form the coding frame (Schreier, 2012, pp.115-120). A point of saturation on which no more new categories appeared was reached after the 9th interview. When revising the coding frame, overlapping subcategories were merged together. The final version of the coding frame is presented in the appendix section.

15.8 Analysis of the data

Qualitative Content Analysis was chosen as method of analysis. QCA is a strategy for giving order and structure to qualitative material such as interviews by producing descriptive systems. In general, this is seen as one of the main tasks of qualitative research (Barton & Larzarsfeld, 1979; Schreier, 2012). Within the logic of this part of the investigation to investigate rather the subjective importance of experience phenomena but objective occurrences of predefined phenomena an inductive (data-driven) category building strategy was chosen.

15.9 Participants and demographics

Ayahuasca tourists who had already booked the seminar had been contacted; they were asked to participate voluntarily in the study and were extensively clarified of the study facts in order to achieve 'enlightened consensus' (Löwer, 2011) and commitment.

Demographic data were collected. Those are pure information, which is best and economically collected with a questionnaire.

The heterogenic structure of the interviewed individuals is presented in table 10. It represents the typical picture of ayahuasca-tourists of such a centre that has been found in previous studies before: mostly male, well-educated, upper middle class. The group also contains contrasting cases such as naïve and experienced, highly educated and moderately educated, non-patient and medically or psychiatrically pre-conditioned participants.

20 Participants were interviewed. During the construction of the coding frame theoretical saturation was reached after the 9th interview was analysed.

Table 10: Demographic data of the Iquitos sample (study about the phenomenology of the ayahuasca experience, Wolff et al., 2019)

No.	Age	Gender	Nationality	Drug experience	Previous medical conditions	Psychiatric conditions	Previous counselling	Profession
1	39	F	Germany	Ayahuasca	-	unknown	Yes	College registerd nurse
2	71	M	USA	-	Hypertension, appendectomy, total knee replacement	-	-	Marine engineer
3	33	M	Canada	Hallucinogens	Drug overdose	-	Yes	17 years of education
4	29	F	Canada	Hallucinogens	Choroid ocular melanoma	Anxiety, Depression	Yes	Registered nurse
5	69	M	Hungary	Ayahuasca	Apendectomy, Hiatal hernia	Depression	Yes	Pharmacist
6	34	F	Turkey	-	Hypothyriodism	-	-	University
7	33	M	Canada	Hallucinogens	Pneumonia	Anxiety	Yes	Registered dietican
8	28	M	England	Hallucinogens	-	-	-	Psychologist
9	27	M	England	Hallucinogens	-	-	-	Physician

The overall age ranged between 27 and 71 (N=9, median=33, interquartile range 10; mean age=40,3 years; +/- 1 SD=17,21 years).

Participants and demographics 151

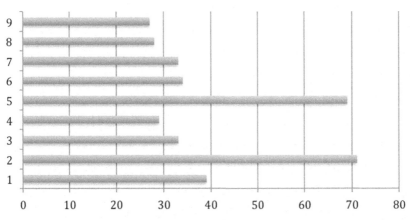

Y-axis: No. of participants; X-axis: age (years) during participation

Figure 8: Age distribution of the Iquitos sample (study about the phenomenology of the ayahuasca experience)

- Gender: 6 male participants, 3 female participants.
- Previous experiences with hallucinogens: 8 participants
  Psilocybin ("magic mushrooms") between one trial and monthly use, for 1 year up to 10 years;
  LSD between one trial and monthly use, since one and 10 years;
  MDMA ("Ecstasy") between one trial and monthly use, for one year up to 10 years.
- History of psychotherapeutic consultations: 5 participants.
- Previous medical conditions such as hypertension, knee replacement, hypothyroidism, pneumonia, appendectomy, choroid ocular melanoma: 6 participants.
- Previous psychiatric conditions such as depression or anxiety disorder: 3 participants.
- 8 of 9 graduated college or university. Reported professions: nurse, dietician, marine engineer, medical doctor, pharmacist, psychologist.

15.10 Answering the research question about ayahuasca phenomenology

How do foreign tourists experience acute ayahuasca effects in the setting of a shamanic jungle retreat in the Amazon rainforest?

15.10.1 The Coding frames

The research question of the second study leads towards the subjective importance of spontaneously mentioned aspects of the experience.

The coding frame represents the common inner structure of the analysed narratives and the coding frequencies represent the subjective importance or relevance for the narrators. The detailed analysis of the entire structure is presented below.

The following 3 figures show the structure of categories and subcategories that were found in the material at the Ayahuasca Foundation centre (taken from Wolff et al. 2019, Creative Commons Attribution-NonCommercial 4.0 International Licence).

Answering the research question about ayahuasca phenomenology 153

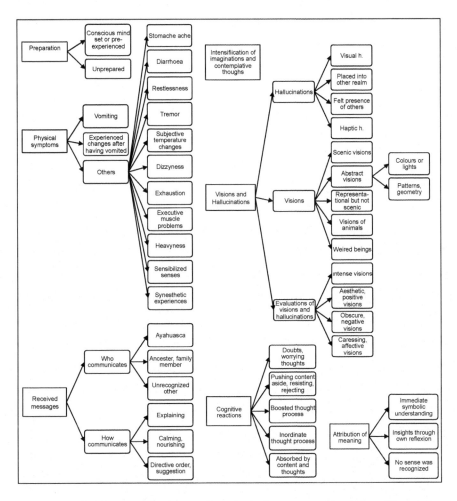

Figure 9: Coding frame part 1 - Preparation, physical symptoms, phantasies, visions, received messages, cognitive reactions and attribution of meaning reported after a shamanic ayahuasca ceremony in the Amazon region (Iquitos, Peru) in narrative interviews of 9 foreign participants using qualitative content analyses (taken from Wolff et al. 2019. All rights reserved.)

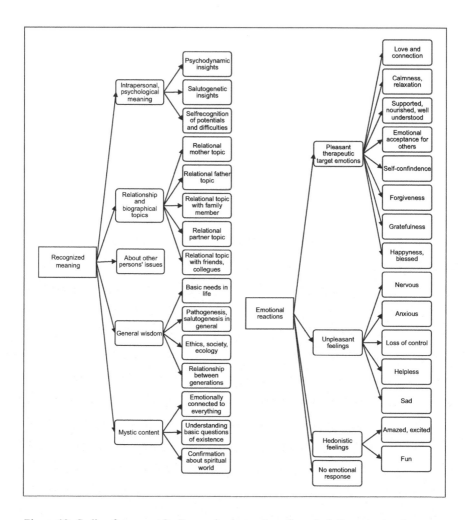

Figure 10: Coding frame part 2 - Recognized meaning of psychedelic content and emotional reactions reported after a shamanic ayahuasca ceremony in the Amazon region (Iquitos, Peru) in narrative interviews of 9 foreign participants using qualitative content analyses (taken from Wolff et al. 2019. All rights reserved.)

Answering the research question about ayahuasca phenomenology

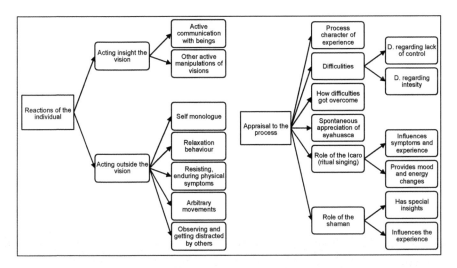

Figure 11: Coding frame part 3 - Appraisal to the process, role of ritual singing and of the shaman, reactions of the individual reported after a shamanic ayahuasca ceremony in the Amazon region (Iquitos, Peru) in narrative interviews of 9 foreign participants using qualitative content analyses (taken from Wolff et al. 2019. All rights reserved.)

16 Expectations, motivation, experiences, meaning and subjective effects

16.1 Research questions

Why are some western people interested in shamanic ayahuasca experiences in South America? How do they experience and how do they interpret their ritual participation in the jungle? Is there evidence that any kind of psychotherapeutic motivation or expectation play a relevant role? How do ayahuasca tourists process and integrate their experiences after the retreat has finished? Do the data support any psychotherapeutic relevance?

16.2 Location and associated institutions

The "intervention" took place in the Amazonas jungle near the Peruvian town Tarapoto. A typical healing and retreat centre was chosen and contacted after a longer period of Internet research. The-Garden of Peace is specialized on western clients (https://www.thegardenofpeace.com). Their web page offers ayahuasca and master plant retreats of different lengths between 7 and 30 days. The main healer was mestizo vegetalista (plant healer) Hegner Paredes Melendez from near Pucallpa. He was employed at the Garden of Peace at the time of the fieldwork and conducted the ayahuasca ceremonies, ayahuasca cooking as well as the application of additional master plants during master plant retreats. The research was approved by the staff and could be done in exchange for work a couple of hours each day in the centre.

16.3 Design

The third study was conducted as a qualitative investigation with the support of quantitative questionnaire data. The connection of both was done through the convergent design strategy of the mixed method research. Such a strategy analyses each database separately and merges the quantitative and qualitative interpretations after (Creswell, 2015, pp. 78-79 and 94). Qualitative interviews were conducted 6 weeks after the retreats had finished.

© The Editor(s) (if applicable) and The Author(s), under exclusive license to
Springer Fachmedien Wiesbaden GmbH, part of Springer Nature 2020
T. J. Wolff, *The Touristic Use of Ayahuasca in Peru*, Sozialwissenschaftliche
Gesundheitsforschung, https://doi.org/10.1007/978-3-658-29373-4_16

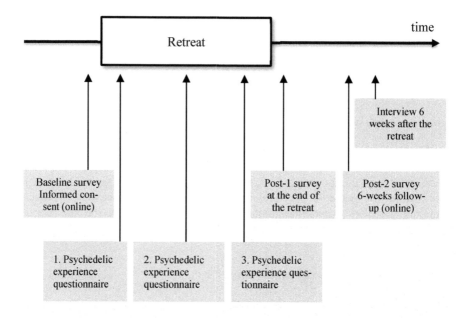

Figure 12: Schematic presentation of the data collection design of the study about expectations, motivations, experiences, meaning and some effects of subjects participating in ayahuasca retreats in Peru

16.4 Methods of the quantitative data collection

For the quantitative part three connected samples were collected. One from before the retreat (baseline) another immediately after the retreat (post-1) and a third one 6 weeks after the retreat had finished (post-2). The baseline set also contained a demographic questionnaire and a personality questionnaire.

Another part of the quantitative research focussed on the actual ayahuasca experiences during the retreats. After every ayahuasca ceremony connected samples data from a questionnaire about altered states of consciousness were collected. The quantitative data collection aims to underpin the qualitative findings.

• Baseline-post1-post2-design:
Variables: Demographic questionnaire
             Personality: NEO-FFI
             Sense of coherence: SOC-29
             Psychosomatic Symptoms: SCL-90-R

- Measurement of dimensions of altered states of consciousness during the retreats – timeline with 3 measurements, each after ayahuasca-ceremony:
Variables: Dimension of altered states of consciousness: 5D-ABZ (English version: 5D-ASC)

16.5 Methods of qualitative data collection

Semi structured guideline-interviews about motivation, expectations, meaning and integration time after the retreat took place 6-weeks after the retreats.

16.5.1 Case selection

There are different sampling strategies found in the literature: The selection of the cases could be done after Lindesmith & Cressey's principles of the search for contrasting counterexamples or Glaser & Strauss's theoretical sampling (Kelle & Kluge, 1999) or with a qualitative sampling plan.

For this investigation I chose the strategy to interview as many participants as possible who had registered for the respective retreat were interviewed. This was repeated in 4 retreats. It was to ensure that a typical mix of clients of the Garden of Peace is depicted. Almost all participants of each group agreed to be interviewed.

After all, there were only 2 participants of all the retreats who previously had decided not to take part in the investigation. They both preferred to focus fully on the experience. They feared being distracted by filling out questionnaires. During the retreats there were two persons who opted out, one of them by leaving the retreat centre. Unfortunately, I lost contact to this person. Three participants could not be contacted for the interview 6 weeks after the retreat, for unknown reasons.

The quasi-experimental design allows accrued samples. An assignment of randomly picked individuals to the ayahuasca group in order to compare with a non-ayahuasca group, as it would be done in a more experimental hypothesis testing design, is not the purpose of this study and would also be ethically problematic. In this naturalistic study participants themselves have done the decision of their individual assignment to the "intervention group" already before the investigation started and the study had no influence on that. With the qualitative examination I tried to expose details of their motivation and with the quantitative part I tested their convergence with mental health variables. In order to fulfil the principles of the convergent mixed methods design the participants of the quantitative and the qualitative databases were from the same population. According to Creswell (2015, pp. 78-79), the sample size does not have to be necessarily the same.

16.5.2 Constructing the interview guideline

16.5.2.1 Methodical considerations about the interview strategy

Helfferich (2011, pp. 37-45) arranges different interview strategies after 5 dimensions, which can be used to reflect why a certain interview strategy was purposefully chosen:

a) One of the main research interests of this investigation are subjective concepts and theories of ayahuasca tourists, their subjective experiences and interpretations. Here, Helfferlich allows a structured strategy like guideline-based interviews (ibid., p. 38). Of further interest are 'subjective or unconscious motives' (ibid., p. 38) which need to be discovered through a more corporate interaction like the problem-centred interview proposed by Andreas Witzel.

As Helfferich (ibid., p. 39) points out, research interests focussion on pure facts rather than on subjective meaning and subjective evaluations of these facts require a more structuring strategy which would reduce the material in early stages of the reseach process. A research interest focussing on the reconstruction of subjective meaning would choose the opposite strategy: a less structuring form in order to generate text.

The research interests of this investigation focus on a combination of reconstructing subjective sense as well as gathering facts. That's why the level of structuring intervention during the narrative process had to be flexible and process orientated.

b) In line with the principles of the problem-centred interview strategy and for the purpose of the disclosure of subjective or unconscious meaning, it can be necessary that the interviewer evaluates the level of earnestness, avoidance and psychological resistance of the interviewee as well as the point of saturation, when no new material is generated but old material is repeated. This includes the right of asking additional questions as well as confrontations with not yet understood contradictions. Pertinent information given by the narrator has to be treated as subjectively true if no other obvious reasons impede this.

c) The chosen interview strategy of this investigation is recommended if, on the one hand, a maximum of openness is needed for the reconstruction of subjective theories and, on the other hand, one has to intervene the open narrative space due to the research interest in particular facts or topics, (ibid., p. 179). The interviewer must be guided by some principles of problem-centered interview. "Comprehension generating strategies" were conducted after a phase of "narration generating strategies" for every guideline question (Witzel 1982, p. 92f). The guideline was used in a flexible way, in order to generate an interview dialogue as open as possible and as structured as necessary.

d) During the interview situation, the interviewer tried to present a position of interested cognitive strangeness as well as emotional friendliness. Between the interviews, he reflected about his own psychological transference and countertransference processes due to the possibility of unconsciously acting out. For this, a transference note with personal impressions was written after every interview.

e) For the interviews, a guideline supported semi-monologue strategy, was selected, as recommended by Helfferich (2011). This was a compromise between a pure monologue-oriented narrative interview strategy and a dialogical focused interview or problem-centred interview strategy. The interviewed person was animated to talk freely about each guideline question. But, other than in a pure narrative interview strategy, in a second phase of each guideline question, the interviewee was 'verbally supported and topically guided' (ibid., p. 43).

16.5.2.2 The construction process

As Helfferich recommends, the construction of the interview guideline followed the so-called "SPSS" principle. SPSS is the acronym for the German words „Sammeln" (collect), "Prüfen" (examine), "Sortieren" (arrange) and "Subsumieren" (subsume) (Helfferich, 2011, pp. 182).

Step one: All possible questions related to the subject of interest were collected from the literature study, discussions and informant talks within the worldwide ayahuasca community:

- Who wants to spend so much money and effort to expose oneself to partly unpleasant and partly non-controllable ayahuasca experiences in a foreign setting?
- What motivates people to ingest ayahuasca?
- What is typical of ayahuasca tourists?
- What do they expect from ayahuasca?
- Are ayahuasca tourists a sort of psychotherapy patients?
- Are there different types of ayahuasca-tourists?
- Are there ayahuasca tourists who experienced negative effects, or nothing happened?
- Are there similarities to meditation deepening levels within the experience of ayahuasca?

- Is it better when the ayahuasca experience is bedded into an on-going psychotherapy or another structured reflection process?
- Are there different processing types of ayahuasca, e.g. the thinker, the visual pattern observer, the hallucinator?
- What do people experience during their experience?
- Is their experience related to what they've expected before?
- How well are people informed about the qualification of the healer, the ritual and the content of the brew?
- What do people do with these experiences afterwards in their life?
- Are the dominant motivations related to neurotic structure of the person?
- Is something of the experience predictable out of their neurotic structure or personality structure?
- Which types or dimensions of motivations can be identified in ayahuasca tourists (inner set)? Hypothetic dimensions: hedonistic (adventure, sensation seeking, its a game), narcissi (cool, dangerous and rare experience), spiritual (what exactly does this mean?), psychotherapeutic, mixed type: spiritual-narcissi.
- How does the neurotic or conflict structure influence the experience?
- Do participants gain psycho-emotional insight, and self-acceptance?
- If there are different types of ayahuasca experiencer, what is particularly helpful for those types?
- Do they need different settings?
- Do people with an affective regulation deficite, e.g. BPD patients, have more problems with their self-regulation when experiencing highly emotional items during the psychedelic ayahuasca-state of consciousness?
- Is ayahuasca better for neurotic patients with a rather rich and conflictual inner word than for low Ego-structure patients with poor phantasy and poor cognitive reflecion processes?
- People who had "bad trips" or problems after their ingestion experience are mostly not reported. They compromise the image of ayahuasca transported in the Internet. There, ayahuasca is often believed to be helpful for everyone and everything. Does ayahuasca help only for certain problems and situations in life and does not for others?
- After many times doing ayahuasca, do you come to a point of qualitative saturation, where you do not discover new personal or psychedelic material but repeat, what you have already experienced before?
- As more neurotic a person is as more psychological, personal items (rather than transpersonal items) a person will experience?
- What do ayahuasca tourists believe how ayahuasca does what it does?
- How did they experience the shaman during their experiences?
- How important do they consider the shaman during the experience?

Methods of qualitative data collection 163

- What makes them know that a shaman is a good shaman?
- What of the experience do participants consider to be helpful?
- Which life experiences lead people to ayahuasca?
- Which elements of the ayahuasca medicine attract western tourists?
- Does the hallucinogenic effect have a special attraction to western tourists? If so – which?
- Is there a desire for spiritual confirmation or a religious prove that drive ayahuasca tourists?
- Is there a desire of clarification and/or integration or acceptance of experienced life events and the hope to do so with the help of ayahuasca in participants of ayahuasca tourism?
- Is there a desire to find solutions for actual problems in the life of ayahuasca tourists?
- Is there a desire for better inner guidance in life through making aware inner preferences, wishes and objectives in life?
- Do ayahuasca tourists differ from average population in aspects of mental health, spiritual and life satisfaction?
- How do the people interpret what they have experienced?
- How is the particular content of the ayahuasca experience related to the expectations of the patient?
- How is the particular content of the ayahuasca experience related to the biography of the patient?
- How does the process of giving sense to the experience work?
- What do they expect?
- Are ayahuasca tourists a sort of drug users, who simply have a better excuse for their consumption than regular drug addicts?
- What does the indigenous setting mean to foreign participants and how does it influence their ayahuasca experience?
- How do paticipants evaluate the quality of their psychedelic experience?
- What is a good trip? Is it possible to identify subjective quality stages in the personal evaluations of ayahuasca trip elements?

Additionally, the previously conducted investigations provided relevant categories. Those categories were used for the development of a concept-driven collection of main topics that served for the construction of interview questions.

Step two: Questions were examined and reduced under the view of openness and pre-knowledge, e.g. doubled questions, fact questions were eliminated as well as very general questions.

Step three: Remaining questions were sorted under useful keywords

Step four: An open invitation question to produce text was developed for every bundle of sub-questions. Different aspects of this were subsumed under this question either as keywords or written out questions.

For every question, the interviewer could explore further aspects that had not been covered by the initial answer. Also, additional questions for better understanding were allowed as well as conducting and continuing questions. Those questions are rather unspecific and facilitate deeper information or boost the flow of thoughts. Different versions of the guidelines were revised and modified.

16.6 Data collection

As done before in the pre-investigation, ayahuasca-tourists, who had already applied for a retreat, were contacted through the cooperating centre and were asked for voluntary participation in the study. This took place weeks before the course started. They were extensively informed of the study facts to achieve the 'enlightened consensus' (Löwer, 2011) and commitment. Baseline questionnaires and demographic questionnaires were collected mainly through the Internet from them. When meeting the retreat groups personally on day 1 in a café in Tarapoto they were again informed about the study and signed an information and commitment paper (see appendix). Participation was voluntary. Opting out was possible at any time during data collection. Anonymisation was assured. All participants agreed to provide data for research and publication under these conditions. During the jungle seminar the contact was reduced as much as possible. This was an agreement with the facilitators in order to maintain their seminar protocol of isolation, solitude and diet between the ayahuasca ceremonies. After the course was finished participants were asked to fill out the post-1 questionnaire. 6 weeks after they were contacted again through Internet and asked for an interview and to fill out the post-2 online-questionnaire before the interview.

This procedure was repeated with four different groups of participants throughout one year.

Table 4: Timetable of a 10-days-retreat at the centre Garden of Peace (Tarapoto, Peru)

Day	Content	Investigation during the retreat
1	Journey to the jungle facility Tobacco purge	
2	Ayahuasca night ceremony	
3	Indicative plant medicine intake	Questionnaire 5D-ASC

	Research interview	
4	Indicative plant medicine intake	
5	Ayahuasca night ceremony	
6	Indicative plant medicine intake Research interview	Questionnaire 5D-ASC
7	Indicative plant medicine intake	
8	Ayahuasca night ceremony	
9	Tobacco ceremony, Breaking the diet with salt and fruits	Questionnaire 5D-ASC
10	Journey back to the town	

16.6.1 Demographic questionnaire

A questionnaire about biography, pre-experiences and personal data was applied through Internet before the retreat together with the other baseline questionnaires.

Demographic variables:
- Age, biological gender, legal status
- Country of childhood
- Education degree and profession
- Baptism, religious education
- Pre-experience with other mind-altering substances
- Addiction issues from previously consumed drugs
- Medicine intake within 12 months before the seminar
- Pre-experience with ayahuasca
- Pre-knowledge about ayahuasca
- Pre-experience with psychotherapy or other psycho-techniques

16.7 Demographic summary

An average participant of the third investigation at the Garden-of-peace centre would be 31 years old, Caucasian, would have experience with cannabis, MDMA, psilocybin. 45% came from the US; 48% hold a college degree; 50% were baptised and raised as Christian and 21% as atheists. 1/3 had experience as psychotherapy/counselling client, but only a minority was currently in therapy. 50% had previous experience with ayahuasca.

16.8 Psychometric Questionnaires

A baseline battery of psychometric questionnaires was given before the ayahuasca experience and another battery was given two times after the retreat. The post1-battery was given immediately after finishing the retreat and the post2-battery was given 6 weeks after the seminars had finished.

16.8.1 NEO-FFI: Personality questionnaire

Personality screening was performed before intervention with the NEO-FFI questionnaire from Paul T. Costa & Robert R. McCrae, which is a short version of the NEO-PI-R. The test is based on the long history of the lexical hypothesis of Sir Francis Galton, Louis Thurstone, Gordon Allport, Henry S. Odbert and others, that common personality factors are reflected in the language. Fife factors have been extracted. They are described by altogether 60 different statements that can be rated on a 5-steps scale between 'strongly disagree', 'disagree', 'neutral', 'agree' and 'strongly agree' (Borkenau & Ostendorf, 2008; Stangl, 2018):

- Neuroticism: confident, secure vs. sensitive, nervous (emotional stability)
- Extraversion: outgoing/energetic vs. solitary/reserved (sociability; confidence; conversationality; activity; optimism; cheerful mood; higher energy level)
- Openness to experiences: inventive/curious vs. consistent/cautious (fanciful life; perceiving own feelings, both positive and negative; accentuated and interested in many personal and public processes; inquisitive; intellectual; imaginative; keen to experiment, and artistically interested; willing to critically scrutinize existing norms and respond to novel social, to ethical and political values; independent in judgment; unconventional behaviour; preference towards variety.
- Agreeableness: friendly/compassionate vs. challenging/detached (altruism; understanding of others; benevolence and compassion; striving to help others and believe in the altruism of others; interpersonal trust; cooperativity; indulgence; need for harmony)
- Conscientiousness: efficient/organized vs. easy-going/careless (purposeful; ambitious; hardworking; persistent; systematic; strong-willed; disciplined; reliable; punctual; orderly; precise and meticulous; related to academic and professional achievements. The negative side is related to exaggerated high standards, compulsive neatness and workaholism.)

The questionnaire is test theoretically evaluated and internationally well established in research.

16.9 SOC-29: Sense of coherence questionnnaire

A mental health related aspect of personality is the Sense of Coherence (SOC), develloped by Aaron Antonovsky. It is defined as the general life orientation. Some researchers see the SOC in a rather reductionist way as a personality trait but ignore cultural and historic contexts of life orientation. A high SOC is seen as protective resource during distress of negative life events. Antonovsky identified three basic dimensions through qualitative methods that were later quantitatively established. The questionnaire reports a general score beside the three sub-scores:

- Comprehensibility: Life is understandable. Because the world works according recognisable rules (11 items).
- Manageability: Life can be shaped; alone or with the help of others (10 items).
- Meaningfulness: It is worth to live. Life is sensible and brings joy (8 items).

Reliability and inner consistence are good, but it was problematic to reproduce the factor solution of these dimensions as independent factors. The questionnaire correlates negatively with anxiety, depression, neuroticism and negative affectivity. It is advisable to use the general score only (see Singer & Brähler, 2014; pp.14-25).

16.9.1 SCL-90-R: Symptom Checklist-90-Revised

The Symptom-Checklist-90-R from Leonard R. Derogatis is a 90 items collection for psychological, social, medical and psychiatric symptoms. Items are rated in self-report manner on a 5-point rating scale. 3 global indices and 9 symptoms dimension are reported (Derogatis, 1994):

- Somatisation
- Obsessive-compulsive
- Interpersonal sensitivity
- Depression
- Anxiety
- Hostility
- Phobic anxiety
- Paranoid ideation

- Psychoticism
- Global severity index
- Positive symptom distress index
- Positive symptom index.

The handbook provides T-scores for both genders and different populations. The questionnaire is internationally recognised and widely used for research and diagnostic. It has been identified as a reliable measure for the global psychic symptom load and there are validity reports. The valid identification of different symptoms through different subscales is problematic (Hessel et al., 2001).

16.9.2 5D-ABZ (5D-ASC)

During the retreats subjective alterations of consciousness were measured after every ayahuasca ceremony night.

The latest version of the questionnaire 5D-ABZ from A. Dittrich, D. Lamparter & M. Maurer (2006) serves for the retrospective scientific investigation of extraordinary states of consciousness. The authors aimed to create an instrument that assesses altered states of consciousness independently from their aetiology. Dimensional analysis was used, and 3 aetiology-independent dimensions were identified:

- Oceanic boundlessness: Enriching aspects of the experience such as experiences of oneness with oneself and the world as well as liberation from the limiting aspects of space and time. Strong 'oceanic' states can also be experienced as mystical or religious.
- Dread of ego dissolution: Fear is central aspect. Feelings of fragmentation of one's own person or the world are in focus. The expression "bad trip" refers to a high level on this dimension.
- Visional destructuralisation: The dimension describes changes in the perception and meaning of perceptual content. These include optical hallucinations and synaesthesia such as seeing sounds in the form of pictures.
- Two further scales report additional aspects of quantitative alterations of consciousness as well as auditory hallucinations:
- Auditory alterations: Perceptual changes and hallucinations of auditory content
- Vigilance reduction: quantitative reduction of consciousness like clouding of consciousness, sleepiness, and drowsiness.

E. Studerus et al. (2010) evaluated the factorial structure and psychometric properties in a large sample of experimental induced altered states of consciousness (ASC) by using structural equation modelling techniques. The original scales were identified as multidimensional constructs. Eleven new scales were constructed and psychometrically tested. They suite better the dimensional structure of induced. The following dimensions were established:

- Experience of unity: oneness, eternity, dissolving conflicts and contradictions
- Spiritual experience: Connected to superior power, impression of awe, religious aspects
- Blissful state: boundless pleasure, profound peace, all-embracing love
- Insightfulness: profound feeling, clarity about connections, original thoughts
- Disembodiment: out of body experience, floating impression, dissolving body
- Impaired control and cognition: paralysed, isolated, disconnected thought process, decision-making problems, felling of being a marionette
- Anxiety: frightened, threatened, terrifyingly distorted, strange and weird surrounding
- Complex imagery: pictures of the biographical past, vivid imagination, seeing rolling scenes with closed eyes
- Elementary imagery: regular patterns with closed eyes, colours in the dark, lights and flashes
- Audio-visual synaesthesia: Noise and sounds influenced the visual perception
- Changed meaning of percepts: special or strange meaning of everything, objects are engaged emotionally.

The questionnaire offers a visual analogue scale for each item. Measures are transformed into %-points from 0 to 100. The items must be grouped and summed for each dimension. For both, the original scales from Dittrich and the new scales from Studerus, means and standard deviations were calculated. For each set of scales, a total number was calculated (Total D and Total S). The scale data can be used for further transformation into percentage of the theoretical scale maximum.

16.10 Methods of data collection and analysis

16.10.1 Qualitative Content Analysis

For analysing the qualitative data, a structuring qualitative content-analysis was applied in a mixed strategy with deductive, pre-knowledge-based main categories and inductive, data-driven subcategories (see Schreier, 2012).

The question clusters for each research question of the interview guideline served as main categories for the initial construction of the coding frame as well as theory-based pre-knowledge and common-sense curiosity. Later the coding frame was inductively modified by a subsuming strategy (Schreier, 2012, pp. 115).

In the process of building the coding frame, categories were defined by name, description of features and, if possible, indicators, typical examples or hypothetical examples and, if necessary, decision rules.

The coding frame was revised by rational re-grouping and partly merging overlapping categories. Differences and conformity of the cases were identified, and context of meaning was constructed.

16.10.2 Methodical considerations: The construction of the coding frame

At first a trial coding was performed with the initial coding frame and matters of reliability and validity were discussed. With this coding frame the same material was recoded. Later the coding frame was tested and modified with other interview material until saturation could be asserted.

The depth and complexity of the coding frame was adjusted to the research question. The coding frame had to serve certain rules to obtain research quality (Schreier, 2012, pp. 71-79):

- Avoidance of confounded dimensions: Signs for mixed dimensions are whe
- subcategories are no example for their main category and names of subcategories appear throughout the coding frame in an identical manner.
- Mutual exclusiveness: One coding unit from the text could only be attached to
- one subcategory of a given dimension. This is important for reliability, especially
- when dealing with categories, which do not exclude
- each other by definition.
- Exhaustiveness: Every coding unit had to be sorted into the coding frame. This is considered to be important for high research validity. "Remains" categories were used sparingly.
- Saturation: It was aimed that every subcategory would be filled at least with one coding unit. This is often the case with pure data driven coding frames. With concept driven coding frames, it can happen that no example is found in the text for certain subcategories. This could be a source of interesting negative findings. That's why empty categories should be kept throughout the research process and should be part of the discussion. Because the constructing

Methods of data collection and analysis 171

process was data-driven on the level of subcategories, no empty categories were left.

The whole material was used, except introductions, goodbyes and parts of Small-talk or technical problems that did not refer to the topic. The coding frame was used for reducing and presenting the relevant material (Schreier, 2012, p. 83).

Subsumption strategy for the construction of the data driven subcategories:

The transcribed material was read through until a concept was found, that related to one of the main categories. It was labelled by a paraphrased name and was sorted under this main category as a sub-category. Continued reading brought up new concepts, which also were labelled and sorted in one of the main categories as new subcategories. Other findings, which were similar to one of the already existing sub-categories as well as and repetitions, were sorted in one of the already existing subcategories. This process continued until the end of the material. The point of saturation, when no other concepts appeared, was noted. Overlapping categories were cleaned before moving on (ibid., pp. 115-120).

16.10.3 Constructing a concept-driven coding frame

Initial attempt to find a theoretical structure for analysing interviews:

The initial attempt of constructing a pure concept driven coding frame is presented below and reflects the making-conscious of pre-knowledge and possibly biased assumptions regarding the theoretical preparation work:

1. Motivation for ayahuasca
1.1 Spiritual/esoteric/religious motives
1.1.1 Belief in spiritual/supernatural phenomena, which can be accessed through ayahuasca
1.1.1.1 Wish for supernatural knowledge or power to communicate with spirits
1.1.2.2 Advice or guidance through ayahuasca or other spirits
1.1.2.3 Connection with nature
1.1.1.1 Sceptical trial or search or doubtful approach for spiritual experiences
1.1.1.1.1 Search for prove or confirmation
1.1.1.1.1.1 Encounter with God
1.1.1.1.1.2 Encounter with ayahuasca, "Pachamama" or others as communicating spirits
1.1.1.1.1.3 After death confirmation
1.2 ayahuasca as psychotherapy
1.2.1 Inner review and correction of personal life-plan
1.2.2 Examination and acceptance of personal biography or ancestral history
1.2.3 Solutions for actual psychological or social problems
1.3. Hedonistic motives
1.3.1 Thrill, kick, angst lust
1.3.2 To be special, "narcissi food"
1.3.3 Discovery of the other culture

1.3.3.1 Authentic native experience
1.3.3.2 Postmodern tourist – does not search for native authenticity
1.4 Solve physical or medical issues
2. Subjective working model
2.1 Shamanic or spiritual model
2.1.1 Personification of ayahuasca and other entities as supernatural beings
2.1.2 Cleaning from negative energies through the shaman
2.1.3 Miraculous interventions through God, Jesus, the Holy Ghost, etc.
2.2 Scientific or western explanations
2.2.1 Biochemical and neurophysiological model
2.2.2 Psychological explanations
2.2.2.1 Psychodynamic model of insight into inner unconscious conflicts
2.2.2.2 Behavioural model of learning new behaviour or thinking
2.2.2.3 Humanistic model of facilitating personal growing and development
2.2.4 Mixed model between biochemical and psychological
3. Ayahuasca-related biographical approaches

16.10.4 Final concept-driven coding frame

The concept-driven plan that was finally used for the construction of the interview guideline is presented here. It consists of the main categories that were operationalised by a question or a set of questions. These main categories also served as starting point for the coding process of the interview material:

1. Retrospective view: before the seminar
1.1 Biographical approach towards ayahuasca
1.2 Preparedness
1.3 Phantasies before the retreat
1.4 Retrospective reflexion on the previous motivation
2. Reflections on the retreat
2.1 Comparison between anticipatory expectations and the actual experience
2.2 Retrospective view on emotionally relevant experiences during the retreat
2.3 Set and setting
2.3.1 Supportive influences during ayahuasca ceremonies regarding the setting
2.3.2 Unhelpful influences during ayahuasca ceremonies regarding the setting
3. Evaluation
3.1 Retrospective interpretative relevance
3.2 Time after the retreat until the interview
3.3 Personal meaning
3.4 Positive effects, life impact, integration
3.5 Satisfaction
3.6 Negative effects
3.7 Lasting effects
3.8 Role of ayahuasca
4. Subjective healing theory
4.1 Healing theory
4.2 Subjective ayahuasca working theory
4.3 Shamanic background belief
5. Religious Experience

Methods of data collection and analysis

In the final interview guideline, a question or in some cases a set of questions were assigned to every point of this concept-driven frame.

16.10.4.1 Interview guideline

Conducting and continuing questions:
- Could you tell me something more about this?
- And then, what happened next?
- How did it go on?
- How was that for you?
- What does it mean to you?
- Did it have any significance to you?
- How exactly?
- Explain this a little more.
- How do you mean this?
- Anything else?

Topic	Questions
	Leading question
	Now the retreat has finished some weeks ago and you might have some distance to reflect about it and how it went on with you after.
	Retrospective view - before the seminar
Ayahuasca focused biographical narrative	Until someone decides to do Ayahuasca there is sometimes a personal history behind this. Please tell me something about this history of yours.
	How did you hear from Ayahuasca the first time?
	Why did you want to do it? (How did you personally come to the idea to do Ayahuasca at all?)
	How was your way until you came to the decision to do this seminar?
Preparedness	Did you prepare yourself before coming to the seminar, how? E.g. did you search for information before? How, where? What else?
Phantasies before	How did you imagine the retreat would be? Did you have any phantasies about it?

Retrospective motivation	If you think back about the time before the seminar started, did you have particular topics, interests or expectations that you wanted to experience or deal with? What exactly brought you to this retreat? Did you want to medicate or treat something with this shamanic experience? If yes, which aspects? If so, how did you imagine that Ayahuasca would solve your issues? (Imagined working mechanism?) Was there any curiosity factor or adventure factor? Tell me something about it? The hosts say that in some cases the actual Ayahuasca-experience would not be the most important healing-part but they emphasize other aspects like the 'dieta' and the other plant medicines. What do you think? Would you have booked the retreat if it had been without Ayahuasca but just dieta and other master-plants?
	Reflections on the retreat
Comparison between anticipatory expectations and the experience	Compare your expectations with the actual experiences. Was it as you had imagined it before or was it different? Explain a bit? Was there something unexpected or surprising? If so, which parts of it were unexpected? How did you deal with those unexpected experiences?
Retrospective emotional relevance	What moved or impressed you the most? How did you feel about it?
	Set and setting
Supportive influences	What was helpful or supportive for you during the Ayahuasca experiences? (Surrounding, people, reactions, ritual, shamanic issues, etc.) How did you take/react to this support?
Unhelpful influences	Was there something unhelpful, difficult or contra productive? How did you deal with it? What did it mean to you?

Methods of data collection and analysis 175

	Evaluation
Retrospective interpretative relevance	If you think now about the experiences during the seminar, was there any experience or topic that you consider relevant for your personal life? If so, what were the most relevant experiences for you in this retrospective view? Why?
Time after the retreat	How did it go on with you after the retreat?
Personal meaning	What does this experience mean to you now?
Positive effects, life impact, integration	Did you benefit from the retreat somehow? Was it helpful in something? Did you take anything with you? Did it have any impact on you or your life? Did the Ayahuasca or other parts of the retreat support or help you with something? Did you change anything in your life or did something change by itself, like e.g. how you treat yourself, your body, situations or other people?
Satisfaction	If you compare your expectations or aims from before the retreat and your situation now? How do you evaluate this? Are you satisfied?
Negative effects	Did you experience any negative effect after the seminar or until now? What does this mean to you?
Lasting effects	If you have noticed any change or effects from the seminar, how lasting, remaining or stable would you consider these effects?
Role of Ayahuasca	Which role does the Ayahuasca experience play in the outcome of the whole retreat? Or in other words how do you see the influence of Ayahuasca on that effects you described - among the other influences and plant medicines of the seminar.
	Subjective healing theory
Healing theory	What is healing and what does it mean to you, personally?

Subjective ayahuasca working theory	What exactly does Ayahuasca do?
	How does it work? (bio-chemical, biographical, psychological, shamanic-magical, insight into symbolic visions)
	Is Ayahuasca really a kind of person? Why do you think so? If yes, please describe him/her/it?
	Did you get new perspectives on your knowledge about how Ayahuasca works?
	If something from the Ayahuasca experience during the seminar was helpful for you, what exactly was that?
	(E.g. the work/presence of spirits (jaguar, eagle, ancestors, etc.),
	the actions of the shaman,
	mystical insight into the oneness or connection of everything,
	the relativisation of your ego problems,
	review of parts of your biographical history,
	the expression of formerly suppressed emotions,
	or something else or a combination of factors?
Shamanic background belief	What do you think about the shamanic background – like the spiritual world, spirits, the explanation about the Dieta, etc.?
	Do you have sometimes doubts about this perspective? If so, about which aspects?
	Could you imagine a western Ayahuasca therapy without the native shamanic setting?
Religious experience	Is Ayahuasca a religious experience?
	Additional comments
	Is there anything else that you want to tell?

16.10.5 Methods of quantitative data analysis

Descriptive statistics were performed on the collected quantitative data. For inference statistics, the aim was to perform the T-test for dependent samples for the pre-post variables if the statistical requirements for parametric testing were met. Otherwise, the nonparametric Wilcoxon-test for dependent pairs was used to analyse differences. For correlation analyses the nonparametric Spearman-Rho test was performed. For depicting causal connections between variables, a linear regression analysis was calculated. All statistical procedures were performed in SPSS-23.

17 Results, conclusions and discussion

17.1 Motivational structure

The sample characteristics show that members of ayahuasca Facebook networks participating in this study were rather well-educated adults. They tended to have had previous experience with other psychedelics or cannabis as well as experience in counselling or other psychotherapies. The interest in ayahuasca experiences among Facebook ayahuasca group members in this study seems not to be a phenomenon of a recreational youth drug culture. They tend towards the intake within organised events such as shamanic healing ceremonies and retreat seminars. Larger samples are needed to generalise to the population level.

It can be assumed that within the motivational structure of the sample there is a stronger group of motivational aspects and a weaker group of motivational aspects. The stronger one contains spiritual interests and the self-exploring motivation. The weaker group contains the intention to solve health issues and to seek interesting sensations.

The two categories, 'self-awareness / self-exploration' and 'spiritual purposes', appeared to be the most relevant in terms of the general motivation for ayahuasca within the sample. 'Self-awareness / self-exploration' also comprises the psychotherapeutic motivation of healing depressive symptoms, social anxiety symptoms and childhood trauma. On the one hand, the motivations subsumed under this item seem to be past-oriented in the sense of biographical understanding, integration and coping with past experiences and, on the other hand, future-oriented in the sense of hoping for guidance, recognition of own preferences in life and meaningful shaping of the future. Another categorization would be possible: psychotherapeutic motivation, personal meaning, adjustment and betterment. A comprehensive qualitative content analysis of the expectations of ayahuasca clients is needed.

'Self-awareness / self-exploration' and 'spiritual purposes' correlated positively with each other in the sample. It is known from European neo-shamanic scenes that previously narrowly defined terms get a changed and sometimes overgeneralized meaning. In neo-shamanic circles, this can be the case with the concept of healing (Morris, 2006). Within those peer groups, the term might overlap with concepts such as "cleansing from civilisation influences" or "personal spiritual development and wisdom". In our sample, there could also be a blurring between 'spiritual purposes' and 'self-awareness / self-exploration'. For this study, the qualitative analysis of the subjective meaning of these predetermined motivational items point towards such a partial overlap when the hope for a 'life changing experience' was expressed that would heal depression (participant 5) as well as the desire to 'reflect the development of the soul' (participant 36) or when ayahuasca was seen as 'another piece ... of the spiritual journey... in the category of how certain plants can heal us' (participant 26).

Since the variable 'spiritual purposes' and 'self-awareness / self-exploration' have similar distributions and are correlated, it would be interesting to further examine similarities and differences in the subjective meaning of them and how they may be connected.

In interviews with curanderos (Spanish: healer) from the upper Amazonas, who work with foreign clients, Stephan V. Beyer reported that they believe that, unlike local clients, foreign ayahuasca drinkers would rather have spiritual and esoteric interests and would rather be confused, tormented and burdened with mental problems, often related to their childhood (Beyer, 2009, pp. 347-348). The higher motivation for spiritual purposes and self-awareness / self-exploration in this sample and their correlation compared with the lower motivation for solving physical issues and the lower interest in interesting or exciting experiences does not contradict this observation.

The wider error bars of the weaker group of variables may show a greater interpersonal diversity in the motivational strength regarding the expectation of healing physical issues as well as to experience an interesting or exciting time with ayahuasca. Here, the motivations seem to be less consistent among the sample than in terms of 'spiritual purposes' or 'self-awareness / self-exploration'.

On the one hand, in terms of solving physical problems, this may also reflect the suggestion from anthropological literature that ayahuasca-interested foreigners may be less interested in actual physical healing than local clients (Beyer, 2009, p. 348). Yet, on the other hand, fantastic rumours about physical miracle healing through ayahuasca are repeatedly transported in the ayahuasca scene, both local and international. This may have led to a wider dispersion of expectations in the interest in physical healing.

The rather low motivational aspect of having interesting or exciting experiences surprised us. But again, the higher deviation in the sample points towards a greater inter-individual variety regarding this motivational aspect.

Statistical group comparisons with larger samples between different types of ayahuasca-drinkers from different settings are needed in order to complete and ensure the knowledge about the motivation of ayahuasca drinkers. Further statistical group comparisons of the motivational structure of local native and mestizo drinkers with non-native ayahuasca-drinkers would be relevant for cultural anthropology to depict the development of possible new traditions in the context of phenomena of the industrialized worlds like the individualization of spirituality and religiosity, patchwork religiosity and how these new developments possibly influence the local motivation and ayahuasca-practise in the upper Amazonas region. Further studies could better detail what ayahuasca-drinkers exactly mean when they report spiritual reasons or self-exploration and how previous motivation and expectation is related to their actual trip experiences. Another promising approach would be the analysis of how possibly the motivation and expectation changes from beginners towards long-term drinkers. (Parts of this chapeter have been published previously under Creative Commons Attribution NonCommercial 4.0 International Licence in Wolff & Passie, 2018.)

17.2 Phenomenological analysis of subjective experiences

How do foreign tourists experience acute ayahuasca effects in the setting of a shamanic jungle retreat in the Amazon rainforest?

The selected group of 9 foreign ayahuasca-tourists in a traditional or "traditionalised" healing centre in the Peruvian rain forest was approximately 33 years old (median), consisted of approximately 2/3 males and 1/3 females, was predominantly experienced in the use of other hallucinatory drugs or ayahuasca, came from a well-educated social background and was heterogenous regarding psychiatric preconditions and pre-experience in psychological counselling.

The narrative structure of ayahuasca experience reports consist of the overarching main topic 'experiences during the ceremony' (figures 9, 10 and 11) and two side-themes: 'preparation' (see figure 9), 'appraisal to the process' (see figure 11). Often, the narratives started with a short sequence about the preparation, then a long sequence about the experiences and finally about appraisal to the process. According to the initial interview question, the most frequent statements made were about the actual experiences. The internal structure, depicted in coding frame, is complex and contains several themes, sub-themes and categories. It is presented category by category and also as a graphical overview (see figures 9, 10 and 11 respectively).

Typical statements of preparedness are about motivation, set of intentions and pre-knowledge.

This side-theme refers to the appraisal and general characterisation of the experience as a dynamic process, which would change in intensity and quality over time. Sometimes difficulties during the process were mentioned such as lack of control, unpredictability and difficulties regarding the intensity or the speed of the perceived flow of psychedelic content.

Although not frequently, more than half of the participants mentioned the role and influence of the shamanic singing on the experience spontaneously. The ritual singing was reported to affect physical sensations within participants' body's and influence visions, as well as help to absorb attention and stimulate mood or energy changes. The shaman himself was experienced as adept at regulating the experience. The singing as a setting variable was experienced as a modulating factor of the process regarding intensity and quality of the psychedelic as well as bodily experience. That's why it was grouped into this category.

The following themes and sub-themes were subsumed under "experiences during ceremony" (see coding frames of the second study, figures 9, 10 and 11). Note that most of the themes contain several sub-categories that are presented later:

- Physical symptoms
- Visions and hallucinations, properties of visions and evaluation
- Intensification of imaginations and contemplative thoughts
- Received messages
- Attribution of meaning (immediate symbolic understanding, insights through own reflection, no sense recognized)
- Different types of meaning recognized within the psychedelic content (intrapersonal, relational, about other people's issues, general wisdom, mystical, spiritual or religious content)
- Emotional and other mental reactions of the individual such as acting inside and outside the visions, cognitive reactions.

Physical symptoms from the ayahuasca ingestion are a common topic that was mentioned by all participants as well as a frequent topic, which took a rather large space during interviews. Of all symptoms, vomiting and nausea are most commonly and most frequently reported. Changes in the quality and intensity of the psychedelic process after vomiting have spontaneously been reported. This points towards a possible bottleneck-like effect during ayahuasca ceremonies, which were previously described by Kjellgren et al. (2009) as sudden transformation of the experience. The typical importance of ayahuasca-vomiting and its relevance in the psychedelic experience and individual meaning-making is discussed in greater detail in the chapter Plateau, peak points and release. Other physical symptoms reported include: stomach pain; diarrhoea; restlessness; tremor; raised temperature; fuzziness; exhaustion; heaviness; executive muscle problems; sensitized senses and synesthetic-like experiences such as visualizing sounds. Our findings are consistent with the previous literature that dealing with physical stresses such as nausea and vomiting is dominant in ayahuascsa trip reports (Shanon, 2014, pp. 62-63). The same applies to ibogaine but not to LSD, mescaline and psilocybin (Schenberg et al., 2017).

Visions have been a common and frequent topic too. They are intended ayahuasca-typical visual perceptions. These qualitative findings are consistent with the quantitative data obtained from the Altered States of Consciousness questionnaire. There, on average, simple and complex visual psychedelic perceptions were highlighted as the dominant feature of the ayahuasca experience, although the scattering is great.

Visions can be of abstract colours and complex geometrical patterns or symmetrical shapes. These types of visions were reported most commonly. Other less common and less frequent types of visions are about representational objects, scenes and people, animals and fantastic or weird creatures. Regarding the visual phenomena, the structuring into abstract, representational (not scenic) and scenic material, as well as animals and weird beings is in agreement with previous reports (Shanon, 2002; Barbosa et al., 2005).

Some of the content seem to have immediate, consciously recognised meaning to the interviewees, some not. Others are interpreted and subjectively understood afterwards, other just remains weird or fascinating but unintelligible.

Hallucinations can appear but are less common and infrequently reported. Haptic hallucinations of being touched or caressed, the presence of other persons or beings and to be entirely dislocated into another realm are such phenomena that had been reported.

The visions and hallucinations were spontaneously evaluated as being intense, aesthetically positive, obscure and affectively kind.

Participants reported that thoughts and imaginations were intensified. They were able to make a distinction between visions and imaginations or fantasies in general. This has been previously described in conjunction with deep self-search and psychological analysis, creativity, metaphysical ideas and new personal perspectives (Shanon, 2014, pp. 69-70).

As already noted by Shanon (2014, p. 67-69), ayahuasca drinkers usually find themselves in the role of spectator of their visual phenomena; however, intense ayahuasca-experiences can involve acting within the visions and even interactions with entities such as relatives, ayahuasca itself and phantasmagoric creatures. Receiving explicit messages from spirits took place subjectively in some narratives but only one participant claimed to have received messages directly from 'mother ayahuasca'. Another received messages from a family member. Receiving direct messages seems not to be a frequent phenomenon, and it seems to be concentrated to some individual narratives so that it was a rather less common phenomenon during the ceremony. Among these few reports, the communication, which took place either in an explaining or teaching style, was a direct therapeutic order or suggestion, or was rather affectively supporting or calming.

Since further detailed inquiry was not allowed for the chosen interview method, it remains unclear to what extent participants really heard a hallucinated voice talking to them or if it rather was a dreamlike phantasy or a metaphoric expression for their own ideas that may have been interpreted as being sent by other entities. Schenberg et al. (2017) see psychotherapeutic potential in such directive messages from entities. The personal long-term impact of those teachings, their uncontrollable nature as well as the possible role of individual expectations and setting influences could be an object of future research.

Making sense of the perceived psychedelic content during an ayahuasca-ceremony is a common phenomenon too. This qualitative finding is in line with the 5D-ASC questionnaire. There, on average, insightfulness was the most dominant dimension of all meaning-making dimensions or less perceptual oriented dimensions. The data is scattered largely around the central tendency, which points towards great inter-individual differences as well as differences from one to another ceremony.

Only a minority reported that they could not understand the meaning of specific content.

The spontaneous recognition of content as symbolic was a rare phenomenon in the qualitative material. Symbolic understanding seems not automatically provided by the ayahuasca-ritual experience, or it is hard to verbalise it.

This may also reflect in the lower scale about change meaning of percepts in the 5D-ASC questionnaire.

Gaining insights through one's own intellectual reflexion during the ceremony was reported more often. This might depend strongly on the predominant cognitive style as part of the cognitive set. Some persons could recognize little sense in psychedelic items. To others, symbolic meaning was immediately evident without having to interpret it intellectually. Some interviewees reported to have gained personal insights through the already mentioned intensified thinking, which Shanon (2014, pp. 69-70) calls "mentation". I did not find this distinction in the previous literature; however, I consider it to be significant because of possible interindividual styles in experiencing ayahuasca inebriations and not least because of the high level of subjective persuasiveness that immediate symbolic understanding can have.

As seen in the retrospective interviews 6 weeks after the retreats, the meaning of the psychedelic content was subjectively evaluated as one of the most impressing phenomena.

The narratives show that a moderate number of participants were able to increase their self-awareness about personal ability, traits and difficulties. However, only one psychotherapeutically pre-experienced participant explicitly reported psychodynamic insights into origins of personal issues, and one other reported salutogenic insight into solving personal issues. It does not appear self-evident in our interviews that ethno-psychedelic ayahuasca-experiences lead to psychotherapeutic insights that would automatically become ingrained in an altered personal narrative about meaning and values in life. For some, it just remained to have been a fascinating or bizarre adventure with no evidence of further impact on self-actualisation, reframed self-view or new narrative about the Self. Although the reasons for its spontaneity in some cases over others is not fully understood, it may be a combination of reasons based on the heterogeneity of tourist participants: intention, cognitive style, personality, life-situation and psychotherapeutic preparedness. Ayahuasca tourism is usually not embedded in post-session or post-retreat care. Subjectively relevant insights occur but immediate symbolic understanding doesn't seem to happen automatically in rather untrained individuals. Individuals who do not experience the immediate emotional and cognitive meaning-evidencing of their inner images and visions may benefit particularly from a post-process questioning in the sense of meaning-making and creating personal relevance during the integration phase.

The particularly used expressions and metaphors can indicate which of the possible explanatory paradigms is dominant in the current state of the interviewee.

The most common one, most often believed by traditional as well as modern ayahuasca drinkers, is a recourse to the paranormal (Shanon, 2014, p. 61), the (neo-)shamanic explanatory model. It claims that an existing, enigmatic 'spiritual world' could be entered or visited through these visions from which 'mother ayahuasca' gives individual teachings or other fantastic beings can be seen and sometimes influence the visitor (e.g. perform healing or harm). Other paradigms operate with psychoanalytic or neurobiological figures. Also, mixed models appear, e.g. in which teaching entities from the spiritual world would reveal psychodynamic insights and perform confrontative trauma healing or models, which claim that ayahuasca would turn the human brain temporarily into a receiver of messages from other paranormal realms. When presenting the results of the part III investigation, I will discuss the different subjective healing-models found in the post-interviews.

The informant, Dr. Eduardo Gastelumendi Dargent (psychoanalyst, professor of the Institute of the Peruvian Society of Psychoanalysis, professor invited in courses in the Pontifical Catholic University of Peru, the National University of San Marcos and the University Antonio Ruiz de Montoya, former president of the Peruvian Association of Psychiatry, member of the Directive Committee of the Psychoanalytic Federation of Latin America), explained in a personal meeting that the psychodynamic explanatory-models reject the traditional shamanic understanding of the visions as an access into a different reality, existing outside of the person's mind, but point to the dreamlike character of the experiences which follows a primary process way. Herewith the qualitative experience is understood as a symbolic energetic drama of desires and fears from the 'Es' as well as an expression of potentials, solutions and the development of propulsions. As postulated by Freud, the symbolisation process of unconscious content in the dreamy state would serve to maintain sleep while at the same time prohibited (sexual) desires would get fulfilled (Freud, 1990, pp. 470). Obviously, the last cannot apply here as main reason for the symbolisation process in visionary ayahuasca-experiences, since at the time of the dreamlike visions the person is already more than awake. C. G. Jung emphasises contrary to Freud the compensatory function of the dream, which would be oriented in the actual life of the dreamer (Jung, 1990, p. 103). The dream is seen as 'a spontaneous self-presentation of the present state of the unconscious in symbolic expression' (ibid., p. 115, translated from German). From a modern perspective of psychoanalysis Gastelumendi Dargent (personal communication, June 19, 2017) gave the following insights:

> 'According to the contemporary perspective the impulses do not only seek their discharge (Freudian perspective) but their development, and in order to achieve this they need to unite with thoughts, to link with them intra-psychically and also with other people. The drives seek to develop in contact with the thoughts.
> The visions during the ayahuasca experience are expressions of the same drives, expressed in physical sensations, emotions, thoughts, visions.
> Some visions are ecstatic, because they connect us with life around, and with the cosmos of which we are part. Much consciousness and feelings for a human being: One enters into panic, or into ecstasy.
> But it also helps us on a more personal, individual level, to walk the path we have made in the bonds with ourselves (our dreams, our potential) and with other people.
> And there, like in a dream, we can remember, reflect, see what we did not see, sustain the pain caused by the mourning of failure, of not having understood. But at the same time, it opens us to the possibility of getting closer to our potential development that our dreams also suggest.'

Here, I present a typical example of recognised symbolic content and subjective sense.

> 'And then the medicine told me, already showed me like there are different energy strings. And one is unconditioned mother love, then next to this, there is expectation and then, next to this, is the own needs, ...' (1: 36-39)

Interviewee no. 1 was thematically concerned with her relationship with her mother, her difficulties in taking love from her and its impact on her present life and her doubts about becoming a good mother herself. From this set-context, she visualised different 'strings.' The psychodynamic symbolism was immediately clear to her. She did not ascribe the deciphering or symbolic meaning to her own realisation but to the teaching or revelation that was given to her by the plant spirit of ayahuasca.

> 'And then suddenly it adorns to me, this is just a symbol for my inner child.' (1: 63-64)

In the same ceremony, the interviewee perceived a scenic vision how she was holding her old dying cat on her lap. First, she felt desperation and panic, but then she realized how childlike and disproportionate these feelings were, being an adult. At this point, it became clear to her that the visualised cat had a symbolic meaning; it represented her feeling of loneliness and desperate search for someone to hold on to. She had understood that it would be impossible to feed and saturate herself with the affective mother-love that she had rejected:

> 'And of course, the medicine was just pointing out: 'this is the place.' You have to connect here, don't connect with the cat. This is just a substitute. It's not really what it is about; don't connect with your husband. Your inner child has to connect with your mum and from this space you get the nourishment that you need, and then you can handle the cat that is dying or whatever. This is a special kind of nourishment; it can only come from there.' (1: 71-80)

In this example the scenic visual content of the dying cat was connected with strong dysphoric feelings. It was understood as a psychodynamic symbol. The insights were attributed to the shamanic model, which proposes a wise ayahuasca spirit that would teach during ingestion.

Since the generation and immediate understanding of symbolic material as meaningful (Belser et al., 2017, p. 372) as well as the later meaning-making (ibid, p. 355) is central in modern psychedelic supported therapy, the categorization of the meaning of psychedelic content in western ayahuasca drinkers is of particular interest: intrapersonal psychological meaning, relationship and biographical topics, other persons' issues, general wisdom and mystic content. These categories, except "other people's issues", seem to relate to the health-related personal values and introspective processes previously mentioned in the literature (Franquesa et al., 2018).

The spontaneous appearance of relationship issues in a scarce majority of participants in this study is in line with previous ayahuasca-reports from Shanon (2003); it was also observed in psychedelic experiences with other substances (Belser et al., 2017).

Social representations, relational conflicts, conflicts of the biographical past and preconscious intrapersonal conflicts are most relevant in modern forms of psychodynamic psychotherapy and counselling. At some point, most therapies try to give the social past relevance for the for the present or have to deal with the regulation of actual or past social relationships. Regarding this, a possible psychotherapeutic benefit of ayahuasca, not least, reflects in the appearance of re-actualized representations of more or less conflicting personal social relationships in the narratives that may indicate a re-actualization and occupation with those topics during the ceremony, according to the common factors of psychotherapy in Grawe (1995). The actualization of conflicting material may also appear in the later discussed emotional variety under ayahuasca.

Insights or solutions into other people's issues were rare among the nine participants. Either, the phenomenon is culturally exaggerated in local healing traditions or it is a highly cultural dependent phenomenon that might be only relevant for native or local protagonists. It is also possible that it may require special personality or extensive experience with such plants, which tourists mostly do not have, as the local perspective of vegetalism would suggest.

A minority reported to have spontaneously processed general topics like, ethical standards, society, life, environmental considerations, generalised healing of mankind and nature that go beyond the just personal issues.

This is astonishing on the one hand, as it is repeatedly and anegdotically reported that ayahuasca would increase ecological consciousness by re-establishing a personal and intensive connection of fraternity with man and with nature. Other findings about the lifetime use of psychedelics point in this direction (Nour at al., 2016). On the other hand, from the perspective of the so-called transpersonal psychology about experiences with mind-altering techniques of the alternative humanistic psychotherapy, it is known that the personal and social realm with its multiple biographical conflicts is often pre-empted before generalized, transpersonal and mystical themes are spontaneously processed. Following this view, it would be to assume that multiple intake in a corresponding therapeutic long-term process could provoke the advertised change in environmental consciousness after the personal and relationship-issues have been processed. Shanon (2003, p. 432) found that personal biographical items would appear less in ayahuasca trips of experienced drinkers, both indigenous or non-indogenous. However, it is possible that psychedelic experiences subjectively confirm tendencies of spiritual ecologic attitudes that might have been previously only present in some individuals, rather than generating them in others.

A scarce majority had mystical experiences of the type that is often reported from higher dosed psychedelic experiences such as being emotionally connected to everything, feeling oneness and a general empathy, understanding metaphysical questions and paradoxes in a state of sudden clarity as well as experiencing confirmation and renewed faith in the existence of a spiritual world beyond the mundaneness of existence. Note, that unlike the definition of mysticism by Walter Terence Stace (1960), which counts only non-sensual and non-intellectual experiences as such, this investigation treats mystical experiences as a collective category for the above-mentioned phenomena. Thus, the study suggests that ayahuasca rituals may have some of the described health related potentials, which are indicated in the previous chapter about mental health, although the conditions of the individual affinity and the inter-individual predictability of mystical experiences under ayahuasca remain unclear. The possible connection between those types of experiences and outcome data should be statistically investigated.

As indicated before, the narratives showed that some participants acted within the so-called visions. Acting inside the visions was related either to the attempt to communicate with ayahuasca as a person, or other subjectively perceived entities, or to the attempt of direct manipulation inside the perceived visionary contends.

Communication with spirits as well as direct manipulations inside the visions were rare phenomena in the narratives about this first ceremony, but it was mentioned.

Direct reactions outside the visions were reported commonly and more frequently. Typical actions were repeating words in a self-monologue, relaxation behaviour, resisting physical distress, arbitrary movements and paying attention to others.

Cognitive reactions were frequent. Doubts and worrying thoughts were moderately common followed by controlling and rejecting content and by getting absorbed. Intensified thoughts or boosted flow of ideas were less common.

Participants reported the spontaneous emotional release, as well as corrective emotional experiences. The high frequency of spontaneous mention of emotional responses in ayahuasca reports points towards a high ly subjective priority of emotions during and shortly after ingestion.

Typical pleasant "target emotions" in this sample were love and connection, calmness and relaxation, secured and nourished, accepting and emotional open, self-confident and proud, forgiveness, gratefulness, blessed and happy.

Typical unpleasant emotions of the narratives were anxious and scared, nervous, loss of control or loss of orientation, helpless and sad.

Typical hedonistic emotions were amazement and enjoyment. Sexual content was not mentioned at all, which may be a result of the setting and set that tabooed sexuality from the therapeutic work.

A majority reported the appearance of pleasant as well as unpleasant emotions. Both seem to be a common part of the ayahuasca experiences. Having "no emotional response" can be interpreted as a defence mechanism in psychoanalytic terminology. Conversely, it could be a sign of having overcome a conflict, emotional exhaustion or of overload inhibition. Subjectively successful ayahuasca-processes appear to be characterised by the presence of unpleasant emotions (as a possible expression of the activation of relevant conflictual material and the inner struggle with it) as well as desirable emotions with possible 'salutatory impact' (Shanon, 2014, p. 64) (as a possible expression of subjective resolution). Hedonistic feelings seem less dominant in those processes as well as emotional blockages or the absence of emotional response to emotionally relevant material. It is worth exploring more deeply the relation of pleasant and unpleasant emotions within the same session as a possible indicator for therapeutically successful ayahuasca processes, possibly described as the before-mentioned "sudden transformation of the experience" by Kjellgren et al. (2009).

It is worth to explore the relation of pleasant and unpleasant emotions within the same session as possible indicator for therapeutically successful ayahuasca processes.

Slightly more than half of the participants mentioned cognitive phenomena such as doubts, worries and sceptical thoughts as well as attempts to control, push aside, reject or endure content. Only a minority reported cognitive phenomena like getting absorbed, agreeing, surrendering to the present moment of the experience or boosted flow of ideas and intensified thinking or inordinate and chaotic thought processes.

Some participants mentioned that the ayahuasca-experience would have a process character of different phases and would be a flow of change from moment to moment. Remembering this during the experience helped some of them through difficult parts of the experience. A minority reported explicit difficulties like the lack of control or the intensity and speed of the experiences.

The singing of the shaman was reported to have affected the visual experience, body reactions (like vomiting), the impression of getting absorbed into the experience as well as mood and energy changes. Likely, that due to the neurochemical stimulation, synesthetic experiences increase.

As mentioned earlier, the role of the shamanic singing is traditionally one of the most important parts of most South-American ayahuasca ceremonies in mestizo-curanderism. In the belief system of South-American curanderos, their singing connects them with the plant spirits. They can invite spirits to the ceremony for help, to protect from bad energies, lower the intensity of the visions or enhance them or induce or lower nausea and the need to vomit.

The state of heightened synesthetic perception seems to allow the shaman to influence the experiences of his clients almost directly through his songs and produced rattling sounds. It is likely that the repeatedly reported and ethnologically described "abilities" of Amazonian shamans to influence the psychedelic experiences through their songs presumably works via the neurochemical stimulation of synesthetic mechanisms, due to pharmaceutical properties of ayahuasca. The data collected with the 5D-ASC questionnaire during ayahuasca retreats supports this. Audio-visual synaesthesia has been one of the most dominant phenomena, along with complex imagery. But, as for most dimensions, the data scatter largely. A majority appreciated spontaneously the experience.

The subjective experience of ayahuasca in the semi-traditional, ethno-touristic setting has great complexity. The inter-individual differences in the phenomena are great as well as the intra-individual differences from one ceremony to another. Vomiting, imagery, meaning and emotional expression seem to be the most common main elements. The phenomenology of experiences of different subgroups and cultures could be systematically investigated by purposeful case selection and by other methods, using greater samples. In general, analysing the possible relation between some of the subjective phenomena of the ayahuasca ingestion and therapeutic outcomes could be helpful in improving ayahuasca supported psychotherapy. (Parts of this chapeter have been published previously under Creative Commons Attribution NonCommercial 4.0 International Licence Wolff et al., 2018)

17.3 Hypothetic psychological working model during flooding and plateau phase

How are elements of ayahuasca experiences, found in the narratives, possibly related to each other?

Individuals react in different ways to the psychedelic changes in the perception of the ayahuasca-specific altered state: physically, perceptually, cognitively, emotionally and behaviourally, in terms of attraction or rejection, in terms of intensity and the duration of attention, etc. The changes in perceptions stimulate or trigger reactions. This seems to depend largely on inner set and outer setting. Interestingly, at the same time these reactions can serve again as stimuli for the perceptual content, especially when much attention is put on those reactions. If a person concentrates on physical reactions of malaise, this might exaggerate those physical symptoms. That generates even more attention. In this way, pleasant as well as unpleasant experiences seem to develop in a circle or spiral form through a resonating cascade effect during the highly suggestive and synesthetic state of the ayahuasca inebriation. Thus, useful psychotherapeutic cathartic reactions and emotional "breakthroughs" that are related to more or less conflictive personal as well as transpersonal material are stimulated. Such processes are often heated up or moderated through external stimuli (like the actions of the healer, his singing, sounds, fragrances, the setting, the group). External behavioural reactions of the experiencing person (like arbitrary movements, relaxation behaviour , self-monologue, paying attention to others, etc.), internal reactions (like communicating with perceived entities and direct manipulations inside the visions as well as cognitive reactions like controlling, resisting or worrying thoughts or surrendering) and the perception of physical sensations can have a self-suggestive and self-hypnotic effect on the specific content material of the trip. They trigger or heat up the described resonating processes and thus become suggestive stimuli and push forward the psychedelic process. The 'heightened powers of suggestibility' (Grob, 1994) under the influence of hallucinogens might serve in the first place as a process of self-suggestion.

The graphic below is illustrated with some quotes from such a psychedelic cascade effect from participant 5. The quotes are taken from a subjectively rewarding experience, spiritually and emotionally. He summarised: 'The universe has been, ... It is not a place to be scared of. It's just a place to be.' (5: 25) and 'I really felt grateful throughout the whole thing, for everything whatever. And all that realisations I had regarding the receiving and not trying to control but just let it happen.' (5: 30).

In summary, internal and external reactions of the individual to the perceived psychedelic contents become suggestive, associative or hypnotic stimuli for changes of the psychedelic contents.

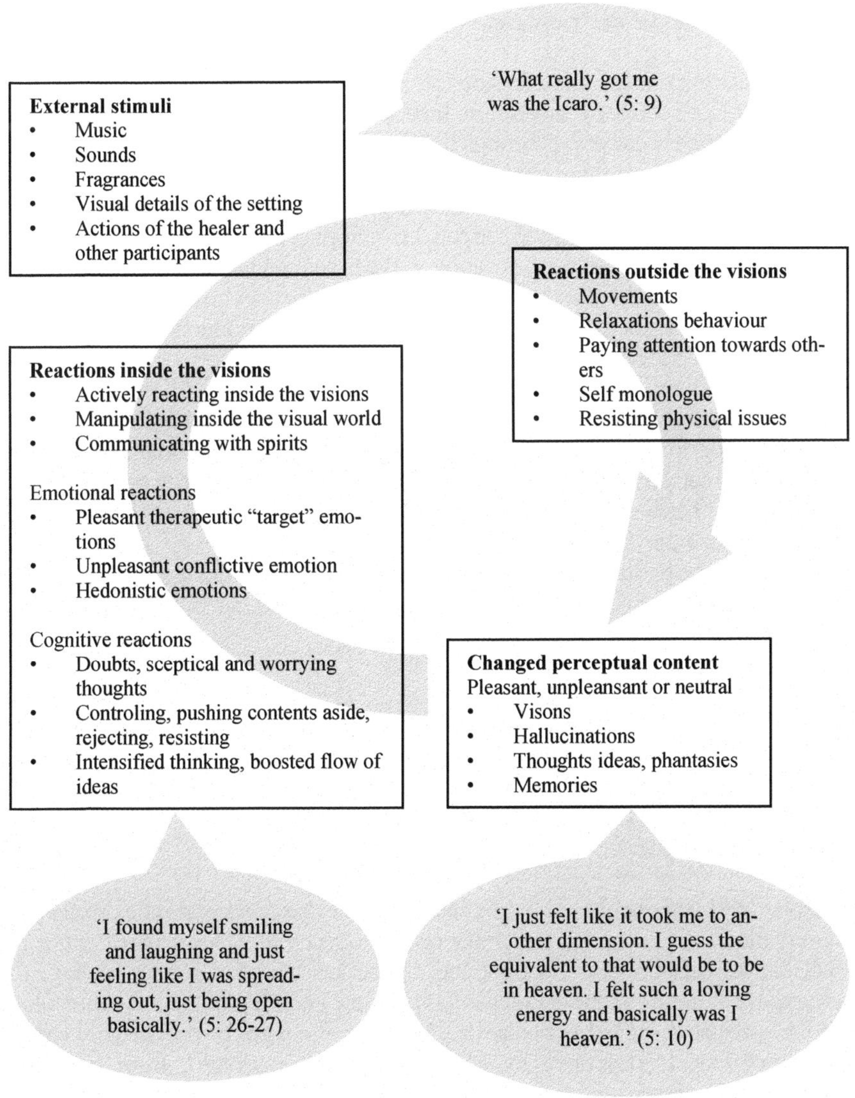

Hypothetic psychological working model during flooding and plateau phase

External stimuli
- Music
- Sounds
- Fragrances
- Visual details of the setting
- Actions of the healer and other participants

'What really got me was the Icaro.' (5: 9)

Reactions outside the visions
- Movements
- Relaxations behaviour
- Paying attention towards others
- Self monologue
- Resisting physical issues

Reactions inside the visions
- Actively reacting inside the visions
- Manipulating inside the visual world
- Communicating with spirits

Emotional reactions
- Pleasant therapeutic "target" emotions
- Unpleasant conflictive emotion
- Hedonistic emotions

Cognitive reactions
- Doubts, sceptical and worrying thoughts
- Controling, pushing contents aside, rejecting, resisting
- Intensified thinking, boosted flow of ideas

Changed perceptual content
Pleasant, unpleasant or neutral
- Visons
- Hallucinations
- Thoughts ideas, phantasies
- Memories

'I found myself smiling and laughing and just feeling like I was spreading out, just being open basically.' (5: 26-27)

'I just felt like it took me to another dimension. I guess the equivalent to that would be to be in heaven. I felt such a loving energy and basically was I heaven.' (5: 10)

Figure 13: Schematic presentation of an amplification circle between subjective psychedelic perceptions and reactions (modulated by external, therapeutic and other stimuli)

17.4 Process model of ayahuasca-tourism experiences

Ayahuasca-tourism can be understood as a modern form of pilgrimage. In addition to curiosity and thirst for adventure, here too it is about self-discovery and self-updating, which is conveyed through the intense self-experience in a non-everyday situation in a non-everyday place. The characteristic of the pilgrimage is often the difficulty. It is important to master a challenge, to pass a personal test, to overcome a bottleneck. In the classical Western Christian pilgrimages, such as to Santiago de Compostela in Spain, this is usually in the arduous hike. The Peruvian healer, Santiago Enrrique Paredes Melendez, mentioned that 'you have to suffer sufficiently for the spirits to have pity on you.' I'll explain the function of tension and suffering within the individual ayahuasca tourism process later.

The motivation of ayahuasca tourists can consist of a (more or less religiously/spiritually coloured) hope for personal change, for clarification and prioritization of desires, for biographical meaning making, for emotional expression as well as for metaphysical confirmation. Sometimes, a desire of liberating healer-qualities or of being recognized and confirmed as a healer by the spirits of the Amazon plants plays a role.

I suggest dividing the process, which ayahuasca-tourists go through, into 3 main phases:

- Attitude and motivation forming phase
- Ingestion:
    - B1. Turning inwards
    - B2. Flooding phase
    - B3. Plateau, peak points and release
    - B4. Reflection and attenuation phase
- Integration phase.

I explain these phases based on the interviews of this investigation as well as the observations of ritual structures at the centres Garden of Peace near Tarapoto and Sanctuario Huishtín near Pucallpa and Ayahuasca Foundation near Iquitos. The interviews at the Ayahuasca Foundation (Iquitos, Peru) about the phenomenology of the ayahuasca ingestion contain elements of all stages of psychedelic experiences, previously described by Masters & Houston (1966), from perceptual changes up to mystical experiences. Unfortunately, the narratives of the subjective phenomenology of the ingestion experience revealed little evidence of temporal sequences of the reported phenomena, so that I can contribute from there only the "building blocks" of the phenomenological picture but not the phase-typical sequence of depth stages regarding ayahuasca. Therefore, further research explicitly about temporal sequences is desirable.

17.4.1 Attitude and motivation forming phase

The attitude and motivation forming phase begins long before the trip. It contains elements that determine the inner mental set: to hear the first time from ayahuasca, the first spontaneous reactions to it, the emerging interest that motivates further information search. When searching for information, the Internet often plays the most important role, in addition to first-hand reports from friends and acquaintances, films and media reports. Often, from the first information to the booking of an ayahuasca trip, less than a year passes, but sometimes the interest can continue to simmer for many years, until someone seizes a concrete opportunity for ayahuasca consumption or actively seeks for it.

Although there is often an interest in an authentic-native experience in the Amazon, the interest in and the knowledge about the actual living conditions and native or mestizo culture is usually quite limited. Anthropological literature on traditional ayahuasca therapy is usually not used in advance. The motivation to acquire knowledge is limited in many cases to trip reports and safety information for ayahuasca consumption, such as the fasting rules established by ayahuasca centres.

In the ayahuasca scene, it is often said that persons would "follow the call from mother Ayahuasca". This already shows an important element of the set: the personification of ayahuasca as a plant spirit. In the further course, it might shape the psychedelic experience as an expectation and interpretation bias. Often, there are recommendations from friends in Internet forums as well as from websites of the healing centres. They recommend a positive, open attitude towards the coming ayahuasca ingestion and are invited to establish an imagined positive relationship with the plant prior the ingestion. Sometimes, they recommend articulating therapy goals and personal questions to be answered by the Ayahuasca entity during ceremony.

Some have doubts about the model of healing plant spirits but are curious to test the model through personal first-hand experience. This probably leads to a certain focus of attention, which later might facilitate the corresponding psychedelic experiences or at least a willingness to allow such experiences or to interpret psychedelic content towards the expectation. Accordingly, it would be interesting to compare ayahuasca experiences from the typical traditionalized jungle setting with those made in a secularized psychotherapy setting. Or conversely, to test other psychedelic substances in the shamanic jungle setting for the appearance of spirits and their teachings.

As already mentioned, there are fasting rules in most healing centres that should be followed in advance of the ayahuasca intake. This usually includes the renunciation of drugs, sex and alcohol, as well as pork a few days before the start of the retreat. Such pre-diets vary in severity and length, depending on the centre.

The sense and nonsense of these pre-diets are sometimes the subject of discussions in Internet forums. In some therapy centres, it is common to perform a cleansing treatment at the beginning of the retreat. For this, tobacco juice, big amounts of water, or other plants or substances are used to cause heavy vomiting and possibly diarrhoea. More recently the use of kambo is observed, which also causes vomiting (skin secretions of the giant leaf frog (Phyllomedusa bicolor), that is applied in superficial minor burns).

Often, on the day of the ayahuasca ceremony, food is completely omitted or greatly reduced.

Perhaps there is a psycho-psychotherapeutic point in the more or less burdensome renunciation of dietary and behavioural habits. Raising the personal costs, it might increase the attribution of importance to the desired ayahuasca experience. To gain access to the desired "real deal" of wisdom and magic, the element of effort may also contribute to the attraction to some western tourists, because it transforms the ayahuasca trip from a purely exotic touristic adventure to a pilgrimage. Also, the initial traditional purging treatment of vomiting from tobacco juice or other substances may have a psychological effect besides any other possible medical purpose. Because it is physically so noticeable, it marks drastically the entry into an extraordinary realm and separates the coming time of the retreat as different from the everyday or worldly realm before. Physical entrance rituals are well known practise of monasteries, sects, armies, and other institutions, such as shaving the hair, undergoing demanding physical entrance tests or tests of courage, putting on uniforms. Often, attendees prepare for their nocturnal ayahuasca ceremonies by putting on special clothing and bringing items of personal symbolic importance to the ceremony.

17.4.2 Ingesting phase

17.4.2.1 Turning inwards

After every participant has found a place in the maloka (rotunda) and the curandero has entered the scene, they are called one by one to the front to drink a cup filled with ayahuasca. The cup is blown with tobacco smoke and handed over to the person. After drinking, one returns to the personal place and the next one is called to appear in front of the curandero. This initial scene reminds me of the Holy Mass. This association seemed even stronger since the wooden cup in which the ayahuasca was served had the form of a chalice in both centres.

In the tradition of Santiago Enrrique Paredes Melendez and Hegner Paredes Melendez, everybody waits in silence and complete darkness until the effects start. In this period, various thoughts or phantasies may cross the minds. Participants might meditate or doze until the first visual effect in the darkness sets in. Then the curandero begins with his songs. During the wait, the far-reaching omission of external perceptual stimuli necessarily leads to an intensified turning inwards towards the mental and imaginative inner world insofar as the ego structure and motivation of the participant allow this.

17.4.2.2 Flooding phase

After the first visual effects set in, the attention is often quickly captivated by colours and patterns. Those can be abstract, geometric patterns, or they can be more representational, scenic or a mixture of them. Often, abstract visual effects or representational images tend to dominate and later, scenic visions. However, there are significant differences between individuals and also between different intakes of the same individual. Sometimes there are no visions at all. In most cases, participants can distinguish between ordinary reality and additional visions. A misjudgement of this difference, which would be typical for real hallucinations, is less common. Some people also describe the visual effects as vivid imaginations, as if they would be seen with the eyes. They also could be described as "waking dreams" or "second screen sight". Sometimes, participants experience visceral or haptic effects and by this some are convinced to have been touched by spirits or at least suppose so. Bright-coloured visions can stand out impressively well from the dark background, but they also can be blurry and pale. Sometimes, participants have no visual effects at all, but they might have them in later ceremonies, or they once had them but lost them. Open-eye visions may occur, when the visual content remains independently from closing or opening the eyes.

Expert informants within the ayahuasca scene occasionally claim that different varieties of the ayahuasca vine would produce different colours and vice versa the perceived colours of the visionary content would indicate which variety was used in the brew. Brilliant and colourful parts of visions are sometimes attributed to the chacruna plant, which provides the DMT to the brew. Local long-term users, who believe in the shamanic world-view, sometimes report that the ayahuasca spirit would be able to hold back vivid colourful visions, if irritations in the relationship to the drinker would give reason to do so That is why they sometimes pray for vivid and meaningful visions, or those prayers are part of the ícaro sung by the curandero (personal message from the visionary artist Mauro Reategui Perez, July 28, 2018 Huishtín centre).

The flooding phase is often accompanied by self-perception of various physiological symptoms. This can be vomiting and feeling sick, dizziness, trembling, feeling cold or hot, sweating, feeling sick, stomach pain, twitching, involuntary movements and others. The variety and intensity of symptoms is great. Sometimes vomiting occurs early, but more often at the end of the flooding phase. However, it is also possible that it happens late in the phase or not at all. During the flooding phase, synesthetic perceptions occur. They can appear as changes of the perceived psychedelic visions that are subjectively caused by sounds, especially the singing of the curandero during ceremony. Often, these changes are attributed towards the shamanic power of the curandero and are subjectively taken as prove of his ability to act or manipulate within the "spiritual world" of ayahuasca.

17.4.2.3 Plateau, peak points and release

Plateau phase is usually reached when the intensity of the psychedelic changes does not increase further. It can be dominated by the changing visual effects of patterns, complex worlds and landscapes, architectures, scenes or people, animals or strange others. The drinker can find himself in the role of an observer of this realm, or he can get the impression of interacting or even communicating. Some participants find themselves entirely disconnected from reality and their physical body, some report to have been placed into another realm or to communicate with other entities. Such experiences are less common than observing visualized scenes. The process or parts of it can also be dominated by an intensified flow of thoughts and can be accompanied by more or less emotional release. Protagonists may believe that thoughts, activated memories and emotional release would be part of salutary purging in line with the vomiting. The intensified thought process, often inspired by visual content, can lead to subjectively significant insights ideas, new convictions or confirmations about different topics. Regarding their own person, the process creates vivid memories of formative key experiences, personal insights about the determinacy of their personality in the past as well as about own abilities, failures, preferences, desires and possible decisions for the future. It can be about the relations and interactions with others, social behaviors, possible conflicts and solutions, family members, partners, children, friends, etc. It can be about the understanding of other people's reasons to act or about solutions for work. It can be about ethical topics, about mankind, the relation between generations, nature, life, ecology, life, death, universe, existence, or paradoxes. The topics are diverse and might depend on personality habits e.g., the affinity to associate in certain directions, the richness of phantasy, inner cognitive and emotional life, inclination to mental argument and ability of wording, etc. Further influences seem to be: interests and convictions, actual psycho-emotional state and life situation. Peak points can occur during the plateau phase when insights or psychedelic experiences release emotions. At times, perceptions can be chaotic, overwhelming, shattering or sickening. Visions are volatile and can sometimes become very fast. Or, certain irritating details attract attention, which can sometimes lead to a turnover of the situation and emotional colouring or create unpleasant or even frightening landscapes. When the shaman, Hegner Paredes Melendez, is asked which attitude is best for being in an ayahuasca ceremony, he usually responds: ¡Concentra te! (Spanish: concentrate!).

To give an example of how it might feel to be in the state of the "visionary ayahuasca world," a painting from José Luis Amaringo can serve as starting point. The picture shows the excerpt of a complex ayahuasca vision.

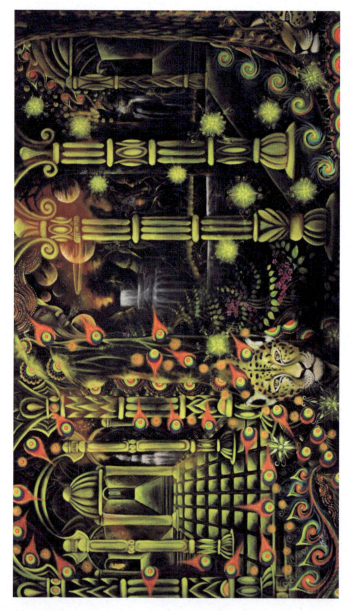

Figure 14: 'El Supay – Temple', oil on canvas (copyright permission granted by © José Luis Vasques Gonzales)

Looking at the painting, abstract, figurative and scenic elements can be recognized. The glowing dots with orange tails on the left side, the "DMT firework", would be expressions of the spirit of the chacruna plant, according to the informant, Mauro Reategui Perez, who is an internationally recognised visionary artist, ayahuasquero and former student of Pablo Amaringo (*1938–+2009) (personal message, July 28, 2018 Huishtín centre, Honoria; confirmed by José Luis Vasques Gonzales, grandson of Pablo Amaringo, Nov 4, 2018 in Pucallpa).

From the viewpoint of a participant under ayahuasca, there would be different opportunities to continue if such a vision emerges. Every detail could alter and open up a new complex scene while interacting with my reactions to it. The process of emerging and changing visions seems to be influenced by the amount of attention which is given to certain details or which may arrise unpurposefully. E.g., I could follow the illuminated way into the temple on the left side and be surprised by what would come behind that door, or I could start thinking about the meaning of this seemingly infinite way of life and maybe discover some insights about the paradox of existence itself, while getting the impression that the tiger is closely watching me. Or, I could explore the darker path on the right side and by that discover the blurry image next to the stairway of – may be – a father and his son. And yes, aren't my remembrances of the few good times with my own father as blurred as this vision? Could this be me, who rejected this troubled relationship for so many years and who also forgot the love and inspiring connection we had? And, by seeing this, I also suddenly see the beautiful colored patterns coming out of my father's mind that made the frightening darkness of the night beautiful when I was a child and couldn't fall asleep. I might remember long forgotten scenes in which he told me fantastic bedtime stories. They made me forget my fear of the night. I may realize that this is my way, not the shiny but empty one on the left side. This was the lesson. I could take this gift from my father and continue that way. I could be the father myself, who shows the fantastic world to his son and by that prepares his way. And, while I have these revelations, the tiger is closely watching....

By having a closer look at the details on the right side, the image of father and son may dissolve into other items that seem meaningful; like faces, inducing or mirroring other faces, smoke and waterfalls, which may evoke other associations and revelations, mysteriously connected to the "teaching" about father and son....

Ayahuasqueros, their clients but also western participants believe that ayahuasca would teach by presenting those picture-images and by giving answers to troubling questions. Ayahuasca and other spirits would be present within those visions. Snakes, hummingbirds, tigers, eyes, fantastic beings would be manifestations of these spirits. The mestizo culture of ayahuasca is full of iconigraphic meaning of elements of visions.

Meaning can be immediately and convincingly clear to the drinker, or it can be interpreted from the symbolic load with more or less personal cogency. As mentioned before, even personal reactions to visions, such as thoughts, questions, emotions and associations can cause (sometimes dramatic) changes in the flow of visions. Also, external stimuli often have influence, like animal sounds, changes in the singing of the curandero, silence between the songs, one's own body reactions and flashlights and sounds from others.

To some participants, it does not make sense at all, and they "just enjoy the show" or are amazed, surprised, scared or tormented until it fades out or until vomiting brings relief.

Vomiting can be a release and turning point. For some participants, the visual psychedelic "firework" calms down after vomiting, and the experience turns to be more reflective, contemplative.

The discharge function of vomiting does not always refer only to the pure physical poisoning symptoms. The unpleasant physical condition can be associated with stressful psychological experiences, which sometimes go along with it. Physical suffering might help to activate relevant, problematic psychological topics in some cases. Probably, that is a phenomenon similar to synaesthesia, and it would be interesting to find out more about it in imaging research, if technically possible. It is likely that different regions of the brain get activated at the same time under ayahuasca, which are normally less connected. Neuropharmacological research about ayahuasca has found unusual activity in visual fields, which are normally not activated when the eyes are closed. This explains the vivid visions under ayahuasca (de Araujo et al., 2012). The associated experience on the psychedelic side before and during vomiting can be an expression of psychic conflicts, e.g., guilt conflicts, shame conflicts, etc., or the increasing sickness can occur along with burdensome biographical memories such as traumatic scenes, or scenes from current relationship conflicts, etc. but also along with more or less symbolic images and "dark visions". The psychic experience can rock along in feedback with the unpleasant physical experience until it comes to heavy relief vomiting. Not in vain is ayahuasca also called la purga (Spanish: the purge) in South America (Beyer, 2009, p. 209 and pp. 213-214; Labate & Pacheco, 2011; Shanon, 2014, pp. 62-63) Not seldomly, the vomiting is subjectively woven into the visions, e.g., when the bucket would turn into a big blossom, a tube or other items or creatures that receive all the suffering which had accumulated over all the year or when the demons of the past are literally puked out, almost in an act of personal exorcism.

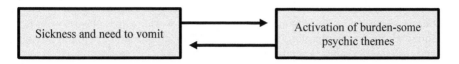

Figure 15: Schematic presentation of the interaction and feedback between physical sickness and the activation of psychological themes

Sometimes vomiting can be triggered by other external stimuli too, e.g., a change in the singing of the curandero, sudden silence or other stimuli, like the smoke of tobacco, or a change in position. Some ayahuasca drinkers and therapists believe that the vomiting itself would be caused by the psycho-spiritual problems like conflicts or traumatic burdens from the past. Other forms of emotional release are crying and laughing.

I have observed ceremonies in which ayahuasca was drunk between one and three times during a ceremony. Sometimes, in more structured ceremonies, another cup is offered to each participant one by one, but in others, more experienced participants can just go in front and ask for another one if needed.

17.4.2.4 Reflection and attenuation phase

In the last part of a ceremony, or even after the official part has ended, the visions are often less, if any at all. They can rather turn into intensified imagination, memories and contemplative thought. Attentive observation of the contents of consciousness can alternate with more unconscious phases of occupied thinking and ideaing as well as sleep and dream. The experience usually shifts towards a thoughtful, associative state of self-reflection or it is simply enjoyed the music. If the ceremony has yet ended, an exchange with others may take place. Good processes can lead to feelings of gratitude, calm and relaxation. Some participants can also go through prolonged processes or disappointment can be felt, if expectations were not met.

17.4.3 Integration phase

The phase of integration begins with the first sharing of experiences, sometimes in the same night after ceremony. Here first narratives are created by verbalisation. During verbalising, some details and single episodes are emphasized and may be defined as significant, others are forgotten. Journaling may support the process of verbalisation and meaning making. Participants may be impressed by the subjectively helpful personal answers, which they may have gained from their ayahuasca experiences, the encounter with a spiritual world, which may serve as personal spiritual confirmation, the recovery of biographic memories, the strength and realism of visions and others.

Different ayahuasca centres advise their clients to maintain a period of reduced post diet. For some participants, this time after the retreat can be marked by difficulties on the one hand and active integration efforts on the other hand. Sometimes, especially after longer and stricter retreats in the nature, the adaptation to the loud, colourful and fast worldliness can be problematic. Some participants experience a personal crisis after such a retreat. Latent inner conflicts can be activated by this, related to anxiety, depression and panic disorders. That is not the rule, but it does happen. Sometimes the gained insights lead participants to make changes in their life, their relationships, their jobs, etc. But without the necessary support, it can also lead to relapses in old behaviour that may bring feelings of guilt, self-criticism and shame. In the ayahuasca tourism encountered in this study, the majority of participants seemed not at all to be prepared in terms of previously organised therapeutic care for the time after the retreat. Nevertheless, active integration effort takes place in different levels extent: Some participants try to apply their insight into daily life and try to life in a more conscious way. They try to improve their relationships and solve conflicts. Some take an extended off time before re-entering their previous every-day life. The integration phase is the most neglected part in ayahuasca health tourism.

These phases should not be understood as a rigid classification but rather as orientation, because individual variations are possible.

17.5 Summary and conclusions about demographics

As shown in the table below, the median age of all persons studied is between 30 and 38 years, with a high interquartile range of 12 years. The hypothesis already developed in the individual investigations that ayahuasca tourism might not be a youth fashion, (such as the MDMA-techno-dance subculture of the 90s and others) gets weight. Although the samples come from different ayahuasca centres and the Internet, the three numbers are quite similar.

The number of male individuals was higher in the ayahuasca centres and a bit lower in the Internet sample.

The higher level of education has been confirmed in all three samples. Previous experiences with counselling or psychotherapy had been reported by 45,1%. There was a also a great variety of alternative therapies and psycho-spiritual techniques. The number of participants of ayahuasca retreats currently psychotherapy was rather low. Pre-experience with other drugs was higher than 50% in all three samples. And pre-experience with ayahuasca fluctuated between 22,2 and 72,5% (total 59,8%).

A typical protagonist of the two centres as well as the participating members of ayahuasca Internet groups would be approximately 34 years old (or between 22 and 46), Caucasian, English speaking, well educated, would have some experiences in other drugs such as Cannabis, MDMA, psilocybin or others and would possibly have experience in other psycho-spiritual offers.

Table 5: Comparison of demographic data of the three samples

	Internet* N=40	Iquitos - Ayahuasca Foundation** N=9	Tarapoto - Garden of Peace*** N=36	Total N=85
Age				
Median	38	33	30	34
IQR	13	25,5	6	12
Range	22 – 67	27 – 71	19 – 46	19 – 71
Gender				
Male	42,1%	66,6%	61%	59.8
Female	57,9%	33,3%	39%	40.2
Education degree Above high school (college, university)	84,2%	100%	76%	81,5%
Experience in counselling, etc.	50%	55,6%	36,4%	45,1%
Drug experience	70%	66,7%	97%	78,6%
ayahuasca pre-experiences	72,5%	22,2%	54,5%	59,8%

IQR = interquartile range
* Study about the motivation of ayahuasca drinkers in social networks (Wolff & Passie, 2018)
** Study about the phenomenology of the ingestion of ayahuasca (Wolff et al, 2019)
*** Study about expectations, motivations, effects and subjective evaluations

The demographic data may be largely determined by the target group of the Peruvian ayahuasca centres and their prices. People who self-organized travel to ayahuasca vendors in the jungle, as well as people who additionally take part in an ayahuasca ceremony during their South American vacation, or spontaneously decide on the spot may have deviant demographic profiles, as such who exclusively come for ayahuasca and book a relatively expensive al-inclusive offer. Also, South American ayahuasca tourists from urban environments have not been systematically mapped and probably represent only a very small proportion of the Internet pilot study. Likewise, local rural drinkers from the Amazon and neo-shaman drinkers attending city ceremonies would be missing if a comprehensive picture of the situation in Peru were to be sought. However, this was not the aim of this study and it should be mentioned here only for the sake of completeness. The persons surveyed thus represent a (albeit most essential) subgroup of ayahuasca tourism in Peru.

17.6 Discussion of quantitative results

17.6.1 Personality

Attendees examined in the study about expectations, motivations, effects and subjective evaluations scored average in most personality dimensions. But the participants of the ayahuasca retreats at the Garden of Peace tended to be more open to experiences than the average. This does not seem surprising, for people seeking such extraordinary experiences.

Additionally, there is evidence from other psychedelic drugs such as psilocybin that even a single high-dose session in an appropriate setting may lead to an increase in the Openness dimension of personality (MacLean et al., 2011). Mystical experiences during psilocybin intake would stabilize such changes even one year after. It is unclear how these findings could be generalised towards other psychedelic drugs or mind-altering techniques of mystic traditions. One explanation for the slightly raised values on the openness dimension in my baseline sample of ayahuasca tourists could be found in previous drug experiences with Cannabis, MDMA and psilocybin (see demographic data). Another factor may be the pre-experience in alternative psycho-techniques and psychotherapies.

17.6.2 Sense of Coherence

I had the hypothesis that ayahuasca experiences could possibly contribute to meaningfulness and comprehensibility. Euphoric case reports repeatedly claim that participants would gain profound insights into the contexts of their lifes and recognize meaning in, for example, stressful life events. Similarly, advertising messages from protagonists of commercial ayahuasca tourism. Would the propagated reconnection with a transcendent reality of nature and universe have a positive effect on the meaningfulness conviction? If the null-hypothesis of no differences of central tendencies between baseline and pre1 and pre2 would be true (as well as all other assumptions of the tested model), the collected data would be would be usual. The sense of coherence as a personality trait was less affected than expected.

This empirical finding seems to be in contradiction to anecdotic reports about possible effects of ayahuasca on the personality and attitude towards life. Studies with rigorous design and better sample selection are needed.

If such an effect would exist, it might not be common, but limited to certain sub-groups of individuals. This idea is supported by some findings of the qualitative interviews about subjective effects: The interest in spirituality was less equally distributed among the sample but rather concentrated in some individuals.

It is also possible that an effect of ayahuasca on the meaning-making in life – if existing – may be rather limited to some specific aspects of the individual's life and not necessarily leading towards an enhancement of generalised meaningfulness as defined by the SOC concept of Antonovsky. This idea is also supported by the qualitative interviews about subjective effects and meaning, which took place 6 weeks after the retreats.

It is also possible that the ayahuasca experience rather confirms transcendental attitudes and convictions in participants that have already been there previously in some individuals. Spiritual confirmation was part of the motivation to participate in an ayahuasca retreat in the part III investigation. However, my results are unclear and vague in this point. More research on ayahuasca and meaning-making is needed.

17.6.3 About psychosomatic symptoms

The ayahuasca tourism and the ayahuasca Internet scene very often use the word healing. Here, as in other neo-shamanism scenes, is a tendency in to criticize modern medicine, especially the pharmaceutical industry. Alternatively, ayahuasca is awarded medicinal healing qualities. Sometimes providers or participants even report cancer treatments with ayahuasca and other traditional vegetalismo methods that should compete with conventional chemotherapy (see Schenberg, 2013). There can be found further testimonials in the Internet, e.g. about curing plaque psoriasis (Internet magazine article by Weiss, 2018), back pain and sarcoidosis (Youtube testimonial from Nimea Kaya Healing Centre, 2016), etc. In the interviews of this study I found expectations in participants about healing from migraine, depression, anxiety or from schizophrenic psychosis. In Facebook I also came across testimonials of curing compulsive behaviours such as drug addiction and eating disorders. Those examples of propagated effects are transported in media and within the ayahuasca scenes and may create expectations in potential participants.

From this the hypothesis arose that ayahuasca tourists might be previously loaded with ailments.

The previous symptom load of the surveyed 34 participants at the centre Garden of Peace showed a slightly raised mean of general symptom distress. The means of levels of obsessive-compulsive symptoms, interpersonal sensitivity and depression are elevated. The inter-individual deviation seems great so that standard deviations of all scales reach above the average range. There is evidence that the investigated group of ayahuasca tourists contains various individuals with significantly elevated levels of distress of clinical nature.

The result supports the hypothesis that persons who are pre-loaded with distress are attracted by the healing offers of international ayahuasca tourism.

There were no changes in the general symptom load between before and after or between before and 6-weeks after the retreats. This tentative general result should be studied with a larger sample, under better controlled conditions and before-and-after comparisons should be broken down into clearly defined symptom areas with diagnosed patient groups. If later studies support this finding, it would contradict the alleged multiple healing claim of ayahuasca.

17.6.4 About altered states of consciousness

ASCs from ayahuasca ceremonies were measured with the 5D-ASC questionnaire. Overall 70 experiences from 34 participants were evaluated. During ayahuasca intake, impaired-control and cognition showed the lowest means. This scale describes severe ego disorders, such as entgleisen or other forms of thought disconnection, the inability to separate important from unimportant thoughts, inability to make decisions, loss of will, paralysis, isolation, feeling of external control. The analysis shows that such experiences were relatively few under ayahuasca.

Also, anxiety was low but with a relatively great deviation. The slightly raised level of Anxiety seems more associated with the psychedelic changes of perception and hallucinations and the likewise raised extent of loss of control than with the insights into inner conflicts, biographical memories and mystical states of oneness. These findings are based on correlation analyses between these scales.

Disembodiment was also relatively low but had a wide deviation. Some individuals experienced this strongly; others did not at all or almost not.

The ayahuasca experience is characterised the most by elementary imagery such as regular patterns, colours, light flashes; complex imagery such as scenes, memories and pictures, vivid imagination; audio-visual synaesthesiae such as noises and sounds influencing visions, shapes and colours. Again, the inter-individual variability between participants in the same ceremony as well as the intraindividual variability of the same person from ceremony to ceremony is great.

During flooding phase, the attention is often drawn towards the visuals by elementary imagery. Participants regularly express how beautiful colours and patterns have fascinated them. Some protagonists of the shamanic belief-system interpret this as if at first ayahuasca would seduce the observer, in order to captivate attention and later mix complex imagery and personal relevant content into the visual flow of events, in order to teach.

Those visual experiences under ayahuasca are most wanted by western tourists and are also probably advertised the most – in combination with personal and spiritual experience or insightfulness. Complex imagery may have a substance-specific psychotherapeutic value, when scenes of personal relevance are visualised. It may make a therapeutic difference whether e.g. a client views the relationship with his deceased grandfather in psychotherapy, or whether he subjectively encounters that ancestor in the form of vivid complex imagery during an ayahuasca ceremony in the rainforest and may have the important conversation that in reality was never possible (Wolff, 2018). I found in the interviews that participants are impressed by the clarity, the realism and the meaningfulness of the imagery when evaluating their experiences.

As shown in a regression analysis, the appearance of complex imagery during ayahuasca ceremonies seems to enhance the appearance of insightful subjective meaning. This supports the psychotherapeutic relevance of complex imagery such as biographical scenes, symbolic representations and interactions within the experienced visionary world. Further studies are needed, to confirm or refute the emerging ayahuasca-specific connection of these two dimensions of altered states of consciousness. Because of the high relevance for psychotherapy it would be worth to further investigate this matter.

Studerus et al. (2010) validated the latest version of the OVA questionnaire (5D-ASC). They used samples of experiences from 3 different substances known to induce altered states of consciousness: psilocybin, ketamine and MDMA. For every substance they reported a distinct profile. Similarities and differences of these effects can be studied in the figure below. E.g. it stands out that all 3 substances showed relatively low mean values on the second dimension 'spiritual experience' and a little higher but still relatively low values on 'insightfulness.' All of them showed very low values on 'anxiety.' There are larger differences on 'disembodiment' as well 'elementary imagery', 'complex imagery' and 'audio-visual synesthesiae' (see figure 16).

Comparing the profile of ayahuasca with the 3 drugs can give an idea of the distinct characteristics. Note, that in the figure 16, the 11 new dimensions from

Studerus et al. (2010) are presented on the left side and the original 4 dimensions of Dittrich et al. (2006) are found on the right side. Figure 17 presents the ayahuasca profile only for the 11 dimensions suggested by Studerus et al. (2010).

First of all, it impresses that all values of ayahuasca seem higher than the ones from psilocybin, ketamine and MDMA. This can be a result of the specific set and setting differences between the traditional ceremonial ayahuasca experience and a more or less artificial clinical setting of Studerus' investigation. Higher self-control of participants in such a setting of objective observation is likely whereas the suggestive setting of traditional ayahuasca night ceremonies tries to maximise the subjective psycho-spiritual effects. It is difficult to compare overall intensities of the four substances because the dose-response relation was uncontrolled in the naturalistic setting of traditional ayahuasca ceremonies. But the specific differences on the different dimensions can still be revealing. Like psilocybin, ayahuasca produces very intense visual effects, both 'elementary' and 'complex.' They both can also produce blissful states as well as experiences of unity. But 'spiritual experiences' as well as' insightfulness' seem to be lower, compared to ayahuasca. Why is that so? Are these differences substance-specific effects or are the effects largely influenced by expectations, belief systems and motivation of the participants as well as by the surrounding situation? All these factors remain uncontrolled when comparing these data from very different settings. That's why, it would not be justified to directly draw in the found ayahuasca profile into Studerus' profile (figure 16). But again, it points towards the question of how set and setting may influence such outcomes. Ayahuasca profiles from larger samples from different settings and from different populations should be investigated under controlled conditions. Note, that I used an unvalidated English version, which was simply translated from German, whereas Studerus et al. (2010) validated the original German version of the OAV. A direct comparison is therefore uncertain, but it may provide an idea, which is worth to be investigated in the future.

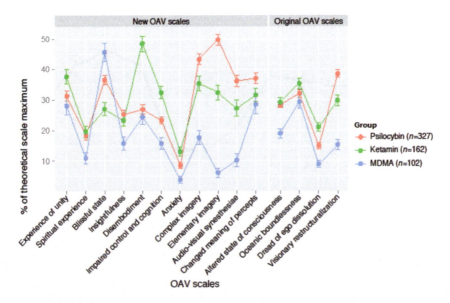

Error bars represent standard errors
OAV is another abbreviation for a former version of the 5D-ABZ questionnaire (translated English version: 5D-ASC)

Figure 16: Known-group validities of the original and new OAV scales (taken from Studerus et al., 2010, http://doi:10.1371/journal.pone.00122412.g002, copyright permission granted. All rights reserved)

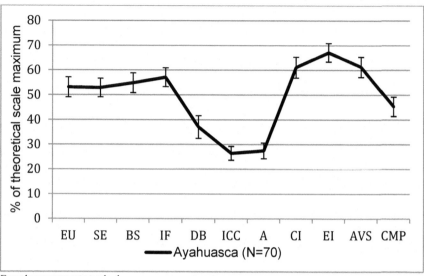

Error bars represent standard errors

Figure 17: Graphic presentation of the 5D ASC ayahuasca-profile, found in the Tarapoto sample

17.7 Discussion of qualitative results

17.7.1 About biographical ayahuasca-related details and motivation

The first knowledge about ayahuasca was usually gained through mouth-to-mouth propaganda, but also through social networks in the Internet, movies and articles. For 70% of the participants, previous knowledge was won from trip reports published in social networks, YouTube, movies and articles as well as from friends and relatives with pre-experience. 45% of the participants reported that the booking decision of the ayahuasca retreat related to a personal crisis, transition time or self-actualisation. For half of the interviewees it took less than one year from the first hearing about ayahuasca until the booking decision.

Without counting the search for information in the media and social networks, 45% admitted a greater attention to the extended personal preparation such as previous- time-out, pre-diet, counselling and journaling (9). Less than half of participants, who had reported a previous crisis that had played a role in the decision to take ayahuasca, also had reported extended personal preparation work previous to the retreat (4 of 9 participants with previous crisis or transition situation in life). More than half of the participants with previous crisis did not report any form of extended personal preparation. This points to a new research question (that has to be answered in another investigation): Why does a part of the mentally loaded sub-population of ayahuasca retreat tourists not actively prepare for the therapy trip, and does this affect their outcome and possible crises after the retreats?

The majority had prepared for the ayahuasca retreat in South America by actively seeking information. However, most of this information was based on testimonials from friends and social media which focused on their own ayahuasca ingestion experience or what they had heard about it from others. The previous search for valid anthropological information about the cultural context was scarce, and the knowledge about local healing methods of traditional Upper Amazon vegetalism was rather low, although the wish for experiencing native authenticity was mostly distinct. The healing expectations were largely focussed on the ayahuasca ingestion in the expected ancestral environment of the rain forest. In some individuals, the focus was shifted more towards the interest in native healing traditions. Most of the time, however, the main motivation was the ayahuasca ingestion itself. 70% of all interviewees stated that they would not have booked the seminar in Peru if it would have been without ayahuasca.

A more detailed analysis revealed that the motivation of ayahuasca tourists had its inherent main aspects that can be pronounced more or less, depending on the individual: psychological interest (inclusive interest in habitual changes), hope for physical relief, general and drug related curiosity as well as spiritual interest.

Intended psychotherapeutic interests in ayahuasca included introspection and self-understanding, guidance and direction in life, unspecific mental and emotional healing, interest in biography-related work and trauma healing, self-acceptance and self-confidence, reduction of depressive symptoms, reduction of anxiety and panic symptoms, clearance of relationship issues, interest in personality development and potentials, increase faith in life as well as purging negative emotions.

Table 6: List of themes and frequencies of expectation about personal treatment in 20 participants of ayahuasca retreats of the Garden of Peace centre (Tarapoto, Peru)

	Expectations about personal treatment	Participant no.	n
Frequent	Ease or cure physical symptoms	4, 5, 12, 14, 15, 16, 18, 19, 20	9
	Self-introspection, self-exploration and greater self-understanding	1, 2, 3, 4, 5, 6, 10, 14	8
	Need for guidance and direction in life	1, 2, 3, 5, 13, 18, 19	7
Typical	Unspecific mental healing, emotional healing and clarification	4, 9, 13, 14, 15, 17	6
	Trauma-healing and biographical memory work	3, 4, 6, 17, 18	5
	Self-confidence, self-acceptance and self-love	5, 12, 15, 17, 18	5
	Alleviation of depressive symptoms	4, 6, 13, 18,	4
	Alleviation of anxiety or panic symptoms	4, 5, 13, 14	4
Variant	Reflection about relationship issues	3, 5, 10	3
	Change negative habits	15, 17	3
	Provide faith in life	6, 12	2
	Unlock personal potentials and stimulate personality development	6, 10	2
	Quit psychiatric medication	9	1
	Purge negative emotions	8	1
	Improve honesty and integrity in life	11	1
	Raise the mood level and increase self control	11	1
	Cure addiction problems	1	1

General curiosity as well as drug-related curiosity were excluded from the category 'psychotherapeutic motivation' and separately analyzed. Psychotherapeutic issues had the highest motivational relevance for almost 85% of the participants. The number of statements is 3 times higher than the number of interviews to which this number refers. This is due to multiple psychotherapeutic motivations that were very common among almost all participants. The high number of statements related to psychotherapeutic themes, the high number of participants who stated psychotherapeutic expectations and the previously reported 45% who related their booking decision to a previous personal crisis, support the conclusion that psychotherapeutic interest was the main motivation in the investigated individuals. This is supported by the quantitative finding of previous psychic symptom distress. The SCL-90-R showed slightly raised means ($\bar{x}$) of obsessive-compulsive symptoms, interpersonal sensitivity (social phobia), and depression with standard deviations, which reached far into the clinically relevant area. The sample means ($\bar{x}$) of the dimension anxiety and (so called) psychoticism borderlined the cut-off T=60. The standard deviations reached above. The global severity index (GSI) as well as the positive symptom distress index (PSDI) were also raised above the average of the normal population. The investigated individuals were partly burdened by psychotherapeutically relevant symptom distress.

45% of the participants had previous physical healing expectations. This number was noticeably lower than the one for psychological healing (85%) but a little higher than the one for spiritual interests (35%). The distribution of 'physical healing expectations' was unevenly distributed among the participants of this study. 9 interviewees focused on physical healing besides other topics. None of them focused exclusively on physical healing.

Physical issues that were hoped to be positively influenced: migraine and headache, gut and stomach issues, menstruation pain and endometriosis, neck and back pain, pain from older injuries as well as food allergies. The section about 'health related insights (below) reports that participant 4 relates her migraine issue to 'stuck emotions' and 'some personal relationship'. She confirmed her personal psychosomatic theory with her purging experiences during ayahuasca ceremonies, where she was able to release some of her restrained emotions and experiencing no migraines afterwards.

The qualitative data about the overall moderate physical healing motivation, which is unevenly distributed among the investigated participants, match the quantitative data of the psychosomatic symptom status. The scale Somatization from the SCL-90-R describes a list of physical symptoms that are known to be affected by the psychological status. The statistical mean of Somatization was raised but still in the average range T<60, although the standard deviation pointed towards individuals that clearly reached above the average of the normal population.

In general, the wish for personal treatment concerned 70,1% of all given statements about motivation. This included psychological interests and issues as well as physiological healing expectations.

Curiosity, as a motivational element, was relevant for 85% of the participants and almost evenly distributed throughout participants. Although it was mentioned by a large majority of participants. It only refers to 17,53% of all statements about motivation. One aspect of the general curiosity was the pre-interest in psychedelics, which partly overlapped with general curiosity. Curiosity, although frequent, was not an exclusive motivation in this sample. Besides their curiosity, participants always reported several other reasons as well.

Table 7: Distribution of motivational elements (motivational subcategories) in 20 participants of ayahuasca retreats at the Garden of Peace centre (Tarapoto, Peru)

Participant	No. of expectations	Spiritual interests	Curiosity	Psychoth. topics	Physical issues	Break out from daily routines
1	5		x	xxxx		
2	3		x	xx		
3	6	x	x	xxxx		
4	9		x	xxxxx	xxx	
5	8		x	xxxxx	xx	
6	6		x	xxxxx		
7	2	x	x			
8	3	x	x	x		
9	3		x	xx		
10	8	xxxx	x	xxx		
11	2			xx		
12	3			xx	x	
13	5		x	xxxx		
14	5		x	xxx	x	
15	5		x	xxx	x	
16	4	xx	x		x	
17	6	x	x	xxxx		
18	5			xxxx	x	
19	4	x	x	x	x	
20	5		x		xxx	x
Sum$_{statem.}$	97	11	17	54	14	1
Sum$_{particip.}$	-	7	17	17	9	1
%$_{statements}$	100%	11,34%	17,53%	55,67%	14,43%	1,03%
				Personal treatment expectation: 68 statements		
%$_{statements}$				70,1%		

Note$_1$: The numbers per category (column) and individual (row) do not refer to the frequency of findings per interview of a category but refer to the frequency of different sub-aspects, which were stated by an individual, belonging to that category. Note$_2$: Only for the column 'Curiosity', no sub-aspects were separately counted - If an interviewee stated general curiosity as well drug-related curiosity, both were merged. Note$_3$: For better visual analysis of frequencies, sub-aspects are not reported as numbers, but every 'x' stands for one particular sub-aspect of the corresponding category that was present in the corresponding interview.

It can be supposed that curiosity might be a rather unspecific element of the motivation that in most cases might accompany the other often more specific elements, such as the desire for personal change, insights and guidance as well as spiritual or mystical experiences and physical healing.

A minority of 35% of the participants had had explicit "spiritual" interests. Spiritual interests were not rare but less frequent than psychological motivational themes or motivation related to general or drug related curiosity. Among participants, spiritual motivation was less equally distributed than curiosity. It was a distinct motivational interest only a part of the ayahuasca tourists. A detail analysis revealed the following aspects: confirmation in spiritual beliefs or spiritual hope, unspecific interest in spirituality, personal spiritual development, finding meaning in life and existence, experiencing a personal connection to the earth and life, breaking through into other dimensions of existence, seeing past lives, and meeting dead relatives.

The prospect of having an authentic native experience played a role in 70% of the analyzed ayahuasca-seekers who traveled to the South American rainforest. This also included the natural habitat of the rain forest that was partly considered a more legitimate place for ayahuasca than northern countries or urban environments.

On the one hand, a cultural idealization and simplified view of the rural life of Peruvian mestizo- and native population, and, on the other hand, a devaluation of western civilization was expressed a minority of the participants.

17.7.2 About previous personal operating concepts

Two main themes of personal operating concepts in ayahuasca tourists were identified:

1. Ayahuasca provides a kind of psychotherapy that mainly gives intensive self-reflection and personal understanding. Sometimes the psychotherapeutic properties of ayahuasca were believed to provide instantaneous and complete change of personality.
2. Ayahuasca operates through magical or esoteric aspects such as personal teaching through spirits or through instantaneous magic that provides whatever is needed or through being a portal into other dimensions or the work of energies. Sometimes desired psychotherapeutic insights were believed to be provided by spirits or entities. This would connect the psychotherapeutic operating model with the magical.

Additional aspects were the idea that ayahuasca would serve as a physical tool for detoxification and that ayahuasca would be like other psychedelic substances.

17.7.3 About previous phantasies and imaginations

Previous phantasies about the coming retreat were stated by 85% when asked about it. Thereby, it has been a common phenomenon. Participants wondered about a) the ayahuasca experience itself, b) the setting and c) the shaman.

Regarding the experience itself, themes of spiritual, esoteric or religious phantasies were the wish to communicate with plants, spirits and Gods, to discover other realms, to see the past or future, to experience revelations about how to become wealthy or have a spiritual journey.

Participants had the idea that they would experience visual phenomena as well as reality shifts.

They expressed the expectation of intense and physically challenging experiences. Anticipated difficulties were related to potentially dark, uncontrollable and threatening psychedelic experiences.

Psychotherapeutic expectations included unrealistic aspects such as the complete change of personality and attitude. Personal growth as well as trauma-healing were also anticipated.

The setting was anticipated in nature with casual dieting rules in a tribal social environment. Occasionally, an esoteric hippy-place was anticipated. The desire for a private, individual ceremony was rare.

The shaman himself was imagined as a good-hearted spiritual hermit, old and experienced and rooted in the traditions of his people.

More than half of the participants claimed to have had no previous imaginations of how the seminar would be, or they actively avoided previous reflexion about their expectation. However, almost all of them reported particular previous imaginations later on.

This may be due to the fact that the direct experience and openness, which would be largely unaffected by the rational mind, has been given a higher priority, which is why the prior deliberate reflection of expectations has not infrequently been avoided.

The contradiction between the statement of no previous phantasies and the later reported particular phantasies is also methodically interesting. It gives some evidence about how the method of data collection may influence the outcome and how inadequate or insufficient collection methods may produce distorted results. A simple questionnaire or a narrative interview without further questioning would have let to the result that more than half of the participants would have had no previous imaginations about the coming retreat.

17.7.4 About unexpected elements of the ayahuasca retreat

There was a greater number and variety of elements that were unexpected or surprising. The most unexpected was and the unpredictable level of intensity of the psychedelic ayahuasca experiences (60% of all participants), followed by challenging physical symptoms (40%), influences of diet, solitude and master-plants (35%), personal insights and visions (25%). Further unexpected elements were reported by few participants (<25%). Such elements were: apects of the shaman, unspecific difficulties, musical influences and housing, life changes after the retreat.

These findings point towards partly unrealistic expectations that seem to be conveyed to a great extent by the propaganda and advertisements from friends and social networks such as Facebook and YouTube. Few have dealt at all with anthropologic literature about Amazonian plant medicine (vegetalismo) and local shamanic practices before coming to South America. The majority of the ayahuasca tourists had a partly distorted image and excessive expectations, which are limited to few aspects – mostly the psychedelic, native-magical, spiritual and introspective. Some participants found their previously unrealistic expectations corrected by the actual experience. Communication with plant-spirits and the "teaching of ayahuasca" was found to be far less direct than expected.

But on the other hand, by some participants were surprised by unexpected mystical experiences and insights, introspective self-understanding as well as emotional activation. Regarding their visions and hallucinations, participants were surprised by out-of-body experiences, the realism of the visions, intra-individual similarities between different ceremonies and clear auditory hallucinations. Regarding the perceived intensity of psychedelic effects, the complexity and diversity of ayahuasca experiences resulted in inter-individual differences within the same ceremony as well as intra-individual differences from one to another ceremony.

Sickness, vomiting, physical pain as well as lack of control were reported to have been stronger than expected by less than half of the participants.

As seen in the interviews, facilitators cannot rely on the fact that the information provided about the setting and procedure was sufficient for all participants of such courses to fully understand what they are getting involved in. A minority was surprised by the challenging and radical nature of the social isolation, the restrictive diet and the very simple accomodation in nature.

Some participants were surprised that the shaman did not fit their image of a hermit or ascetic as they had thought before. A minority indicated that the facilitators and staff of the center were unexpectedly perceived to be non-natives, young and inexperienced.

This meets with previous findings, described in the literature, that ayahuasca tourists tend to look for such conflicting attributes as a transcendent monk and selfless, global, world-teacher in very local or primitive clothing.

Further elements of the setting caused surprise in a few interviewees.: the surprising effects of the master-plants throughout the diet and ayahuasca-ceremonies, the influence of the singing and music during ceremonies on the psychedelic content and the process was also unexpected. For some participants, a greater variety of music and singing might help better to activate associated personal meaning than exclusively singing or music from only one local style. This might apply especially when working with foreigners.

In humanistic psychotherapies, in psychedelic therapies, as well as in traditional shamanic ethno-therapies, music plays an important role for the activation and modulation of emotional-cognitive, qualitative contend. In the belief-system of traditional Amazonian medicine and especially in the psychedelic ayahuasca-therapies, the singing of the shaman is traditionally considered to be one of the most important elements, as he calls allied entities for healing, protection or attacking purposes and modulates the process during ceremony. The psychedelic state is known to be especially sensitive to all kinds of suggestive influences. In general, the answers of the participants underline the therapeutic value of music in the ayahuasca ceremonies. They also point towards the use of music, not only from the tradition of mestizo shamanism, but also from the cultures of the participants.

17.7.5 About what impressed the most

More than half of the participants described helpful personal answers as the most impressive aspects of taking ayahuasca in such a setting. This points towards the great importance of the introspective qualities of ayahuasca for the participants of this study.

Some participants were impressed that they personally encountered spirits and extra-terrestrials within the psychedelic experiences. These were the same participants who had stated their motivation to seek confirmation of a spiritual world beyond the ordinary reality.

A close examination of a possible relationship between expectations and experience with a large sample might be of interest. Does the desire for affirmation of fantastic realities affect the psychedelic experience of it?

Others claimed to have been impressed by clear biographical memories of long past events and childhood memories.

Some mentioned the realitstic character, strength and clarity of the visual content.

Only one participant mentioned amazement about open-eye visions. Open-eye visions sometimes occur but are not as common as visions with closed eyes. Most often, the perception and distinction between ordinary reality and the visual world remains intact.

Differences between ceremonies related to the intensity, or process fluctuations between ecstatic and challenging states, as well as the influence of additional master-plant diet were aspects that caused astonishment.

The work of the shaman caused astonishment, especially the influence of the shamanic singing. Facilitators were confirmed to have good balance, standing between freedom and mothering, and to be able to withstand well the emotional intensity and organizational duties involved.

Mystical or spiritual experiences were reported to have been impressive; in particular, to meet God and to receive proof for the existence of a meaningful spiritual world behind the ordinary reality as well as to receive helpful messages from the surrounding.

The close contact to nature and the minimalist lifestyle had been reported to be impressive to some participants.

17.7.6 About the time after the retreat

An analysis of the time between the end of the retreats and the interview 6 weeks after, indicates that there was no general narrative for the time after that would apply for all of the interviewees. Two tendencies of experiencing the time after, however, could be extracted: On the one hand, paticipants reported difficulties and, on the other hand, active personal efforts to integrate their experiences. Some participants clearly reported signs of post-crisis or experienced relapses into old behaviour and former drug use. After the retreats in deep solitude and internal activation., some reported that it was difficult at first to re-adapt to the noisy world, full of sensations. Some consciously took a time-off for the re-adaptation into their normal life, others immediately continued with their former routines. Some mentioned that they would try to keep their personal insights or advice in mind and apply them into their daily life, or they would try to implement a more consciously healthy life-style. For some of them, the last included the active solving of relationship issues.

The post-diet, with the spiritual explanation of a "sacred treaty" that one would take with the master-plant consumed beside the ayahuasca, may provide western participants with a powerful reframing of renunciation that should facilitate the alteration of undesirable behaviors. On the other hand, there is also a psychological pressure that pushes for compliance and can trigger fear of failure or feelings of guilt.

Some participants found themselves unable to sustain new behaviors or implement a stable, new, healthier lifestyle on their own.

Although the concept of the post-diet and its explication model has its own internal logic, and should encourage the implementation of a behavioral change, for some of the participants, it obviously means a systematic, excessive demand, which sometimes can hardly be met without further help.

17.7.7 About retrospective life relevance and subjective effects

A large majority was generally satisfied with the retreat. The few expressions of dissatisfaction were less about criticizing the retreat or setting itself but rather about realising how much therapeutic work is still to come or that they might have benefited more if they would have been able to meet the suggested diet regulations.

Four topics were isolated, outlining the subsequent subjective relevance assessment 6 weeks after ayahuasca intake: changed life quality, insights about their own personality, spirituality-related relevance and, finally, relationship-related insights, clarifications or improvements.

Regarding the changed life quality after the ayahuasca retreat, more than half of the participants perceived improvements in self-esteem, I-strength or self-compassion, and they found themselves more self-aware, sensitive, self-caring and selective regarding their decisions in everyday life. Almost half of them found themselves calmer, more relaxed, more satisfied and in a more positive attitude towards life. Single individuals found themselves more open for creativity, more hopeful to solve their problems and more able to enjoy music.

Symptom reduction was mentioned about a variety of different areas, but only by 30% of the participants. Physical symptom reduction was reported explicitly only by 2 participants about circulation issues, knee pain and weight loss. They might partly be related to the strict diet restrictions of the retreat as well as possibly to higher stress tolerance or relaxation and self-care, which also were reported in the previous chapter.

Reduction in craving behavior, increased clarity of thinking, loss of social fears, increase of emotional responsiveness, control over negative thoughts as well as the reduction of anxiety were reported.

This rather diffuse picture may have been caused by the self-selection of a very heterogenic sample of ayahuasca-tourists, of which only a minority suffered from abnormal health status. The study can only contribute with heuristic ideas about which pathologies might be worth examining in relation to traditional ayahuasca therapy. It does not provide any kind of evaluation of effects.

A minority of 20% reported that changes of their life style were related to the ayahuasca retreat. Such changes were the reduction of drug use and compulsive behavior such as work addiction, changing the job, moving into another place, relationship changes and changes towards healthier nutrition. For some of the participants, the retreat seems to have played its role in changing their focus or priorities in life, as participant 20 puts it in words, "the context of life has changed" (20: 43 - 43). For some, it seems to have subjective value for support during a transition time in life.

Insights into their own person were reported by a majority of 85%. This theme focused either on the possible personal future or on elements of the past development of the personality or on the understanding and improvement of the present situation.

The most frequent sub-category of this theme relates to insights about possible future directions in life and inner clarity and guidance about what to do, how to be or who to be. The concept of self-actualization, especially the one suggested by Carl R. Rogers, seems to be appropriate to describe these processes of finding new meaning through self-concept adjustments in line with inner preferences, life directions and identity. The ayahuasca therapy seemed to have provoked or helped in already on-going processes of self-actualisation in the majority of participants. As Rogers points out, the development towards self-enhancement and growth does not go smoothly but rather progresses in struggle and pain (Rogers, p. 490). According to Roger's theory of personality, self-actualization and corresponding personal crises are based in psychological maladjustments between organismic needs and their representations in the self. They are expressed in anxiety, the feeling, of inner lack of integration' (ibid., p. 511) or the feeling of being unsure of direction. On the conscious level, they provoke the individual not to know what he wants, not to be able to make decisions, not to know what he may be afraid of (ibid., p. 511). As shown, participants have again found direction in life, which consists in becoming aware or "updating" their needs. Some described this as a form of deepened, emotionalized reflection. Others symbolized vivid scenes that allowed them to gain access to their desires and needs through fantasized or dreamlike experience, making those organismic needs verbalizable and part of the personal narrative about the self.

A minority of 20% explicitly mentioned self-understanding and insights into their own personality. Actual behavior was sometimes related to biographical memories gained during the ayahuasca retreat, or a further acknowledgement of their own personality traits was indicated. Due to the many other questions in this interview, the answers rather have the character of a brief overview. For economic reasons, a further in-depth survey on this topic was waived, and it was postponed to possible later investigations.

Some interviewees explicitly reported to have benefitted from accessing biographic content and from reflecting about memories (20%). At this point, it can only be speculated why this number is rather low. Either the focus of the ceremonies for most participants turnd towards other themes or possible memory related outcome was included into other reported benefits, such as insights into their own person without specially mentioning it. For the few who did have subjective benefits from accessing biographic content, it was mostly marked as highly impressive. One participant gained subjective psychodynamic insights into the relation between biographic childhood events and actual behavioral patterns. Another one found a new perspective about subjectively traumatic events. On the one hand, the responsibility for onerous events and a resulting problematic family relationship could be re-directed towards the adults and guilt could be rejected by shifting the perspective towards the mental issues related to the problematic background of the offender. The person entered the retreat cognitively prepared for such a shift of perspective. That participant specifically mentioned the difference between the theoretical knowledge and the confirmation through her actual, vivid experience under the psychedelic alteration of consciousness. It can be supposed that such productive psychotherapeutic processes under ayahuasca therapy would occur more often in a specific population of carefully selected and prepared psychotherapy patients than under rather heterogenic or unprepared ayahuasca tourists.

Some interviewees found themselves more open to new perspectives and experiences in life (20%). One interviewee, for example, described how he opened himself up for getting a dog, although he had some previous phobia issues. Another one used the personal findings under ayahuasca to change her job. Another one reported to have become more mind-open after experiencing something that would not match his worldview and personal explication models.

Health related insights were reported by 15%. These included the confirmation of a personal psychosomatic etiology, the observation of body-sensations related to unpleasant habitual emotions such as anxiety and hate as well as insights about the psychodynamic functionality of self-protective and anxious self-observational illness behavior.

In the distant review 6 weeks after, 65% of the participants found the ayahuasca experience in this setting as personally relevant in terms of spirituality. This shows an increase of 30% compared with the previous motivation to take ayahuasca for spiritual reasons.

The themes that were found and subsumed as indicating spiritual personal relevance of the ayahuasca retreat were the confirmation or dispersal of spiritual doubts, an increase of basic trust in life, a renewed connection with nature and existence, the impression of gratitude and acceptance with life.

Half of all interviewees reported insights and clarifications of their relationships from the ayahuasca retreat or improvements of their relationships that were related to their ayahuasca experience. Insights gained during ceremony influenced their behaviour towards the other after the retreat. Some also had clarifying talks and expressed their feelings towards the other. Insights, clarifications and improvements were related towards family members (such as parents, children, ancestors), partners (such as girlfriend, boyfriend, wife, husband) or friends. It was reported that changes in the relationship after the retreat were sometimes initiated by a shift of the perspective towards the other and a relativization or dissolution of a formerly fixed, personal position during the ayahuasca ceremony.

17.7.8 About adverse effects after the retreat

Although there was a diversity of 12 different themes of adverse effects, they mostly seemed to be related to single cases. No subcategory building was possible with the low frequency of cases per theme. The most severe was a panic attack after the retreat had finished, when participants were dropped off in town and left for themselves. Another participant experienced an aggravation of depression and anxiety symptoms in the context of a post crisis and integration problems. Other problems after the retreat had finished were oversensitivity against negative thoughts of others, relapse into old behaviors, physical weakness and temporary sleeping disorder.

17.7.9 About the characterization of ayahuasca by the participant's personal working theories

Several statements were made about the role of ayahuasca and how it does what it does. Such personal working concepts, action mechanisms, models or theories could be logically closed systems or could be incomplete or fragmentary. Missing links could be neglected or overbridged by a number of additional assumptions. Explanations could focus solely on selected themes and neglect others. However, all participants made some attempts to find personal explanations about how ayahuasca would work in different levels of elaboration and complexity. I define a personal theory as a detailed system of consciously elaborated elements that stand in a mostly logical connection to each other. A theory does not have to be necessarily rational. Whereas I use the term "personal model", for less elaborated and less logically connected or incomplete explanatory elements. And finally, the term "concept" is used for mental descriptions that have not been elaborated much in a verbal or rational manner. I use this distinction for the sake of intelligibility.

1. Most participants focussed on a psychotherapeutic action mechanism of gaining relevant personal psychological information, experiencing emotional catharsis and relief as well as on a re-evaluation of personal convictions, beliefs and attitudes.

2. The second big theme of personal theories, models and concepts was the idea of gaining access to another realm behind or within the ordinary reality, often called the spiritual world. Ayahuasca would be a medium to access this world. Once opened through the acute perceptual effects of ayahuasca, spiritual entities would reach out towards the person and teach or heal the mind or body, either by influencing the process of the intensified inner monologue towards emotionally relevant insights or by influencing the psychedelically enriched process of visual perception or by direct visual manifestation or by dialogic telepathy-like communication or by physical manipulation of certain parts of the body (feeling ayahuasca or other supposed spirits 'working' in the body). More often than experiencing a direct communication with other entities, ayahuasca itself was attributed as the communicating and teaching entity.

This view is more or less compliant with the local view. Participants have often learned in advance about the local shamanic worldview and are often looking for confirmatory experiences. Thereby, they may be more willing to attribute elements of psychedelic experiences and visual effects accordingly. Such beliefs may possibly have a protective role against re-traumatization and negative processing of psychedelic experiences when associated with trust, care, and protection. Common elements of the local worldview as well as globalized ayahuasca neo-shamanism seem to possess such elements. For example, ayahuasca itself is often believed to be a loving mother (madre ayahuasca), who would be at the same time confrontative and protective. Typical phrases that can be heard throughout the ayahuasca scenes and retreat centers are: 'you get whatever you need' and 'she does not confront, what you would not be able to take'. Another flanking element is the role of personified tobacco as a protective paternal or grandfather-spirit. The black tobacco (nicotiana rustica) called mapacho played an important role as guardian spirit in all the South American ayahuasca ceremonies I attended. Smoking mapacho before, during or after the ceremonies as prayer for protection is a common practice among ayahuasqueros. (The insufflation of rapé is also becoming popular among Peruvian healing centres). Another element may be the belief that the shaman could "see", what is going on in the person's psychedelic process as well as influence parts of it. This, in addition, may give a feeling of security to those who consider it possible, namely not to be entirely at the mercy of the arbitrary moods of cerebral dysfunction due to the acute ayahuasca intoxication.

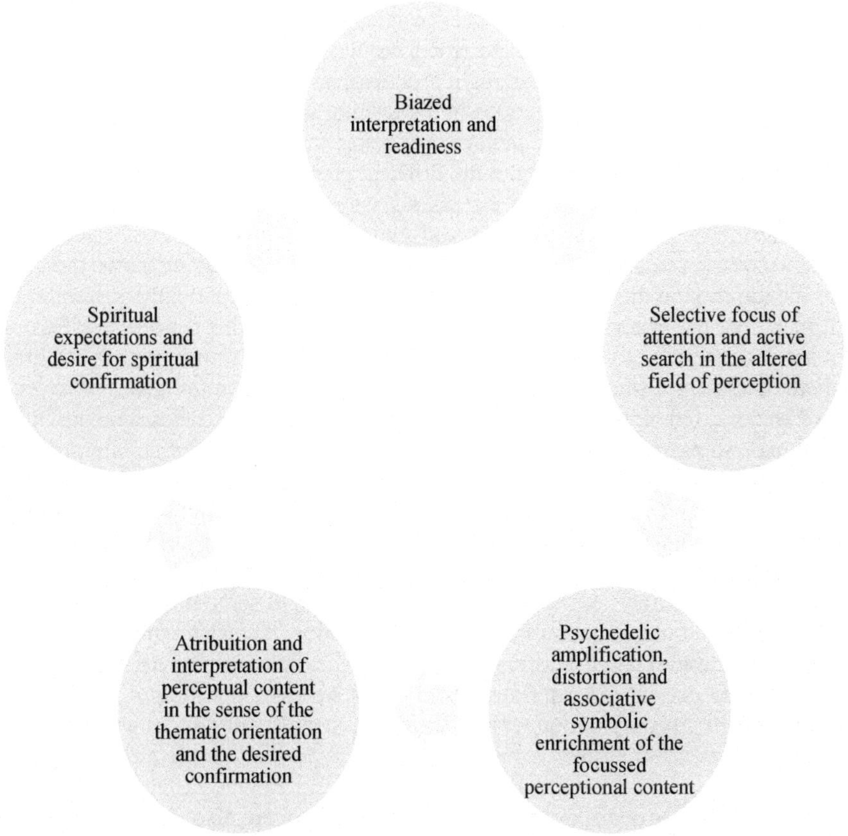

Discussion of qualitative results 225

```
                    ┌─────────────────┐
                    │     Biazed      │
                    │ interpretation and │
                    │    readiness    │
                    └─────────────────┘
   ┌─────────────┐                       ┌─────────────────┐
   │  Spiritual  │                       │ Selective focus of │
   │ expectations and │                  │ attention and active │
   │ desire for spiritual │               │ search in the altered │
   │  confirmation │                     │ field of perception │
   └─────────────┘                       └─────────────────┘
   ┌─────────────┐                       ┌─────────────────┐
   │ Atribuition and │                   │   Psychedelic   │
   │ interpretation of │                 │  amplification, │
   │ perceptual content │                │  distortion and │
   │ in the sense of the │               │   associative   │
   │ thematic orientation │              │    symbolic     │
   │  and the desired │                  │ enrichment of the │
   │  confirmation │                     │     focussed    │
   └─────────────┘                       │ perceptional content │
                                         └─────────────────┘
```

Figure 18: Schematic presentation of a theoretical circle of subjective confirmation of the "spiritual world" among tourists consuming ayahuasca in shamanic South American jungle settings

The figure above illustrates how possibly spiritual preconceptions are confirmed during the acute ayahuasca process. This may occur from active confirmation seeking, corresponding selective attention on certain perceptual content, amplification, distortion and symbolic-associative enrichment by ayahuasca-induced cerebral hyper-stimulation in the serotonergic system and corresponding attribution of the psychedelic perceptual content in the sense of the spiritual anticipation.

Connections between cerebral processes that are less correlated in the functional modes of normal waking consciousness can lead to increased evidence on the qualitative side of the subjective experience, for example, when perceptual contents react associatively to analytic thought processes and produce appropriate visual or other hallucinogenic confirmations in the form of images, scenes or symbols. Examples include: the haptic hallucination of being comforted and caressed by spirits or ancestors when thinking about the difficult present family situation; the visual presentation of different strings that would represent basic human needs when reflecting the personal lack of emotional nourishment and aggrieved rejection of one's mother; voice-like therapeutic thoughts that differ from one's own thoughts, or the impression that one's own thoughts would be therapeutically guided.

It may give the experiencing person the impression that this process itself would react concordantly to the inner monologue or the inner thinking process. From there, it is only a small jump to the idea that an external intelligence intervenes and teaches. Often, this leads to the use of phrases like "and then ayahuasca has told me / showed me that ..." The thinking activities like insights, interpretation and emotion from such (mostly) visual experiences again might lead to other perceptual content that associatively "comment" on details of this inner monologue. However, a majority of over 70% confirmed that ayahuasca would have given the subjective impression of an intelligence or interacting personality.

Of course, this is only one theoretical approach to some possible psychological interaction mechanism of spiritual confirmation. The shamanically prepared set of expectations and the corresponding ritual may have impact on such confirmatory experiences of the "spiritual world". A systematic variation of such set-setting variables in combination with different psychedelic substances would provide some empiric information.

3. Biochemical or neurological models and theories were also used for the explanation of how ayahuasca would work. Participants referred a) to the reversible biochemical alternations in the brain made by the DMT substance, b) to a deconditioning of inappropriate reactions learned by strong biographic triggers (trauma model) by deactivating corresponding synaptic pathways, c) to a perceptual filter of the ordinary consciousness that would be reversibly removed by ayahuasca. The filter-model appeared in two versions: either ayahuasca would provide the possibility of receiving revelations by unfiltered information from the outside or the removal of such a filter would enable the person to access a huge amount of knowledge that would be already there within.

4. Another element of subjective working theories, models and concepts is the attributed physical healing property. Physical healing was explained a) through the biochemical properties, b) purging or cleansing or c) through the physical work

of either various spirits or through ayahuasca itself. Some participant felt physically scanned during ayahuasca ceremony. The last is an overlap between physical healing elements and spiritual elements.

Sometimes, contrasting elements of different working concepts were combined in a surprisingly creative way. Participant 3 combined elements of a biochemical or neurological working theory with a spiritual working model by theorizing that there would be "a higher order of brain functions" (see below) that would act as a receiver for messages or beings from another (spiritual) realm, when activated through the DMT. The brain would be physiologically able to switch from a conductor mode to receiver mode through adequate stimuli. Those higher brain functions would be the product of human evolution, which itself would be modified by those spiritual beings in order to be able to access and understand the physical world.

> Participant 3: 'It seems to me like a product of the spiritual world like having some control over human evolution and basically the higher order of brain functions that allow the spirits that inhabit the spiritual world to access and understand the physical world. And in that moment, when you intake that substance like DMT or ayahuasca your brain function basically switches to like leaving this world to connect with the collective consciousness and may experience the non-physical realm. And in that moment, the beings that experience the non-physical realm come into your body to experience the physical realm. And, it seems like that some of our higher purpose, I cannot really explain that.'
> Interviewer: 'Biochemical mechanism?'
> Participant 3: 'Yeah, on one end of it. Biochemical mechanism that switches your brain from the conductor mode to the receiver mode. Instead of creating and maintaining your own consciousness like from within your brain based on biochemical reactions it kind of switches mode to taking in information from the non-physical realm and become more like a ...[?] or receiver for that information.' (03: 69 - 71)

17.7.10 About other elements of the retreat and their supposed relation with ayahuasca

Most participants (95%) felt there was a benefit in the connection of ayahuasca and other elements of the retreat such as diet restrictions, solitude in nature, master-plant diet. The diet and solitude in nature were considered generally helpful, e.g., the first would be good for detoxing the body, and the last would help avoiding distractions. Various effects were attributed to the master-plant diet. Ingesting additional plant medicines between the ceremonies, would modulate, soften or deepen the ayahuasca experience or master plants would interact with the person and activate unconscious feelings. Although there was such great acclaim in those elements beside ayahuasca, 6 participants (30%) were in doubt of the effects of their ingested master plant on the ayahuasca experience or that of the strict diet.

17.7.11 About the question 'what is healing?'

Health was described either as a state or as a process. Health, as a state, was characterized as life satisfaction, being content, having a social orientation, having gained a deeper understanding of life, having adequate coping strategies and living a mindful lifestyle as well as the absence of pain and illness. Other elements, which, however, represent only individual opinions, were self-love, resilience by an unconditioned mind, having a purpose in life, having chosen a personally appropriate environment, having an inner relationship with the planet and being critical to civilization.

Healing, as a process from illness to health, has been more related to emotional healing. Sometimes physical healing was seen as an effect of emotional healing. Characterizations of the healing process are related to the understanding of basic causes of problems, expelling negative emotions and old conditionings, confronting and accepting past experiences and future experiences as possibly self-made carmic fate, understanding diseases and problems as messengers or teachers, overcoming growth blockages of self-actualization, doing hard work, refusing and resisting consumerist attitudes of industrialized civilization. Healing was also seen as a complex or holistic process on many levels of existence.

Five different aspects of disease and healing were inherent the material. Those elements of disease are subsumed under 1. Container metaphor, 2. Trauma metaphor, 3. Balance metaphor, 4. "Update-from-an-incomplete-state" metaphor and 5. Plant metaphor. In some interviewees, these models were incomplete or rather remained as implied concepts or overlapped with each other without noticing possible logical contradictions. Inconsistency, instability, context-dependency, psychodynamic defence, coping and magical thinking are functions and elements of personal health theories identified by Verres (1986).

The container metaphor that was found in the material seems very similar to the storage basin theory, which was one from three subjective health theories proposed by Herzlich (1973). The balance metaphor is similar to Herzlich's equilibrium theory as well as the theory of equilibrium or adjustment of Faltermaier, Kühnlein & Burda-Viering (1998). Vacuum theories that define health as absence of disease (Herzlich, 1973) were rare in the material (see also the chapter 'subjective health and disease theories'). Plant and update metaphors may represent a therapeutic understanding towards the concept of self-actualization.

The theory of risk (Faltermaier, Kühnlein, Burda-Viering, 1998) was clearly found among many of the subjective health and disease concepts of ayahuasca tourists, e.g., in the idea that modern, industrialized civilization and consumerism would make people sick, and a simple rural lifestyle would lead to more happiness. Container model, trauma model, balance model and plant model contain elements of the theory of risk. They all claim external causes that either would be collected throughout one's lifetime, or would damage, would threaten equilibrium or block natural growth. Disease was widely understood as a task to either empty negative loads or to remove traumatic scars (or to accept them), to forgive and reorientate, to question, change and to actively rebalance one's own lifestyle, to understand hidden messages from diseases in order to resolve blockages of self-actualization. Ayahuasca was seen as an agent to support or enable such processes in the individual. Disease was not understood or welcomed as liberation from demands and duties. Disease theories of fate (see Faltermaier, Kühnlein, Burda-Viering, 1998) were rare in the material. They were sometimes found in the trauma model when used in the context of carmic fate.

The demographic profile of the observed ayahuasca tourists shows that many have tried various kinds of self-improvement or self-help techniques. The desire for self-improvement, self-awareness and self-understanding was one of the main reasons for their motivation to participate in an ayahuasca-retreat. It was hoped that ayahuasca would play its role within their individual healing concepts. But, at the time of the retreat, few were in active psychotherapeutic care. This discrepancy may possibly be due to subjective health theories that are incompatible with those officially represented in the health care systems. At least, this possibility should be examined more closely. As one example, here I am thinking of the criticism of civilization, especially against the pharmaceutical industry and the symptom-oriented conventional medicine, which is more widespread in the ayahuasca scene and was also expressed by the participants examined here. container

17.7.12 About opinions regarding the shamanic belief system

The belief system that forms the background of the ayahuasca retreats refers to the Upper Amazonian mestizo-vegetalism. This is subject to no dogma or unity among mestizo population, since the ayahuasca shamanism is carried most often by individual professionals rather than by tribe traditions. However, some shared beliefs are also conveyed in the retreat center via introductory speeches, web-site information, Facebook posts, YouTube videos and Skype talks to Western participants. Plants would have spirits or energies which would communicate, heal or harm. They could be contacted through extensive fasting in solitude in nature, drinking decoctions or else preparations. Ingesting them would require the personal preparation of fasting, cleansing and retreat. Drinking decotions from master plants during fasting (Spanish: dieta) would mean to enter into an agreement with such spirits, a "holy contract" (expression used by the facilitators Lara and Ashley in the Garden of Peace). Some plant spirits would be easy handle during and after the dieta; others would have rather "difficult personalities". Breaking such contracts with spirits could potentially be dangerous. Spirits would present themselves to apprentices in dreams, phantasy and ayahuasca visions, mostly during extensive fasting and retreat times in solitude. Sometimes they would present a healing song (ícaro) to the apprentice, which would appear in the mind during retreat. Such songs would be suitable to call spirits when sung with the right intention, especially during ayahuasca ceremonies. Ayahuasca would be a gateway or a window into the spiritual world, and, at the same time, it would be a plant spirit within that world, which has the qualities of a wise teaching mother, a cleaner and healer from within. Healers, such as ayahuasqueros (Spanish: ayahuasca healers), would be able to call spirits and energies with their songs, ask them for their service, as well as, be able to send others away. They would understand visions and patterns and would also be able to moderate the ayahuasca experiences of their clients. This might be the most commonly shared base between local vegetalismo and the one deputized in centers for western clients. Spiritual wars between different brujos (Spanish: sorcerer), curanderos (Spanish: healer) and ayahuasqueros, as reported by anthropologists from traditional local Peruvian curanderismos (Spanish: healing provided by folk healers), are not emphasised nor mentioned in the tourist healing centers that I visited or contacted during 3 years of fieldwork in Peru. Those very traditional elements of curanderismo that are practiced among Peruvian people can be e.g., the shooting and removing of magic darts, identifying attackers from the social field of a client, folk theories about pathogenesis such as susto (Spanish: soul-loss by fright), daño (Spanish: harm from the attack of a sorcerer) and mal ojo (Spanish: evil eye). But, ayahuasca centers that focus on foreign clients promote an adapted form of 'reduced tourist shamanism' as the German psychologist Frank Pfitzner said (personal statement, 4.8.2017, also see Pfitzner, 2008). Some centers focus almost exclusively on the consumption of ayahuasca as 'the medicine' and gateway into direct experience of the spiritual world. Others focus on master plant diets. Generally, they all focus on personal development. Ayahuasca always serve as the cornerstone and flagship of their offers.

The local beliefs about the mode of action of (plant)-medicine, disease and healing processes are in strong contrast to scientific explanatory models (which might be quite irrelevant to rather poorly educated rural clients of curanderism in Peru). The same seems to apply for the convictions of the facilitators and promoters of the centers for westerners. I was interested in this contradiction, from my own background in western, Euro-American education, and I suspected such conflicts in at least a part of western participants of shamanic ayahuasca ceremonies.

Surprisingly, a majority of participants did not express doubts when asked about their opinion of the shamanic worldview, even when I later offered them the possible contradiction in a more confrontational inquiry. A minority did express scepticism or internal conflict. One possible explanation could lie in the "going-native" characteristic of this form of tourism. In order to experience the spiritual world of the shamans as true and to subjectively make authentic first-hand experiences, excessive doubt and distancing criticism may be counterproductive. Participants pay a lot of money, travel long ways and expose themselves to adventurous, often unknown psychedelic situations in the jungle for this. Cognitive dissonance is not only harder to bear, it may also disrupt the process.

17.7.13 About openness for a "secular" ayahuasca-psychotherapy

Half of the group expressed openness to the idea of possible ayahuasca-supported, western psychotherapy. A guide with plenty of personal ayahuasca experience and a supportive, emotionally warm setting was usually seen as important prerequisites. Other settings would produce other experiences. Typical arguments against western, ayahuasca-supported psychotherapy were that the native origin and primordial knowledge would have been passed from generation to generation and that experiences of communication with nature-spirits would go missing in a "secularized," western-style ayahuasca therapy.

17.7.14 About ayahuasca and religious experience

A possible connection between the ayahuasca experiences and religion was often rejected by participants of this study. The reasons had to do with their definition of religion and their criticism of the concept. The term religion was usually associated with an institutional form of religion that would focus more on imparting rigid belief dogmas rather than on personal spiritual experience and, therefore, be seen as inappropriate. In opposition, ayahuasca would provide direct spiritual, mystical, personal and healing experience.

But, some reflected the dependence of one's own response to the personal definition of religion. They admitted that the experiences made under ayahuasca could also be personally interpreted as religious experiences with a corresponding interpretive background.

Generally, they all held in common that ayahuasca would enable personal spiritual experiences, independently from defining this as religious or not. This, in combination with the criticism of institutional religion, apparently may reflect a trend that has already been described in religious studies as a 'fluid religion' (Lüddeckens & Walthert, 2010): Institutional religion loses its interpretative sovereignty and authority for the individual, and personal, experiential interpretations are preferred; religion is radically individualized. Personal religious assumptions and convictions are then fed from different sources and are subjectively confirmed in the course of the 'situational event communitization' (Gebhardt, 2010, p. 175). This new form of a 'hybridization of the cultural framework' (ibid.) contains loose, network-like connections, in contrast to the former rigidity of confessionality. As a 'popular spirituality' (Knoblauch, 2010), it no longer represents an alternative to social reality, neither as an established institution nor as a new religious movement.

Perhaps, the following characteristics of commercial ayahuasca-tourist shamanism are contributing to its present success as a provider of religiosity in the current field of transformation of religion:

- No obligations
- No institutionalisation
- Event character of the personal intense experience
- Focus on individualism not on society change
- Loose networked communitization of (former) participants
- Belief in access to uncorrupted authenticity and spiritual first-hand truth.

17.8 Stress-theoretical considerations

Several studies have suggested that meaning-making as an element of coping may serve as a mediator between stress and emotional well-being (Folkman & Greer, 2000; Knoll et al., 2005; Tuck at al., 2006; Mihaljevic et al., 2016).

According to the post-interviews of the 3rd study (Tarapoto sample), the ayahuasca retreats have helped some individuals to overcome spiritual doubts, which were part of their previous motivation. They reported that they had learned greater acceptance and gratitude for life, basic trust in life, as well as renewed connection with nature and existence. However, this was not limited to persons who had expressed a previous corresponding spiritual expectation. As mentioned earlier, a sense of connectedness with the surrounding world is believed to be a key factor of mental health, well-being and an anti-depressive mood by some researchers.

Modern transactional stress theory emphasises the personal interpretation of stimuli during the process of stress generation. In general, acceptance, basic trust in life and sense of connectedness can be considered as results or conclusions of such personal interpretation activity in life, and again they may positively modulate the process of stimuli interpretation in everyday life and, thus, have relevance for mental health. However, these points need more research and empirical evidence.

Although some participants clearly described the influence of the ayahuasca experience in this setting on the identified variables, 'acceptance and gratitude with life', 'basic trust in life', as well as 'renewed connection with nature and existence', no general direct influence of the experience on the trait, Sense of Coherence, could be shown.

This contradiction could either point to the multidimensional nature of the SOC construct or to the possibility that the relevant participants previously already had a higher level of basic trust and connectedness as their conviction of meaningfulness. Thus, they may have experienced the ayahuasca experience merely as a confirmation of it.

However, the results show that in this particular setting, ayahuasca is able to affect the relation between the self-image and a personal, larger frame of reference and, thus, personal meaningfulness in some individuals.

In the evaluation of the subsequent interviews (part III investigation), some influences of the ayahuasca experience on environmentally focussed regulatory activity (alloplastic adaptation) as well as self-focussed regulatory activity (autoplastic adaptation) could be found.

Examples of subjective effects found in the interviews:

- Alloplastic regulation activity: changing the job, moving into another place, active clarifying talks and relationship changes, trying to maintain structure in life and diet.
- Autoplastic regulation activity: reduction of drug use and compulsive behavior such as work addiction, biographic memories or trauma related memory work, self-understanding and rejection of guilt as a victim, improvements in self-esteem, I-strength, self-compassion, self-awareness, sensitivity, self-caring, calmness, relaxation, satisfaction, positive attitude towards life, openness for creativity, confidence to solve problems, and better able to enjoy music.

Not all the reported benefits could be clearly sorted into either alloplastic or autoplastic regulation activity but had aspects of both. For example, the reported reflections and insights about relationship issues and family members during the ceremonies would have reframed the personal attitude of the participant toward the other person and by that would have increased understanding, compassion and more inner peace towards the other (autoplastic emotional regulation activity), but would also have led towards clarifying talks, changed social behavior and improvements in the social family network.

Regarding the interview statements of participants, ayahuasca ritual therapy seems to have a potential influence on both alloplastic and autoplastic regulation activities.

The conditions under which autoplastic processes (self-regulation) and alloplastic processes (person-environment-regulation) are initiated or facilitated by ayahuasca ritual-therapy can be the object of future research.

17.9 Model of supply and demand interaction in ayahuasca tourism

Acording to the previous literature about tourism as well as own field observations, I developed a general model of ayahuasca tourism. It explains how typical standarts develop through an interaction process between demand side (tourists) and supplier side (healers and centre owners). Expecations and imaginations about the respective other side shape the development of this touristic phenomenon.

The international ayahuasca tourism is mostly offered by touristic lodges around the touristic centres of the Peruvian rain forrest (Iquitos, Pucallpa, Taraporo), as well as other touristic areas ("sacret valley" near Cuzco). It is characterised by the following attributs:

Traditionalization: The aquitecture of healing lodges, clothing and appearance of healers often follow a folkloristic indigenous image and symbolize an unbroken connection to very local traditions of the past of the Amazon rainforest and the nature. This is supported by the absence of signs of the modern industrialised lifestyle as well as the absence of Christian symbols. Certain standarts of a touristic shamanism have developed, on the one hand, from local traditional healing elements and, on the other hand, from the desires and limitations in time and knowledge of the foreign clients. Shaman tourism meets the healing practice of the local mestizo population only in parts, but it gives the impression of an unbroken tradition, sometimes supposedly thousands of years old. Tourists are usually not able to recognize such differences and are left unclear about it.

Globalization: Many healing lodges and healers are focused especially on wealthy clients from abroad. On the one hand, they follow the expectations and the images of their international clientele about a native culture which is supposed to be very local and preferably uncontaminated by modernity. On the other hand, they convey a patchwork philosophy of global liberation, purification and harmony of mankind, which consists of non-local secular takeovers of different religious pieces. Ayahuasca tourism carries elements of Buddhism, Yoga as well as secular "updates" of Christianity. Often, other activities such as Yoga, hiking or souvenir shoping is offered. Indigenous and mestizo culture is usually not based on the global paradigm of individual accumulation of wealth but on the principle of exchange and balance, either by appropriate forms of participation of the community in the economic success or by stealing and defamation by neighbors. Local clients

of curanderos usually can not pay much. In serious cases, the rather long treatment in the house of the healer, can be a burden for the healer. In oppositon to this, as longer the foreign clients stay as more money can be accumulated in the touristic setting.
Professionalization: Healing centres tend to advertise in the Internet through professional web pages in English and in social medias like Facebook. The high price of most centres – compared to local economic standarts – often between 100 USD and 200 USD per night, also points towards the foreign or at least wealthy urban clientele.

Reduction: In the Shipibo-tradition, which has opened up the most for ayahuasca tourism in Peru, it is usually not common that the local patient drinks the ayahuasca but the curandero. He usually drinks ayahuasca searching for information about the causes of the patient's issues and the appropriate healing strategy or to initiate healing activities through plant spirits or magic warfare or other shamanic practices. In opposition to that, the expectation of most foreign clients lies on personal, meaningful, visual experiences during their own ayahuasca ingestion. The complex healing system of various healing plants, diets and magic elements, of which ayahuasca is only a part of, is often (but not always) neglected or marginalised in the ayahuasca shamanism-tourism. In any case, ayahuasca serves as the cornerstone of this kind of tourism. For a greater number of foreigners, ayahuasca tourism can be interpreted as a modern form of pilgrimage which is free of institutional integration of the individual into a given religion. In the same manner, an ayahuasca ceremony can be interpreted as a modern church service without a church.

Exaggeration: Along with the reduction of the vegetalismo and the focus on the psychedelic ayahuasca experience, supposed healing properties of ayahuasca are stressed. Within the short time of the average touristic stay in a healing centre, between one or two weeks, far more ayahuasca ceremonies are attended than what would be appropriate for the local practice.

Foreign tourists have specific expectations about their stay regarding the traditional native setting, the legitimation of the shaman, the nature surrounding of the jungle, the safety, hygiene and housing standart, the ceremonies, the power of the ayahuasca, about the philosophy and wisdom communicated by the healer, about their personal motivation. Such expectations may not always be fully conscious or reflected by tourists. But to meet such expectations may decide over the satisfaction in the narratives which they will transport home. In general, the expectations of tourists may be shaped not only by their personal motivation but also by the cultural phenomena and paradigms of belief of which the tourist's life may be part of. In the case of ayahuasca tourists who attend retreats in healing lodges, this background often seems to consist of the trend of fluid religiosity and patchwork philosophy, the trend of individualistic self-optimising, alternative medicine and popular psychology, the romantic images of "Indian" culture and critics on moderity as well as neoshamanistic beliefs. The, often unspoken, expectations shape the decision-making when booking an ayahuasca retreat or when getting hooked up by a "shaman" on the street.

On the suppliers' side, such expectations may not remain unnoticed. Healers have their own theories and expectations about their "gringo" clients. As pictured earlier, healing centres and curanderos adapt to some of the expectations so that the touristic shamanism differs from the local vegetalism. A circle of mutual expectations surrounds the interactions between supply and demand side in the ayahuasca tourism. This might be the motor which drives forward the process of shaping the standarts in ayahuasca tourism which are believed to be traditions.

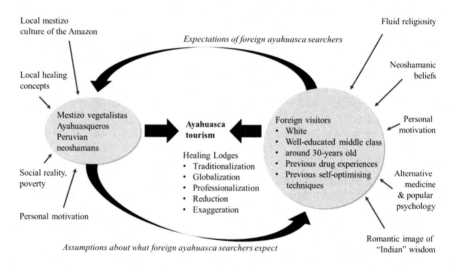

Figure 19: Schematic presentation of mutual expectations between demand side and supply side, which shape ayahuasca tourism

18 Limitations

The generalizability of these findings towards the whole population of non-native ayahuasca drinkers is statistically uncertain due to the active self-selection of participants within this non-experimental design without randomization and rather small sample seizes. The generalization towards the whole population of ayahuasca -experimenting non-locals should, therefore, be avoided for the present.

Regarding the ayahuasca-motivation: The representativeness of the sample for the targeted population of western ayahuasca users is limited to active members of the international ayahuasca Facebook scene, who are willing to take part in such a study. It is unknown if the self-selected sample, which is small compared to the great number of members of the selected of Facebook groups, over-represents a particular part of the ayahuasca community, who might have a particular intrinsic motivation for partaking in such a study that may have affected the results. Since the qualitative description of the given motivational categories was not mandatory, a complete picture of their subjective meaning could not be given, especially the variable "spiritual purposes" might be overlapping with "self-awareness / self-exploration". This may have partly contributed to the correlation of the two. A better validation of the four motivational categories beforehand would be important. Validity and reliability are unknown for these 4 items. Correlation hypotheses were developed after the data had been collected and analysed and were not part of the original conceptual design.

More statistical data from different sources and from different types of ayahuasca-drinkers is needed for a general picture of the motivational structure of ayahuasca-tourism as well as its effects, integration efforts and subjective evaluation.

Regarding the subjective phenomenology of the ayahuasca ingestion: In general, items which had been mentioned during the narrations are believed to have more subjective importance to the teller than those possibly not mentioned.

There might be exceptions from this logic, if material would be held back because of possible doubts, embarrassment or other motivations. However, I consider this possibility as very low. Participants showed a great desire to expound upon their experiences during the interviews. It seems more likely that some important items from the ayahuasca experience might have been forgotten, possibly under the influence of preconscious and unconscious defence mechanisms. This is a common phenomenon known from dream contents. In contrast to previous studies on phenomenology, which queried the already finished narratives of recent ayahuasca experiences, I tried to counter this by performing the interviews as early as possible after the ceremony. Nevertheless, this must be accepted as a possible limitation.

The indication of the frequencies at the level of analysis units (interviews) is subject to restrictions with regard to their informative value. Since many questions were relatively openly formulated, in line with the interview technique of the structured interview, a low frequency of a category does not automatically mean that it would be less subjectively relevant or less common. It is possible that low-frequency categories were less prevalent in the interviews because interviewees might have believed that these contents were trivial to the interviewer or that some of the content seemed too trivial to some to mention it separately. However, in the case of frequent occurrence of a topic, it may well be assumed that this was also of more common subjective relevance within the group of interviewees.

Also, in terms of the very large diversity among participants, demographic variables, motivation, expectations, and mental-health data, it is understandable that responses were often scattered into many low-frequency subcategories.

It is important to emphasize that frequencies and percentages of numbers of interviewees regarding specific categories are given mostly for the sake of completeness. However, the qualitative parts of the work should not be treated as results obtained from a statistical sample. No such statistical generalizations may be derived. Extreme frequencies or the extreme absence of these I regard as hypothesis-generating interpretable. The purpose of this study is to show what subjective phenomena exist and how they can be experienced and evaluated by participants without telling how often such phenomena may exist. The last would be next steps for future hypothesis-testing studies.

Although theoretical saturation of the coding frames was reached for the subjective phenomenology investigation and the investigation about subjective effects and subjective evaluation, the small number of participants, for each study one only from one retreat center, may be a limitation since other participants might provide new aspects not yet covered in the coding frame. On the other hand, it could be argued that the natural selection of tourists in this study already provides a large heterogeneity of relevant demographic and mental health related variables such as age, educational level, physical and mental preloading, previous experience with psychotherapeutic thinking. Dose, amount and ratio of the pharmacological components remained uncontrolled. An interpretative uncertainty when defining categories and subsuming units of meaning to it lays in the method of QCA (Qualitative Content Analysis). I met this with a determination of reliability (stability in time). Another limitation can be seen in the chosen narrative interview method. Although, on the one hand, an interviewer bias is largely avoided by means of a narrative interview strategy; on the other hand, the method has the disadvantage that additional interesting aspects cannot be particularly asked for and may, therefore, not be reported.

19 Closing words

There are still strong concerns, prejudices and fears about the use of psychedelics. Fortunately, taking ayahuasca is psychologically too demanding, physically too challenging and uncomfortable for becoming globally interesting as recreational drug. Furthermore, it has almost no addictive potential because there is no physiological tolerance.

Although ayahuasca tourists in South America, as far as seen in my studies, are not seldomly people who have previous experience with psychedelics, ayahuasca tourism is usually neither addiction tourism nor recreational drug tourism, as my research and those of others have repeatedly shown. The vast majority of participants I met in ayahuasca centres in the rainforrest wanted to change something in their lives.

Probably the most fundamental difference between the exclusively local ayahuasca curanderismo and ayahuasca shaman-tourism is that the focus of the latter is usually the experience itself. In contrast, local mestizo-clients tend to focus more on getting rid of their often very tangible problems when hiring a curandero. The ayahuasca experience itself is rather secondary or even undesirable, at least it is just a means to an end.

The ayahuasca tourism is probably part or product of larger movements of our industrialized, cultural landscape and globalizing media-world. Maybe a happy coincidence that only became possible because several things came together at the right time. Some believe that it is a gift from Mother Earth to global mankind, a return to the right path of life in harmony with the earth, the cosmos, the living and non-living beings. I would like to abstain for now, and only mention this as it often encounters you when you are moving through the ayahuasca scene.

Some elements that may be responsible for the current international success of ayahuasca in South America and beyond are these:

- The individualization of biographies of metaphysical conviction. A reasonable number of persons move away from denominational religions or at least become interested in other influences. The traditional churches suffer for many years under membership loss. It shifts towards a fluid or patchwork-spirituality, which is more an expression of the biography of the individual development of spiritual interests, than an ideological, denominational affiliation (Lüddeckens & Walthert, 2010, pp. 9-18). It lets a large number of people develop their own religious beliefs, which they acquir from own life experiences and search for knowledge.

- Affordable opportunities for long-distance tourism for many people. The non-ordinary is longed for as something special which is sought in the distance. One can experience the non-ordinary in a rather controlled way for a limited time, without being completely torn out of the ordinary, as it would be the case with for example war experiences, migration, social crash or bad illnesses. One hopes to be able to take the experience of the non-ordinary back into everyday life.

- No obligations or liabilities. The ayahuasca offers have event character. The result is a casual social network, which often remains connected only through a few final photos and some more or less active Facebook contacts. It is not political and asks for no membership or further restrictive rules to follow in life (apart from the limited time of post diet).

- Romanticizing and historizing use of stereotypes by the mass media. Ayahuasca-tourists, as many other people, obtain ethnographic opinions and knowledge from film and television. So that opinions of what is original and authentic are a mixture of fiction, selective facts and desires.

- The touristic design of a contradictory stage authenticity of all-inclusive offers and their strangely uncritical acceptance by the tourist audience. Did not it want to escape of what has been made up, longing for an environment of naïve truth that leads back to the essential truth in one's own life? Shaman tourism creates tourist shamanism. Ethnographs have lamented this reduced and contaminated form, which relatively quickly represses what has been there before. When replacing the word "tourist" by "visitor", the phrase does not sound so very bad any more. Now, we can say, "Visiting shamans creates visitor shamanism." That is what mestizo shamanism always has been in the dwelling cultures along the Amazonian rivers, even before foreign tourism had started. Whenever the needs change, an adaptation of the offers will follow. But to use exclusively the term "staging" for a general description would include the danger of being misunderstood, as it would suggest a willful manipulation in the sense of a honey trap without having more than commercial meaning to the healer. Staging may be an important aspect of shamanism in general, even without having rich clients from foreign places. In the jungle, a feather crown might help as much as a long white doctor's coat in a hospital. As so often in South America, intentional staging and authenticity can coexist. It remains open, who is more responsible for the publicity-compliant design of the touristic offer, the local healers or their employers and foreign business partners. Sometimes this is the same person. It also remains unclear how much the curandero perceives his chosen form of acting as self-congruent and in harmony with his internal healing motivation (clothing, appearance as a shaman, architecture, etc.). Is he aware that, in the touristic context, he is always on a stage? Anyway, none of the healers I've met and interviewed have indicated a corresponding inner conflict here. Maybe it is nothing to share with a stranger. Another aspect: There is this way of acting, in which the actor becomes so engrossed in the moments of his play that he stops pretending. He becomes authentic. When he cries, he feels the pain, and because he feels the pain he cries. When he laughs, he feels the joy, and then, he laughs because he feels the joy. For the moment, the stage is forgotten, and the drama is real. There are also these moments in theater, in movies and books, when the recipient forgets the fact of being deceived. That is another kind of authenticity. It is always possible, even on artificial stages. You can not really be sure about which play is going to be performed, but you can be sure that the drama that follows the ingestion of ayahuasca in ceremony always has this form of authenticity.

- The mixing of fragments of different traditions from East and West, North and South. There is a broadly shared conviction that in this colourful collage of ignored incompatibilities, one finds the supposedly red thread of a pure doctrine of unbroken global truth, which redeems from everything and heals of everything.

The ayahuasca tourism may take part in a greater societal movement of secularized religiosity (I mean predominantly dechristianised Christianity). As earlier mentioned, I also see ayahuasca tourism as a modern equivalent to pilgrimage. For participants, the journey can provide orientation in a state of upheaval, search of meaning and confirmation of spiritual hopes. Psycho-spiritual self-improvement can be considered as the main motivation. Since Arnold van Gennep (*1873 – +1957), the cross-cultural function of rites of passage in societies has been described. In the case of ayahuasca pilgrimages, there is no institutional social form and no definite societal transitional stages, as may be in denominational pilgrimages such as e.g. in the case of Islamic hajj. From the viewpoint of the participating individuals, the journey can often be considered a personal rite of passage, from the first recognition, the motivation development and decision making, the travel preparation and personal preparation (goal setting, pre-fastening, etc.), the actual journey to the edge of industrialised civilization, the central phase in the ayahuasca centre and the subsequent integration efforts afterwards into everyday life when coming back. Accordingly, the ayahuasca journey can be understood in particular as a liminal phase in the sense of the ethnologist Victor Turner (*1929 – +1983). Social norms and statuses are temporarily suspended during such a journey. It creates its own comunitas with own group standards of behaviour and beliefs. Own hierarchies, e.g. between the master and the disciple develop, who may lose their importance for the individuals after departure.

The setting is loaded with its strong neo-shamanic suggestions, its pantheon of ghosts and plant personalities, its ceremonial dramaturgy, its strange sounds and smells of the jungle, the fasting procedure and social withdrawal. How does the specific rainforest setting in connection with expectations and previous phantasies contribute to the subjective and may be psychotherapeutic value of ayahuasca? I think I threw some light on this question so that the evidence I found provides a basis for the empirical testing of more detailed hypotheses. Would it make any difference to either ingest ayahuasca as part of such a personal pilgrimage or within the setting of a therapist office at home? The term pharmahuasca was invented for a standardized ayahuasca analogue, which is used in experimental laboratory settings. Of course, such a setting is more oriented towards European psycholysis or North-American psychedelic therapy. In examining the subjective effects of psychedelics, particularly when studying their potential psychotherapeutic effects, the context or environment in which the substance was administered must be considered as an independent variable.

As shown in my data, participants have a great desire for spiritual experiences. The spiritual interest is mixed in many cases with a psychotherapeutic interest. The subjective belief that the altered state of consciousness with its distorted and productive changes would provide insight into a hidden spiritual world behind normal reality, as well as the occasional subjective encounter with teaching or else communicating entities during this ayahuasca state, be it plant spirits, extra-terrestrials, family members or whatever, fulfils that spiritual desire. The often visual ayahuasca experiences impress with a high realism character and therefore provide a great deal of affirmation. This applies at the same time not only to the mystical or spiritual experience complex, but also to psychotherapeutic insights of the personal history, the clarification of current personal situations and relationships as well as future orientation.

Psychoanalytic and humanistic psychotherapeutic approaches were not developed on the academic drawing board but by practicing physicians out of their healing pragmatism. Their modifications and secessions had always taken place since the beginning, and academic or statistical credentials came later. The situation is similar with the South American ayahuasca-vegetalismo and its touristic form, but with the difference that the founders, bearers and continuators of these practices and beliefs are not academic physicians, trained in scientific, deductive method of thought but mostly simple peasants or fishermen at the edge of industrialised civilisation. They did what they could with their own means to deal with problems and diseases, and the methods are often not gentle. You have to keep in mind that even what seems scientifically untenable or absurd, can have significance in everyday life and can even be salutary. We have our own examples. Psychoanalysis, for instance, has made realities describable with terms that carry meaning in everyday life. But these terms can be useless or untenable from a perspective of hard science, e.g. the concept of the ego. In our normal lives, such terms make sense and people (even experimental psychologists) believe in it as a matter of course. From a certain perspective, behavioural therapy might do nothing more than skilfully convincing their phobic clients of not being afraid any more. Subsequently, from the viewpoint of a psychotherapy client, believing enough into being healed may already be the healing. I try to indicate that even in our world subjective convictions determine our expectations and reality. With these thoughts I do not want to claim that psychedelic psychotherapists working with ayahuasca should convince their clients of the existence of wise plant spirits when such concepts are alien to them. But what can we do when we meet people in rural South America for whom these things are everyday reality or when meeting clients coming back from an ayahuasca journey who are convinced of having received highly important personal teachings from 'mother ayahuasca' or other spirits? I believe that such convictions and experiences are fully justified in the subjective context of South American curanderismo. Even while I do not necessarily share them as a belief in an objective reality. My research suggests that they can play a helpful role to non-local customers in the context of this setting. In respect of the impressive subjective effects I have experienced and accompanied, and the deep devotion and self-sacrifice of Peruvian vegetalistas, I support the idea that ayahuasca, used by modern psychedelic therapists as interchangeable psychedelic substance among other serotonergic drugs, should better be named differently than 'ayahuasca'. It runs the risk of marginalizing the complex system of Amazonian herbs, beliefs, and practices, of which ayahuasca is only one, albeit important part. I have met doctors, psychoanalysts and academic psychotherapists in South America who respect the traditional use of ayahuasca and even practice co-operation with local healers as a possible option for psychotherapeutic processes. Why not?

References

Abegleen, R. (1996). Psycholytische Psychotherapie. Katamnestische Auswertung von Psycholyseprotokollen und Fragebögen von Ausbildungskandidaten mit Bezugnahme zu Ergebnissen aus der Klinischen Literatur [German: Psycholytic Psychotherapy. Catamnestic evaluation of psycholysis protocols and questionnaires of training candidates with reference to results from the clinical literature]. Unpublished thesis, University of Zürich, Zürich, Switzerland.

Abramson, H. A. (1967). The use of LSD in psychotherapy and alcoholism. New York, USA: Bobbs Merrill.

Adamson, S., Metzner, R. (1988). The Nature of the MDMA Experience and its Role in Healing, Psychotherapy and Spiritual Practice. Revision Vo. 10, No. 4, 10, pp. 59-72.

Agurell, S., Holmstedt, B., Lindgren, J. E. (1968). Alkaloid content of Banisteriopsis rusbyana. Am J Pharm, 140(5), pp. 148-151. PMID: 5698439.

Airaksinen, M. M., Lecklin, A., Saano, V., Tuomisto, L., Gynther, J. (1987). Tremorigenic effect and inhibition of tryptamine and serotonin receptor binding by beta-carbolines. Pharmacol Toxicol. 1987 Jan;60(1), pp. 5-8. PMID: 3562389

Albani, C. (2008). Beziehungsmuster und Beziehungskonflikte: Theorie, Klinik und Forschung. Göttingen, Germany: Verlag Vandenhoeck & Ruprecht, p. 139.

Allport, G. W. (1951). The individual and his religion. USA, New York: Macmillan.

Amelang, M., Bartussek, D., Stemmler, G., Hagemann, D. (2006). Differentielle Psychologie und Persönlichkeitsforschung. Stuttgart: Kohlhammer.

Amirkhan, J. H., Greavessense, H. (2003). Sense of coherence and stress: The mechanics of a healthy disposition. Psychology and Health, 18(1).

Antonovsky, A. (1979). Health, stress, and coping: New perspectives on mental and physical well-being. San Francisco, USA: Jossey-Bass Inc.

Antonovsky, A. (1987). Unravelling the mystery of health: How people manage stress and stay well. San Francisco, USA: Jossey-Bass Inc.

Antonovsky, A. (1996) The salutogenic model as a theory to guide health promotion. Health Promotion International, 11(1).

Axelrod, J. (1961). Enzymatic formation of psychotomimetic metabolites from normally occurring compounds. Science 134 (3475): 343, DOI: 10.1126/science.134.3475.343. PMID 779022

Balzer, C. (2003). Wege zum Heil: Die Barquinha. Eine ethnologische Studie zu Transformation und Heilung in den Ayahuasca-Ritualen einer brasilianischen Religion. Aspekte der Brasilienkunde, Bd. 26. Mettingen, Germany: Institut für Brasilienkunde.

Barbosa, P., Giglio, J., Dalgalarrondo, P. (2005). Altered States of Consciousness and Short-Term Psychological After-Effects Induced by the First Time Ritual Use of Ayahuasca in an Urban Context in Brazil. Journal of Psychoactive Drugs. Jun 2005;37, 2; ProQuest Ledical Library, pp. 193.

Barbosa, P., Cazorla I. M., Giglio, J. S., Strassman, R. (2009). A six-month prospective evaluation of personality traits, psychiatric symptoms and quality of life in ayahuasca-naïve subjects. J Psychoactive Drugs. 2009 Sep;41(3), pp. 205-12. PMID: 19999673, DOI: 10.1080/02791072.2009.10400530

Barbosa, P., Mizumoto, S., Bogenschutz, M., Strassmann, R. (2012). Health status of ayahuasca users. Drug testing and analysis, DOI: 10.1002/dta.1383.

Barker, S. A., Borjigin, J., Lomnicka, I., Strassman R. (Jul 2013). LC/MS/MS analysis of the endogenous dimethyltryptamine hallucinogens, their precursors, and major metabolites in rat pineal gland microdialysate. Biomed Chromatogr. 27(12), pp. 1690-1700, DOI: 10.1002/bmc.2981. PMID 23881860.

Baroni, D. (1931). Geständnisse im Meskalinrausch [German: Confessions in the mescaline inebriation]. Psychoanalytische Praxis, 1, pp. 145-149. In T. Dürst (2005). Veränderungen im Verlauf psycholytischer Therapie aus der Sicht von Patienten. Unpublished theses. Germany: Freie Universität Berlin.

Bastiaans, J. (1983). Mental liberation facilitated by the use of hallucinogenic drugs. In: L. Grinspoon, J. B. Bakalar (eds.). Psychedelic Reflections. New York, USA: Human Sciences, pp. 143-152.

Bastiaans, J. (2000). The use of hallucinogenic Drugs in Psychosomatic Therapy. In M. Schlichting (Ed.). Welten des Bewusstseins. Pränatiale Psychologie und psycholytische Therapie. vol. 10. Berlin, Germany: VWB.

Batthyany, A., Russo-Netzer, P. (2014). Meaning in Positive Existential Psychology. New York, USA: Springer, DOI: 10.1007/978-1-4939-0308-5

Baudrillard J. (1988). Selected Writings. ed. Mark Poster. Stanford, USA: Stanford University Press, pp. 166-184.

Becker, H. (1984). Die Bedeutung der subjektiven Krankheitstheorie des Patienten für die Arzt-Patienten-Beziehung. Psychotherapie, Psychosomatik. Medizinische Psychologie 34.

Belser, B., Agin-Liebes, G., Cody Swift, T., et al. (2017). Patient Experiences of Psilocybin-Assisted Psychotherapy: An Interpretative Phenomenological Analysis. Journal of Humanistic Psychology 2017, 57(4), pp. 354-388.

Bensheim, H. (1929). Typenunterschiede bei Meskalinversuchen [German: Type differences in mexcaline trials]. Zeitschrift für die gesamte Neurologie und Psychiatrie 121, pp. 531-543.

Benz, E. (1989). Halluzinogen-unterstützte Psychotherapie. Erhebung bei der Schweizerischen Aerztegesellschaft für Psycholytische Therapie [German: Hallucinogen-assisted psychotherapy. Survey at the Swiss Physicians Association for Psycholytic Therapies]. Unpublished dissertation, Zurich, Switzerland: University of Zurich.

Benzenhöfer, U. & Passie, T. (2006). The early history of Ecstasy. Nervenarzt 77, pp. 95-99. PMID 16397805.

Beringer, K. (1927). Der Meskalinrausch. Seine Geschichte und Erscheinungsweise [German: The mescaline inebriation. His history and appearance]. Berlin, Germany: Springer.

Beyer, S. V. (2009). Singing to the Plants: A Guide to Mestizo Shamanism in the Upper Amazon. Albuquerque, USA: University of New Mexico Press.

Beyer, S. V. (2012a). On the Origins of Ayahuasca. Online article recived May 17, 2016, Web site: http://www.singingtotheplants.com/2012/04/on-origins-of-ayahuasca/

Beyer, S. V. (2012b). Special Ayahuasca Issue Introduction: Toward a Multidisciplinary Approach to Ayahuasca Studies. Anthropology of Consciousness, Vol. 23, Issue 1.

Biniecki, S., Krajewski, E. (1960). Production of d,1-N-methyl-beta- (3,4-methylenedioxyphenyl)-isopropylamine and d,1-N- methyl-beta-(3,4-dimthoxyphenyl)-isopropylamine. Acta Polon Pharm 1960; 17, pp. 421-5.

Bird, J. B. (1943). Excavations in northern Chile. Anthropological Papers of the American Huseum of Natural History, vol. XXXVIII, part IV, New York, USA.

Bischoff, C., Zenz, H. (1989). Patientenkonzepte von Körper und Krankheit. Bern-Stuttgart-Toronto: Huber.

Bogenschutz, M., Pommy, J. (2012). Therapeutic mechanisms of classic hallucinogens in the treatment of addicions: From indirect evidence to testable hypotheses. Drug Testing and Analysis, 4(7-8), pp. 543-555.

Bonn-Miller, M., Rousseau, G. (2015). Web site of the U.S. Department of Veteran Affairs. Retrieved June 1,2018 from http://www.ptsd.va.gov/professional/co-occurring/marijuana_use_ptsd_veterans.asp

Boorstin, O. J. (1964). The Image: A Guide to Psycho-events in America. New York, USA: Harper and Row.

Borkenau, P., Ostendorf, F. (2008): NEO-Fünf-Faktoren Inventar nach Costa und McCrae (NEO-FFI). Manual (2. Aufl.). Göttingen, Germany: Hogrefe.

Boskin J., Rosenstone R. A. (1969). Protest in the sixties. Annals of the American Academy of Political and Social Science 382. Philadelphia, USA, pp. 1-219.

Bouso, J. C., González, D., Fondevila, S., et al. (2012). Personality, psychopathology, life attitudes, and neuropsychological performance among ritual users of ayahuasca: a longitudinal study. PLOS ONE 7:e42421. Retrieved August 1, 2016 from the Web site: http://journals.plos.org/plosone/article?id=10.1371/journal.pone.0042421

Bouso, J. C., Fábregas, J. M., Antonijoan, Rodríguez-Fornells, Jordi Riba, J. (2013). Acute effects of ayahuasca on neuropsychological performance: differences in executive function between experienced and occasional users. Psychopharmacology (Berl). 2013 Dec;230(3): 415-24, DOI: 10.1007/s00213-013-3167-9. Epub 2013 Jun 21. Retrieved August 1, 2016, from the Web site: http://www.neip.info/upd_blob/0001/1287.pdf

Bouso, J. C., Riba, J. (2014). Ayahuasca and the treatment of drug addiction. In B. Labate, C. Cavnar (eds.), The therapeutic use of ayahuasca. Heidelberg, Germany: Springer, pp. 95-109.

Bouso, J. C., Palhano-Fontes, F., Rodríguez-Fornells, A., Ribeiro, S., Sanches, R., Crippa J. A., Hallak, J. E., de Araujo, D. B., Riba, J. (2015). Long-term use of psychedelic drugs is associated with differences in brain structure and personality in humans. Eur Neuropsychopharmacol. 2015 Apr;25(4), pp. 483-92, DOI: 10.1016/j.euroneuro.2015.01.008. Epub 2015 Jan 16. PMID: 25637267, DOI: 10.1016/j.euroneuro.2015.01.008

Bower, T. (1988). Verschwörung Paperclip: NS-Wissenschaftler im Dienste der Siegermächte. [German: Paperclip conspiracy: Nazi scientists in the service of the victorious powers.] München, Germany: List.

Brabec de Mori, B. (2011). Tracing hallucinations: Contributing to a critical ethnohistory of ayahuasca usage in the Peruvian Amazon. In B.C. Labate, H. Jungaberle (eds.), The internationalization of ayahuasca, pp. 23-47. Zürich, Switzerland: Lit Verlag.

Brabec de Mori, B. (2013). Die Psychologisierung der Funktionen von Musik und Drogen in westlichen Interpretationen indianischer Magie [German: Psychologizing the functions of music and drugs in Western interpretations of Indian magic]. In J. A. v. Belzen (Ed.). Musik und Religion, psychologische Zugänge. Wiesbaden (Germany): Springer.

Bresnick, T., Levin, R. (2006). Phenomenal qualities of ayahuasca ingestion and its relation to fringe consciousness and personality. Journal of Consciousness Studies. 13, pp. 5-24.

Brewer, J. A., Worhunsky, P. D., Gray, et al. (2011). Meditation experience is associated with differences in default mode network activity and connectivity. Proceedings of the National Academy of Sciences of the United States of America 108, pp. 20254–20259, DOI: 10.1073/pnas. 1112029108 PMID: 22114193

Bucher, A. (2007). Psychologie der Spiritualität. Handbuch. [German: Psychology of spirituality: Handbook]. Weilheim, Germany: Beltz.

Buckholtz, N. S., Boggan, W. O. (1977). Monoamine oxidase inhibition in brain and liver produced by beta-carbolines: structure-activity relationships and substrate specificity. Biochem Pharmacol. 1977 Nov 1;26(21), pp. 1991-6. PMID: 921812.

Bourguignon, E. (1973). Religion Altered States of Consciousness and Social Change. Columbus, USA: Ohio State University Press. ISBN-13: 978-0814201671

Burkert, S., Knoll, N., Daig, I. (2012). Laienätiologie, subjektive Krankheits- und Gesundheitstheorien [Laity etiology, subjective disease and health theories]. In E. Brähler, B. Strauß (eds.). Grundlagen der Medizinischen Psychologie. Göttingen, Germany: Hogreve Verlag, p. 399. ISBN: 9783840905773

Bustos, S. (2008). The healing power of the icaros: a phenomenological study of Ayahuasca experiences. Dissertation thesis. San Francisco, USA: California Institute of Integral Sudies.

Califano, M., Fernandez Distel, A. (1982). The Use of a Hallucinogenous Plant Among the Mascho (southwestern Amazonia, Peru). Zeitschrift Für Ethnologie 107 (1982), pp. 129-143.

Callaway, J., Airaksinen, M., McKenna, D., et al. (1994). Platelet Serotonine Uptake Sides Increased in Drinkers of Ayahuasca. Psychopharmacology, 116(3), pp. 385-7.

Callaway, J. C., McKenna, D. J., Grob, C. S., et al. (1999). Pharmacokinetics of Hoasca alkaloids in healthy humans. Journal of Ethnopharmacology 65 (1999), pp. 243-256.

Carod-Artal, F. J. (2011). Hallucinogenic drugs in pre-Columbian Mesoamerican cultures. Neurologia. 2015 Jan-Feb;30(1): 42-9, DOI: 10.1016/j.nrl.2011.07.003. Epub 2011 Sep 3.

Castelan Felipe, A. (2015). Ayahuasca, Um Enigma Contemporâneo: Produção Científica Do Uso Terapêutico Do Chá. [Portugese: Ayahuasca, A Contemporary Enigma: Scientific Production of Therapeutic Tea Usage]. Bachelor thesis. Universidade do Extremo Sul Catarinense for biological sciences. Brazil. Retrieved August 6, 2016, Web site: http://repositorio.unesc.net/bitstream/1/3726/1/Amanda%20Castelan%20Filipe.pdf

Casullo, M. M., Castro, A. (2000). Evaluación del bienestar psicológico en estudiantes adolescentes argentinos. Revista de Psicología. Lima, Peru: Pontificia Universidad Católica del Perú XVIII, pp. 35-68.

Carhart-Harris, R. L., Erritzoe, D., Williams, T., et al. (2012). Neural correlates of the psychedelic state as determined by fMRI studies with psilocybin. Proceedings of the National Academy of Sciences of the United States of America 109, pp. 2138-2143, DOI: 10.1073/pnas.1119598109 PMID: 22308440.

Carhart-Harris, R. L., Goodwin, G.M. (2017). The therapeutic potential of psychedelic drugs: past, present and future. Neuropsychopharmacology, 42, pp. 2105-2113.

Carhart-Harris, R. L., Erritzoe, D., Haijen, E., et al. (2018). Psychedelics and Connectedness. Psychopharmacolog, 235, pp. 547-550.

Cervinka, R., Roderer, K., Hefler, E. (2012). Are nature lovers happy? On various indicators of well-being and connectedness with nature. J Health Psychol 17, pp. 379-388.

Chabrol, H. & Oehen, P. (2013). MDMA assisted psychotherapy found to have a large effect for chronic post-traumatic stress disorder. J Psychopharmacol 2013(27), pp. 865-866, DOI: 10.1177/0269881113495119

ClinicalTrials.gov (2018). A Multi-Site Phase 3 Study of MDMA-Assisted Psychotherapy for PTSD. ClinicalTrial.gov Identifier: NCT03537014. U.S. National Library of Medicine. Retrieved Dec 16, 2018, Web site: https://clinicaltrials.gov/ct2/show/NCT03537014

Cohen, E. (1988). Authenticity and Commoditization in Tourism. In Annals of Tourism Research, Vol. 15(3). New York, USA: Pergamon Press, p. 380.

Cole, J. M., Pieper, W. A. (1973). The effects of N,N-dimethyltryptamine on operant behavior in squirrel monkeys. Psychopharmacology 29, pp. 107-112.

Conrad, K. (1960). Die symptomatischen Psychosen. In W.H. Gruhle, R. Jung, W. Mayer-Gross, M. Müller (eds.), Psychiatrie der Gegenwart, Band 2, pp. 369-436. Berlin, Germany: Springer.

Creswell, J. W. (2003). Research design: Qualitative, Quantitative, and Mixed Methods Approaches. Thousand Oaks, CA, USA: SAGE Publications. ISBN 0761924426, 9780761924425

Creswell, J. W. (2015). A Concise Introduction to Mixed Methods Research. Los Angeles, USA: SAGE Publications. ISBN-13 978-1-4833-5904-5

Crumbaugh, J. C., Maholick, L. T. (1964). An experimental study in existentialism: The psychometric approach to Frankl's concept of noogenic neurosis. Journal of Clinical Psychology, 20, pp. 589-596.

Cuatrecasas, J. (1965). Banisteriopsis caapi, B. inebrians, B. rusbyana. Journald'Agri- culture Tropicale et de Botanique Appliquée 12, pp. 424-429.

D'Andrade, R. G. (1987). A folk model of the mind. In D. Holland, N. Quinn (eds.), Cultural Models in Language and Thought. Cambridge, UK: Cambridge University Press.

D'Andrade, R. G. (1995). Models and theories. The development of cognitive anthropology. Cambridge, UK: Cambridge University Press, pp. 150-176.

Da Silveira, D. X., Grob, C. S., de Rios, M. D., et al. (2005). Ayahuasca in adolescence: a neuropsychological assessment. J Psychoactive Drugs 37, pp. 129-133, DOI: 10.1080/02791072.2005.10399792

Dann, H.-D. (1983). Subiektive Theorien: Irrweg oder Forschungsprogramm? Zwischenbilanz eines kognitiven Konstrukts. In L. Montada, K. Reusser, G. Steiner (eds.), Kognition und Handeln. Stuttgart, Germany: Klett-Cotta.

De Alarcón, H. R. (1629). Tratado de las supersticiones y costumbres gentilicias que hoy viven entre los indios naturales de esta Nueva España. Retrieved August 17, 2016, from the Web site: http://www.cervantesvirtual.com/obra-visor/tratado-de-las-supersticiones-y-costumbres-gentilicas-que-hoy-viven-entre-los-indios-naturales-de-esta-nueva-espana--0/html/cf187f38-7e62-49f7-bcf3-71d3c710fe4e_2.htm

De Araujo, D. B., Ribeiro, S., Cecchi, et al. (2012). Seeing with the eyes shut: Neural basis of enhanced imagery following ayahuasca ingestion. Human Brain Mapping 33(11), pp. 2550-60. PMID: 21922603. DOI: 10.1002/hbm.21381

Demange, F. (2002). Amazonian Vegetalismo: A study of the healing power of chants in Tarapoto, Peru. Unpublished M.A. thesis in Social Sciences by Independent Studies. London, UK: University of East London. Received September 26, 2016, from the Web site: http://neip.info/novo/wp-content/uploads/2015/04/demange_icaros_peru.pdf

De Mille, R. (1976). Castaneda's Journey: The Power and the Allegory. Santa Barbara, USA: Capra Press. ISBN 978-0-88496-067-6.

De Mille, R. (2000). The Don Juan Papers: Further Castaneda Controversies. iUniverse, ISBN 0-595-14499-3

Demyttenaere, K. Bruffaerts, R., Posada-Villa, et al. (2004). Prevalence, severity, and unmet need for treatment of mental disorders in the world health organization world mental health surveys. Journal of the American Medical Association, 291(21), pp. 2581-90.

Deperu (2016). Toe. Retrieved July 20, 2016, from the Web site: http://www.deperu.com/abc/plantas-medicinales/4196/toe

De Rios, M. D. (1972). Visionary vine: Hallucinogenic healing in the Peruvian Amazon. San Francisco, USA: Chandler Publishing.

De Rios, M. D. (1994). Drug Tourism in the Amazon, Antropology of Consciousness 5(1), pp. 16-19.

De Rios, M. D., Grob, C. S., Lopez, E., da Silviera, D. X., Alonso, L. K., Doering-Silveira, E. (2005). Ayahuasca in adolescence: Qaualitative results. J Psychoactive Drugs. 2005 Jun;37(2), pp. 135-9. PMID: 16149325, DOI: 10.1080/02791072.2005.10399793

Derogatis, L. R. (1994). SCL-90-R Symptom Checklist-90-R – Administration, Scoring and procedures manual. Minneapolis, MN, USA: NCS Pearson.

Dittrich, A., Scharfetter, Ch. (1987). Ethnopsychotherapie. Psychotherapie mittels außergewöhnlicher Bewußtseinszustände in westlichen und indigenen Kulturen [German: Ethno psychotherapy. Psychotherapy through exceptional states of consciousness in Western and Indigenous cultures]. Stuttgart, Germany: Enke Verlag.

Dittrich A. (1975). Zusammenstellung eines Fragebogens (APZ) zur Erfassung abnormer psychischer Zustände [Construction of a questionnaire (APZ) for assessing abnormal mental states]. Z Klin Psychol Psychiatr Psychother 23, pp. 12-20.

Dittrich, A. (1998). The Standardized Psychometric Assessment of Altered States of Consciousness (ASCs) in Humans. Pharmacopsychiatry 1998; 31(S02), pp. 80-84. DOI: 10.1055/s-2007-979351

Dittrich A., Lampartner, D. Maurer, M. (2006). 5D-ABZ. Fragebogen zur Erfassung Außergewöhnlicher Bewusstseinszustände. PSIN PLUS Publications c/o Dr. M. Mairer, im oberen Boden 140, 8049 Zürich, Swizerland.

Domínguez-Clavé, E., Soler, J., Elices, M., Pascual J. C., Álvarez, De la Fuente, M., Revenga, M., Friedlander, P., Feilding, A., Riba, J. (2016). Ayahuasca: pharmacology, neuroscience and therapeutic potential. Brain Research Bulletin. Retrieved July 6, 2016, from the Web site http://dx.DOI.org/10.1016/j.brainresbull.2016.03.002

Dörfler, H. (2015). Indigene Medizin im ärztlichen Umfeld Kolumbiens - ayahuasca-Rituale in der Großstadt [German: Indigenous medicine in the medical environment of Colombia - ayahuasca rituals in the big city]. Dissertation. Halle, Germany: Martin-Luther-Universität Halle-Wittenberg.

Dörner, K. (1975). Wie werde ich Patient oder Sozialisation zum Patienten. In: K. Dörner (Ed.). Diagnosen der Psychiatrie. Frankfurt am Main, Germany: Campus.

Dos Santos, R. G., Strassman, R. J. S. (2011). Ayahuasca and psychosis. In R.G. Dos Santos (Ed.), The Ethnopharmacology of Ayahuasca. Trivandrum, Kerala: Transworld Research Network, pp. 97-98. Retrieved July 20, 2016, from the Web site: https://www.researchgate.net/publication/216385597_Ayahuasca_and_psychosis

Dos Santos, R. G., Grasa, E., Valle, M., Ballester, M. R., Bouso, J. C., Nomdedeu, J. F., Homs, R., Barbanoj, M. J., and Riba, J. (2012).

Pharmacology of ayahuasca administered in two repeated doses. Psychopharmacology (Berl.), 219(4), pp. 1039-1053, DOI: 10.1007/s00213-011-2434-x

Dunckel, H. (1991). Mehrfachbelastung und psychosoziale Gesundheit. In S. Greif, E. Bamberg, N. Semmer (eds.), Psychischer Stress am Arbeitsplatz, pp. 154-167). Göttingen, Germany: Hogrefe.

Eco, U. (1986). Travels in Hyperreality. Orlandu, USA: Hartcout Brace & Company.

Elder, G., O'Rand, A. (1995). Adult lives in a changing society. In K. S. Cook, G. A. Fine, J. S. House (eds), Social perspectives on social psychology Boston: Allyn and Bacon, p. 465.

Eliade, M. (1964 [1951]). Shamanism: Archaic Techniques of Ecstasy. London, UK: Routledge.

Elkins, D. N., Hedstrom, L. J., Hughes, L. L., Leaf, J. A., Saunders, C. (1988). Toward phenomenological spirituality: Definition, description, and measurement. J Humanist Psychol 28, pp. 5-18, DOI: 10.1177/0022167888284002

Engel, F. (1963). A preceramic settlement in the central coast of Peru: Asia, Unit 1. Transactions of the American Philosophical Society, new series, vol. 53, part 3, Philadelphia, USA.

Fábregas, J. M., González, D., Fondevila, S., Cutchet, M., Fernández, X., Barbosa, P. C., (2010). Assessment of addiction severity among ritual users of ayahuasca. Drug and Alcohol Dependence, 111(3), pp. 257-261.

Faller, H. (1998): Krankheitsverarbeitung bei Krebskranken [German: Disease processing in cancer patients]. Göttingen, Germany: Verlag für Angewandte Psychologie.

Faller, H., Schilling, S. Lang, H. (1991). Die Bedeutung subjektiver Krankheitstheorien für die Krankheitsverarbeitung [The importance of subjective disease theories for disease processing]. In U. Flick (Ed.), Alltagswissen über Gesundheit und Krankheit: Subjektive Theorien und soziale Repräsentationen. Heidelberg, Germany: Asanger, pp. 28-42.

Faltermaier T., Kühnlein I., Burda-Viering, M. (1998). Gesundheit im Alltag. Laienkompetenz in Gesundheitshandeln und Gesundheitsförderung [German: Health in everyday life. Laity competence in health activities and health promotion]. Weinheim, Germany: Juventa.

Faltermaier, T. & Kühnlein I. (2000). Subjektive Gesundheitskonzepte im Kontext. Dynamische Konstruktionen von Gesundheit in einer qualitativen Untersuchung von Berufstätigen [German: Subjective health concepts in context. Dynamic constructions of health in a qualitative study of working people]. Zeitschrift für Gesundheitspsychologie, 8, pp. 137-154.

Faltermaier T. (2005). Gesundheitspsychologie [German: Psychology of health]. Stuttgart, Germany: Kohlhammer.

Feifer, M. (1985). Going Places. London, UK: Macmillan.

Feigin, R., Sapir, A. (2005). The relationship between sense of coherence and attribution of responsibility for problems and their solutions, and cessation of substance abuse over time. Journal of Psychoactive Drugs, 37(1).

Feldt, T., Lintula, H., Suominen, S., Koskenvuo, M., Vahtera, J., Kivimäki, M. (2007). Structural validity and temporal stability of the 13-item sense of coherence scale: prospective evidence from the population-based HeSSup study. Quality of Life Research 16(3), pp. 483-493.

Ferenczi, S. [1919] (1982). Hysterische Materialisationsphänomene. Gedanken zur Auffassung der hysterischen Konversion und Symbolik [German: Hysterical materialization phenomena. Thoughts on the concept of hysterical conversion and symbolism]. In: S. Ferenczi, Schriften zur Psychoanalyse, Bd. II. Frankfurt am Main, Germany: Fischer, pp. 11-24.

Fiedler, L., Jungaberle, H., Verres, R. (2011). Motive für den Konsum psychoaktiver Substanzen am Beispiel des Ayahuasca-Gebrauchs in der Santo-Daime-Gemeinschaft [German: Motives for the use of psychoactive substances using the example of ayahuasca use in the Santo-Daime community]. Zeitschrift für Medizinische Psychologie, 20(3), pp. 137-144, ISSN: 0940-5569

Filipp, S.-H. (1995). Kritische Lebensereignisse (3. Auflage) [German: Critical life events]. Weinheim: Psychologie Verlags Union.

Filipp, S.-H., Ferring, D. (1998). Who blames the victim? – Kausal- und Verantwortlichkeitszuschreibungen im Umfeld einer Krebserkrankung. In U. Koch, J. Weis (eds.), Krankheitsbewältigung bei Krebs und Möglichkeiten der Unterstützung. Stuttgart, Germany: Schattauer.

Fish, M. S., Johnson, N. M., and Horning, E. C. (1955). Piptadenia alkaloids. indole bases of P. peregrina (L.) benth. and related species. Jour Amer Chem Soc, 77(22), pp. 5892-5895, DOI: 10.1021/ja01627a034

Flick, U. & Niewiarra, S. (1994). Alltag, Lebensweisen und Gesundheit [German: Everyday life, ways of life and health]. Bericht 94-5 from the Institut für Psychologie, Ms. Berlin, Germany: Technische Universität Berlin.

Flick, U. (1998). Subjektive Vorstellungen von Gesundheit und Krankheit [German: Subjective ideas of health and illness]. in U. Flick (Ed.), Subjektive Vorstellungen von Gesundheit und Krankheit. Wann fühlen wir uns gesund?. Weinheim, Germany: Juventa, p. 7-32.

Folkman, S., Greer, S. (2000). Promoting psychological well-being in the face of serious illness: when theory, research and practice inform each other. Psychooncology 9.j

Fotiou, E. (2010). From Medicine Men to Day Trippers: Shamanic Tourism in Iquitos, Peru. Doctoral dissertation. USA: Department of Anthropology, University of Wisconsin-Madison.

Fotiou, E. (2012). Working with "La Medicina": Elements of Healing in Contemporary Ayahuasca Rituals. Anthropology of Consciousness 23 (1), pp. 6-27.

Frank, L. (1927): Die psychokathartische Behandlung nervöser Störungen [The psychokathartic treatment of nervous disorders]. Leipzig, Germany: Thieme.

Frankl, V. E. (1986). The doctor and the soul: from psychotherapy to logotherapy. NY: Vintage Books.

Franquesa, A., Sainz-Cort, A., Gandy, S., Soler, J., et al. (2018). Psychological variables implied in the therapeutic effect of ayahuasca: a contextual approach, Psychiatry Research (2018), DOI: 10.1016/j.psychres.2018.04.012

Frecska, E. (2007). Therapeutic guidelines: Dangers and contraindications in therapeutic applications of hallucinogens. In M. J. Winkelman, T.B. Roberts (eds.), Psychedelic medicine: New evidence for hallucinogenic substances as treatments. Vol. 1, pp. 69-96. Westport, CT, USA: Praeger.

Frecska, E. (2011). The Risks and Potential Benefits of Ayahuasca Use. In B. C. Labate, H. Jungaberle (eds.), The Internationalization of Ayahuasca. Zurich, Switzerland: LIT.

Frederking, W. F. (1953). Über die Verwendung von Rauschdrogen (Meskalin und Lysergsäurediäthylamid) in der Psychotherapie [German: About the use of intoxicants (mescaline and lysergic acid diethylamide) in psychotherapy]. Psyche, 7.

Frenz, A., Carey, M., Jorgensen, R. (1993). Psychometric Evaluation of Antonovsky's Sense of Coherence Scale. Psychological Assessment 5(2). DOI: 10.1037//1040-3590.5.2.145

Freud, S. [1924] (1982). Der Realitätsverlust bei Neurose und Psychose [German: The loss of reality in neurosis and psychosis]. In: A. Mitscherlich, A. Richards, J. Strachey (eds.), Sigmund Freud-Studienausgabe, Bd. III: Psychologie des Unbewußten. Frankfurt am Main, Germany: Fischer, pp. 355-361.

Freud, S. (1990). Die Traumdeutung [German: The Interpretation of Dreams]. Frankfurt am Main, Germany: Fischer.

Freudenmann, R. W., Öxler, F., Bernschneider–Reif, S. (2006). The origin of MDMA (ecstasy) revisited: the true story reconstructed from the original documents. Addiction 101, 2006, pp. 1241-1245. DOI: 10.1111/j.1360-0443.2006.01511.x PMID 16911722

Furst, P. T. (1976). Hallucinogens and Culture. Novato, CA, USA: Chandler & Sharp.

Gable, R. S. (2006). Risk assessment of ritual use of oral dimethyltryptamine (DMT) and harmala alkaloids. Addiction, 102, pp. 24-34, DOI: 10.1111/j.1360-0443.2006.01652.x. Retrieved July 25, 2016, Web site: https://www.iceers.org/docs/science/ayahuasca/ayahuasca-paper-addiction-ja07.pdf

Gashemi, A., Zahediasl S. (2012). Normality Tests for Statistical Analysis: A Guide for Non-Statisticians. International Journal of Endocrinology and Metabolism. 2012 April; 10(2), pp. 486-489, DOI: 10.5812/ijem.3505. Retrieved July 27, 2016, Web site: http://www.ncbi.nlm.nih.gov/pmc/articles/PMC3693611/

Garratt, A., Schmidt, L., Mackintosh, A., & Fitzpatrick, R. (2002). Quality of life measurement: bibliographic study of patient assessed health outcome measures. BMJ: British Medical Journal, 324(7351), p. 1417.

Gasser, P. (1996). Die psycholytische Psychotherapie in der Schweiz von 1988-1993. Eine katamnestische Erhebung [German: Psycholytic psychotherapy in Switzerland from 1988-1993. A catamnestic survey]. Schweizer Archiv für Neurologie und Psychiatrie 147(2)96. Bern, Switzerland: Verlag Bäbler.

Gasser, P. (2008). Über verschiedene therapeutische Rollen bei der Arbeit mit psychoaktiven Substanzen [German: On various therapeutic roles in working with psychoactive substances]. In H. Jungaberle, P. Gasser, J. Weinhold, R. Verres (2008), Therapie mit psychoaktiven Substanzen, Praxis und Kritik der Psychotherapie mit LSD, Psilocybin und MDMA. Bern, Switzerland: Hogrefe.

Gasser, P., Holstein, D., Michel, Y., Dolbin, R., Yazar-Klosinski, Passie, T. Brenneisen, R. (2014a). Safety and Efficacy of Lysergic Acid Diethylamide-Assisted Psychotherapy for Anxiety Associated With Life-threatening Diseases. The journal of nervous and mental diseases. volume 00, number00, month 2014. Retrieved November 13, 2016, Web site: http://journals.lww.com/jonmd/Documents/90000000.0-00001.pdf

Gasser, A., Kirchner, K, Passie, T. (2014b). LSD-assisted psychotherapy for anxiety associated with a life-threatening disease: A qualitative study of acute and sustained subjective effects. Journal of Psychopharmacology 2015 Jan;29(1), pp. 57-68, DOI: 10.1177/0269881114555249.

Gastelumendi Dargent, E. (2017). Personal communication. June 19, 2017. Lima, Peru.

Gebhardt, W. (2010). Flüchtige Gemeinschaften: Eine kleine Theorie situativer Event-Vergemeinschaftung [German: Volatile communities: a small theory of situational event communitization]. In D. Lüddeckens, R. Walthert (eds.), Fluide Religion, Neue religiöse Bewegungen im Wandel, Theoretische und empirische Systematisierungen. Bielefeld, Germany: transcript Verlag, pp. 175-188.

Geyer, S. (1997). Some conceptual considerations on the sense of coherence. Social Science & Medicine, 44(12), pp. 1771-1779. Retrieved January 12, 2017, Web site: https://www.sciencedirect.com/science/article/pii/S0277953696002869

Gillin, J. C., Cannon, E., Magyar, R., Schwartz, M., Wyatt, R. J. (1973). Failure of N-N-dimethyltryptamine to evoke tolerance in cats. Biological Psychiatry, 7: 213-220.

Gillin, J. S., Kaplan, J., Stillman, R., Wyatt, R. J. (1976). The psychedelic model of schizophrenia: the case of N,N-dimethyltryptamine. Am J Psychiatry 1976; 133, pp. 203-8.

Gisinger, C. (2007). Seelsorge und Spiritualität bei Krankheit und Pflege [German: Pastoral care and spirituality in sickness and care]. Österreichische Ärztezeitung 15/16, pp. 28-29.

Gläser, J., Laudel, G. (2010). Experteninterviews und qualitative Inhaltsanalyse. Wiesbaden, Germany: VS Verlag Springer, pp. 95-102.

Glaser, B. C., Strauss, A. L. (1998). Grounded Theory. Strategien Qualitativer Forschung. Bern, Switzerland: Huber, pp. 51-83.

Goeldner, Ch. R., Brent Ritchie, J. R. (2003). Tourism, Principles, Practices and Philosophies. Newjersey, USA: John Wiley & Sons. Retrieved August 18, 2016, Web site: https://archive.org/stream/TourismPrinciplesPracticesAndPhilosophies/TourismConceptPrinciplesPractices_djvu.txt

Golden, C. J. (1978). Stroop color and word test. A manual for clinical and experimental uses. Illinois, USA: Stoelting Co, Wood Dale.

Goldscheider. (1892). Freiherr von Schrenck-Notzing: Die Bedeutung narkotischer Mittel für den Hypnotismus mit besonderer Berücksichtigung des indischen Hanfs [German: Baron von Schrenck-Notzing: The importance of narcotic remedies for hypnotism with special consideration of Indian hemp]. Schriften der Gesellschaft für psychol. Forschung, 1891(1), pp. 1-73.

Gomes, M. M., Coimbra, J. B., Clara, R. O., Dörr, F. A., Moreno, A. C., Chagas, J. R., Tufik, S., Pinto, E. Jr., Catalani, L. H., Campa, A. (2014). Biosynthesis of N,N-dimethyltryptamine (DMT) in a melanoma cell line and its metabolization by peroxidases. Biochemical Pharmacology 88(3), pp. 393-401, DOI: 10.1016/j.bcp.2014.01.035. PMID 24508833.

Grawe, K. (1995). Grundriss einer Allgemeinen Psychotherapie [German: Ground plan of a general psychotherapy]. Psychotherapeut, 40, pp. 130-145.

Greenwood, D. J. (1977). Culture by the Pound: an Anthropological Perspective on Tourism as Cultural Commoditization. In V. L. Smith (Ed.), Hosts and Guests: the Anthropology of Tourism. 1989. USA: University of Pennsylvania Press, p. 137.

Greif, S. (1991). Streß in der Arbeit – Einführung und Grundbegriffe [German: Stress at work – Introduction and basic terms]. In S. Greif, N. Semmer, E. Bamberg (eds.), Psychischer Streß am Arbeitsplatz. Göttingen, Germany: Hogrefe. In Udris, I., Frese, M. (1999). Belastung und Beanspruchung. In C. Hoyos, D. Frey, (eds.), Arbeits- und Organisationspsychologie. Weinheim, Germany: Beltz, pp. 429-445.

Griffiths, R. R., Richards, W. A., McCann, U., Jesse, R. (2006). Psilocybin can occasion mystical-type experiences having substantial and sustained personal meaning and spiritual significance. Psychopharmacology 187. pp. 268-283. DOI: 10.1007/s00213-006-0457-5. Retrieved August 24, 2016, Web site: https://www.hopkinsmedicine.org/Press_releases/2006/GriffithsPsilocybin.pdf

Grob, C. S. (1994). Psychiatric research with hallucinogens: What have we learned?. Yearbook for Ethnomedicine and the Study of Consciousness, Issue 3. VWB – Verlag für Wissenschaft und Bidung.

Grob, C. S., Bravo, G. L. (1996). Human research with hallucinogens: Past lessons and current trends. In M. J. Winkelman & W. Andritzky (eds.), Jahrbuch für transkulturelle Medizin und Psychotherapie 1995 (Vol. 6), pp. 129-142. Berlin, Germany: Verlag für Wissenschaft und Bildung.

Grob, C. S., McKenna, D. J., Callaway, J. C., Brito, G. S., Neves, E. S., Overlaender, G., Salde, O. L., Lablgalini, E., Tacia, C., Miranda, C. T., Strassman, R. J., Boone, K. B. (1996). Human psychopharmacology of Hoasca: A plant hallucinogen used in ritual context in Brazil. The Journal of Nervous and Mental Disease, 184(2), pp. 86-94, DOI: 10.1097/00005053-199602000-00004.

Groeben, N., Wahl, D., Schlee, J., Scheele, B. (1988). Das Forschungsprogramm Subjektive Theorien. Eine Einführung in die Psychologie des reflexiven Subjekts [German: The research program Subjective Theories. An introduction to the psychology of the reflexive subject]. Tübingen, Germany: Francke.

Grof, S. (1976). Realms of the Human Unconscious: Observations from LSD Research. New York, USA: Dutton

Grof, S. (1980). LSD-Psychotherapy. Pomona, CA, USA: Hunter House Publishers.

Groffman, E. (1959). The Presentation of Self in Everyday Life. New York, USA: Anchor Books. ISBN-13 978-0-14-013571-8

Grom, B. (2011) Spiritualität – die Kariere eines Begriffs: Eine religionspsychologische Perspektive. In E. Frick, T. Roser (eds.), Spiritualität und Medizin: Gemeinsame Sorge für den kranken Menschen. Germany: Kohlhammer, pp. 12-17.

Grunwell. J. N. (1998). Ayahuascatourism in South America. MAPS Buletin 8(3), pp. 59-62.

Guzman, G., Allen, J. W., Gartz, J. (1998). A worldwide geographical distribution of the neurotropic fungi, an analysis and discussion. Ann. Mus. Civ. Rovereto 14, pp. 189-280.

Halberstadt, A. L. (2016). Behavioral and pharmacokinetic interactions between monoamine oxidase inhibitors and the hallucinogen 5-methoxy-N,N-dimethyltryptamine. Pharmacol Biochem Behav. 2016 Apr; 143, pp. 1-10, DOI:10.1016/j.pbb.2016.01.005.

Halifax, J. (1979). Shamanic voices - a survey of visionary narratives. New York: Dutton.

Halpern, J. H., Sherwood, A. R., Hudson, J. I., Yurgelun-Todd, D., Pope, H. G. Jr (2005). Psychological and cognitive effects of long-term peyote use among Native Americans. Biol Psychiatry. 58(8), pp. 624-631, DOI: 10.1016/j.biopsych.2005.06.038.

Halpern, J. H., Sherwood, A.R., Passie, T., Blackwell, K. C., & Ruttenber, A. J. (2008). Evidence of health and safety in American members of a religion who use a hallucinogenic sacrament. Medical Science Monitor, 14(8), pp. 15-22.

Harner, M. (1990). The Way of the Shaman. New York, USA: HarperOne. ISBN: 0-062-50373-1.

Hausner, M., Segal, E. (2009). LSD: the highway to mental health. Malibu, CA, USA: ASC Books.

Havelock, E. (1897). Mescal. A new artificial paradise. Ann. Rep. Smithsonian Institute, 1897, I, 537. In Smythies, J. (1953). The mescaline phenomena. The British Journal for the Philosophy of Science 3(12), pp. 339-347.

Heider, F. (1958). The psychology of interpersonal relations. New York, USA: Wiley & Sons.

Heinz, W. (2000). Selbstsozialisation im Lebenslauf: Umrisse einer Therapie biografischen Handelns. In E. Hoernig (ed.), Biografische Sozialisation. Stuttgart, Germany: Lucius & Lucius, pp. 165-186. In A. Witzel (2010), Längsschnittdesign. In G. Mey, K. Mruck (eds.), Handbuch Qualitative Forschung in der Psychologie. Wiesbaden, Germany: VS Verlag. p. 291.

Helfferlich, C. (2011). Die Qualität qualitativer Daten, Manual für die Durchführung qualitativer Interviews. Wiesbaden [German: The quality of qualitative data, manual for conducting qualitative interviews]. Wiesbaden: Germany: VS Verlag.

Hendricks, P. S. (2014). Back to the future: A return to psychedelic treatment models for addiction. Journal of Psychopharmacology 28(11), pp. 981-982, https://DOI.org/10.1177/0269881114550935

Herbert, A. (2010). Female Ayahuasca Healers Among the Shipibo-Konibo (Ucayali- Peru) in the Context of Spiritual Tourism. Núcleo de Estudos Interdisciplinares sobre Psicoativos, NEIP. Retrieved August 19, 2016, Web site: http://neip.info/novo/wp-content/uploads/2015/04/herbert_female_ ayahuasca_healers_shipibo_spiritual_tourism.pdf

Hermle, L. (2008). Risiken und Nebenwirkungen von LSD, Psilocybin und MDMA in der Psychotherapie. In H. Jungaberle, P. Gasser, J. Weinhold, R. Verres (eds.), Therapie mit psychoaktiven Substanzen. Bern, Switzerland: Huber, pp. 147-164

Herzlich, C. (1973). Health and illness. A social psychology analysis. European monographs in social psychology 5. European Association of Experimental Social Psychology by Academic Press. London. In Burkert, S., Knoll, N., Daig, I. (2012). Laienätiologie, subjektive Krankheits- und Gesundheitstheorien. In E. Brähler, B.Strauß (eds.), Grundlagen der Medizinischen Psychologie. Göttingen, Germany: Hogreve Verlag, p. 389. ISBN: 9783840905773

Hess, P. (2008). Bedeutung und Variationen des Settings in der Substanz-unterstützten Psychotherapie [German: Meaning and variations of the setting in substance-assisted psychotherapy]. In H. Jungaberle, P. Gasser, J. Weinhold, R. Verres, (eds.), Therapie mit psychoaktiven Substanzen: Praxis und Kritik der Psychotherapie mit LSD, Psilocybin und MDMA. Bern, Switzerland: Huber.

Hessel, A., Schumacher, J., Geyer, M., Brähler, E. (2001). Symptom-Check-Liste SCL-90-R: Testtheoretische Überprüfung und Normierung an einer bevölkerungsrepräsentativen Stichprobe. Diagnostica 2001;47, pp. 27-39.

Hoffer, A., Osmond, H. (1967). The hallucinogens. New York, NY: Academic Press.

Highpine, G. (2012). Unreveling the mystery of the orign of ayahuasca. Núcleo de Estudos Interdisciplinares sobre Psicoativos, NEIP. Retrieved may 20, 2016, Web site: http://neip.info/novo/wp-content/uploads/2015/04/ highpine_origin-of-ayahuasca_neip_2012.pdf

Hochstein F. A., Paradies A. M. (1957). Alkaloids of Banisteria caapi and Prestonia amazonicum. Journal of the American Chemical Society 79(21), pp. 5735-36, DOI: 10.1021/ja01578a041.

Hoffer, A. (1967). A Program for the Treatment of Alcoholism: LSD, Malvaria and Nicotinic Acid. In: H. A. Abramson (Ed.), The Use of LSD in Psychotherapy and Alcoholism. Indianapolis, New York, Kansas City, USA: Bobbs Merill, pp.343-406.

Hofmann, A. (2001). LSD – Mein Sorgenkind, die Entdeckung einer Winderdroge. [German: LSD - My problem child, the discovery of a miracle drug]. München, Germany: DTV.

Holman, Ch. L. (2010). Spirituality for Sale. An Analysis of Ayahuasca Tourism. Doctoral dissertation. USA: Arizona State University.
Holman, Ch. L. (2011). Surfing for a Shaman. Analyzing an Ayahuasca Website. Annals of Tourism Research 38(2011), pp. 90-109.
Holt, C. L., Clark, E. M., Kreuter, M. W., Rubio, D. (2003). Spiritual Health locus of control and cancer beliefs among urban African American women. Health Psychology. 22(3), pp. 294-9, DOI: 10.1037/0278-6133.22.3.294. PMID 12790257.
Horsley, J. S. (1943). Narco-analysis. Oxford, UK: Humphrey Milford.
Hudson, J. (2011). Ayahuasca and Globalization. Undergraduate Honors Theses. Retrieved September 15, 2016, Web site: http://scholar.colorado.edu/honr_theses/625
Hunt, L. (1991). Secret Agenda. The United States Government, Nazi Scientists, and Project Paperclip, 1945-1990. New York, USA: St. Martins Press.
Hunter, R. (1971). The storming of the mind. Toronto, Montreal, Canada: Doubleday.
Hurrelmann, K. (1983). Das Modell des produktiv realitätsverarbeitenden Subjekts in der Sozialisationsforschung. Zeitschrift für Sozialforschung und Erziehungssoziologie 3, pp. 91-103.
Incayawar, M. (2007). Indigenous peoples in South America – inequalities in mental health care. In K. Blui, D. Bhugra (eds.), Culture and Mental Health – A Comprehensive Textbook. London, UK: Holder Arnold. pp. 185-190.
Inquisition in Mexico (1620). Edict of Faith concerning the Illicit Use of Peyote. Archivo General de la Nación, Ramo de Inquisición, vol. 289, exp. 12. Quoted and translated into English in J. F. Chuchiak IV. (Ed.) The Inquisition in New Spain, 1536–1820: A Documentary History. 2012. Baltimore, MD, USA: Johns Hopkins University Press. pp. 107-121.
International Narcotics Control Board (1971). Convention on Psychotropic Substances, 1971. Retrieved Augunst 22, 2016, Web site: http://www.incb.org/documents/Psychotropics/conventions/convention_1971_en.pdf
International Narcotics Control Board (2015). List of Psychotropic Substances under International Control in accordance with the Convention on Psychotropic Substances of 1971. Retrieved Augunst 22, 2016, Web site: http://www.incb.org/documents/Psychotropics/greenlist/Green_list_ENG_2015_new.pdf
Jakobsen, M. D. (1999). Traditional and Contemporary Approaches to the Mastery of Spirits and Healing. New York, USA: Berghahn Books.
Jing, J., Sklar, G. E., Min Sen Oh, V., Chuen Li, S. (2008). Factors affecting therapeutic compliance: A review from the patient's perspective. Therapeutics and Clinical Risk Management, 4(1), pp. 269-286.

Johnson, F. G. (1969). LSD in the treatment of alcoholism. American Journal of Psychiatry, 126(4).
Joint Appendix, O Centro Espirita Beneficiente Uniao Do Vegetal et al. v. John Ashcroft, no. CV02-2323, on Writ of Certiorari to the US Court of Appeals for the 10th Circuit, New Mexico, 2002.
Jørgensen, C. R. (2004). Active ingredients in individual psychotherapy. Searching for common factors. Psychoanalytic Psychology, 21, pp. 516-540.
Jung, C.G. (1990). Traum und Traumdeutung. München, Germany: DTV.
Kahoe, R. (1974). Personality and achievement correlates of intrinsic and extrinsic religious orientations. Journal of Personality and Social Psychology. 29 (6), DOI: 10.1037/h0036222.
Kaluza, G. (1996). Gelassen und sicher im Stress. Psychologisches Programm zur Gesundheitsförderung (2. Aufl.). Berlin, Germany: Springer.
Kamppinen, M. (1989) Cognitive Systems and Cultural Models of Illness. A Study of Two Mestizo Peasant Communities of the Peruvian Amazon. Doctoral dissertation. FF Communications No. 244, Helsinki, Finland: Academia Scientiarum Fennica.
Kanner, A. D., Coyne, J. C. Schaefer, C., Lazarus, R. S. (1981). Comparison of two modes of stress management: daily hassles and uplift versus major life events. Journal of Behavior Medicine, 4, pp. 1-39.
Kärkkäinen, J.; Forsström, T.; Tornaeus, J.; Wähälä, K.; Kiuru, P.; Honkanen, A.; Stenman, U.-H.; Turpeinen, U.; Hesso, A. (2005). Potentially hallucinogenic 5-hydroxytryptamine receptor ligands bufotenine and dimethyltryptamine in blood and tissues. Scandinavian Journal of Clinical and Laboratory Investigation 65(3), pp. 189-199, DOI: 10.1080/00365510510013604. PMID 16095048.
Karp, D. A. (2017). Speaking of sadness: depression, disconnection, and the meanings of illness s. Oxford, UK: Oxford University Press.
Kaufmann, I., Pornschlegel, H., Udris, I. (1982). Arbeitsbelastung und Beanspruchung. In L. Zimmermann (Ed.), Humane Arbeit – Leitfaden für Arbeitnehmer, Band 5: Belastungen und Stress bei der Arbeit. Reinbek, Germany: Rowohlt, pp. 13-48.
Kavenská, V., Simonová, H., (2015). Ayahuasca Tourism: Participants in shamanic rituals and their personality styles, motivation, benefits and risks. J Psychoactive Drugs. 47, pp. 351–359, DOI: 10.1080/02791072.2015. 1094590
Kawulich, B. B. (2005). Participant Observation as a Data Collection Method. Forum Qualitative Sozialforschung / Forum: Qualitative Social Research, 6(2), Art. 43. Retrieved June 11, 2018, Web site: http://nbn-resolving.de/urn:nbn:de:0114-fqs0502430.

Kelle, U, Kluge, S. (1999). Vom Einzelfall zum Typus: Fallvergleich und Fallkontrastierung in der qualitativen Sozialforschung. In R. Bohnsack, Ch. Lüders, J. Reichertz (eds.). Qualitative Sozialforschung; Band 4. Wiesbaden, Germany: Springer Fachmedien, p. 54.

Kelly, G. A. (1955). The psychology of personal constructs. vol. I, II. New York, USA: Norton.

Kivimäki, M., Feldt, T., Vahtera, J., Nurmi, J. (2000). Sense of coherence and health: Evidence from two crosslagged longitudinal samples. Social Science & Medicine, vol. 50.

Kjellgren A., Eriksson A., Norlander, T. (2009). Experiences of Encounters with Ayahuasca - "The Vine of the Soul". Journal of psychoactive drugs, 2009, 41(4), pp. 309-315. ISSN: 0279-1072

Knauer, A., Maloney, W. J. (1913). A prelimnary note on the psychic action of mescaline, with special reference to the mechanism of visual hallucinations. Journal of Nervous and Mental Disease 40, pp. 425-436.

Knoblauch, H. (2010). Vom New Age zur populären Spiritualität. In D. Lüddeckens, R. Walthert (eds.). Fluide Religion, Neue religiöse Bewegungen im Wandel, Theoretische und empirische Systematisierungen. Bielefeld, Germany: transcript Verlag, pp. 175-188.

Knoll, N.; Scholz, U.; Rieckmann, N. (2005). Einführung in die Gesundheitspsychologie [German: Introduction to health psychology]. München, Germany: Ernst Reinhardt Verlag.

Koenig, H. G., King, D. E., Carson, C. B. (2012). Handbook of Religion and Health. UK: Oxford University Press, p.37.

Kohn, E. O. (1992). Some observations on the use of medicinal plants from primary and secondary growth by the Runa of eastern lowland Ecuador. Journal of Ethnobiology 12(1). pp. 141-152.

Konttinen, H., Haukkala, A. & Uutela, A. (2008). Comparing sense of coherence, depressive symptoms and anxiety, and their relationships with health in a population-based study. Social Science & Medicine (1982), 66(12).

Krebs, T. S., Johansen, P. O. (2012). Lysergic acid diethylamide (LSD) for alcoholism: Meta-analysis of randomized controlled trials. Psychopharmacology, 26(7), pp. 994-1002, DOI: 10.1177/0269881112439253.

Kristensen, K. (1998). The Ayahuasca Phenomenon: Jungle Pilgrims: North Americans Participating in Amazon Ayahuasca Ceremonies. MAPS. Retrieved October 5, 2016, Web site: http://www.maps.org/articles/5408-the-ayahuasca-phenomenon

Kurland, A. A., Grof, S., Pahnke, W. N., Goodman, L. E. (1973). Psychedelic Drug Assisted Psychotherapy. In Patients With Terminal Cancer. In I. K. Goldberger, S. Malit, A. H. Kutscher (eds.), Psychotheramacological

Agents for the Terminally Ill and Bereaved 1973. Columbia University Press, New York, NY, pp. 86-133.

Küsters, I. (2009). Narrative Interviews: Grundlagen und Anwendungen [German: narrative interviews. basics and applications]. Wiesbaden, Germany: VS Verlag für Sozialwissenschaften.

Labate, B. C., MacRae, E. (2010). Ayahuasca, ritual, and religion in Brasil. London, UK: Equinox.

Labate, B. C., Jungaberle, H. (eds.), (2011). The internationalizitation of ayahuasca. Zürich, Switzerland: LIT.

Labate, B. C., Pacheco, G. (2011). The Historical Origns of Santo Daime. In B.C. Labate, H. Jungaberle (eds.), The internationalizitation of Ayahuasca. Zürich, Switzerland: LIT Verlag.

Labate, B. C., Santos, B. C., Strassman, R., et al. (2013). Efectos de la afiliación al Santo Daime sobre la dependencia a sustancias [Spanish: Effects of Santo Daime affiliation on substance dependence]. In: B. C. Labate, J.C. Bouso (eds.), Ayahuasca y Salud. Barcelona, Spain: Los Libros de La Libre de Marzo.

Lademann-Priemer, G. (2000). Schamanismus. Internet article. Retrieved November 7, 2016, Web site: http://www.glaube-und-irrglaube.de/index2.htm

Landsverk, S. S., Kane, C. F. (1998). Antonovsky's sense of coherence: Theoretical basis of psychoeducation in schizophrenia. Issues in Mental Health Nursing, 19(5), pp. 419-431.

Langdon, E. J. (1986). Las clasificaciones del yagé dentro del grupo Siona. Etnobotánica, etnoquímica e historia. América Indígena 46(1). pp. 101-116.

Laplanche. J., Pontalis, J.-B. [1967] (1972). Das Vokabular der Psychoanalyse [German: Vocaburary of psychoanalysis]. Frankfurt am Main, Germany: Suhrkamp

Lazarus, R. S. (1974). Cognitive and coping processes in emotion. In B. Weiner (Ed.), Cognitive views of human motivation. New York, USA: Academic Press.

Lazarus, R. S. (1975). A cognitively oriented psychologist looks at biofeedback. American Psychologist 30, pp. 553-561.

Lazarus, R. S., Folkman, S. (1984). Stress, Appraisal and Coping. New York, USA: Springer.

Lazarus, R. S. (1990). Streß und Streßbewältigung – Ein Paradigma [German: Stress and stress coping: a paradigm]. In S.-H. Filipp (Ed.), Kritische Lebensereignisse. Weinheim, Germany: Beltz, Psychologie Verlags Union, pp. 198-229.

Lazarus, R. S. (1999). Stress and Emotion: A New Synthesis. New York, USA: Springer.

Leary, T. (1966). Programmed communication during experiences with DMT. Psychedelic Review, 8, pp. 83-95. Retrieved May 10, 2017, Web site: https://web.archive.org/web/20170107010902/http://deoxy.org/h_leary.htm

Lee, M., Shain, B. (1985). Acid Dreams: The complete social History of LSD. New York, Germany: Grove Weidenfeld.

Leitner, K., Lüders, E., Greiner, B., Ducki, A., Niedermeier, R., Volpert, W. (1993). Analyse psychischer Anforderungen und Belastungen in der Büroarbeit. Das RHIA/VERA-Büroverfahren. Handbuch – Manual und Arbeitsblätter [German: Analysis of mental demands and burdens in office work. The RHIA / VERA office procedure. Manual and Worksheets]. Göttingen: Hogrefe. In Udris, I., Frese, M. (1999). Belastung und Beanspruchung. In C. Hoyos, D. Frey, D. (eds.), Arbeits- und Organisationspsychologie. Weinheim, Germany: Beltz, p 431.

Leuner, H. (1959). Psychotherapie in Modellpsychosen [German: Psychotherapy in model psychoses]. In E. Speer (Ed.), Kritische Psychotherapie. München, Germany: J. F. Lehmanns Verlag, pp. 94-102.

Leuner, H. (1962). Die experimentelle Psychose: Ihre Psychopharmakologie, Phänomenologie und Dynamik in Beziehung zur Person [German: The experimental psychosis: psychopharmacology, phenomenology and dynamics in relation to the person]. Berlin, Germany: Springer.

Leuner, H. (1981). Halluzinogene: Psychische Grenzzustände in Forschung und Psychotherapie [German: Hallucinogens: Psychic limit states in research and psychotherapy]. Bern, Swizerland: Huber.

Leuner, H. (1987). Die psycholytische Therapie: Durch Halluzinogene unterstützte tiefenpsychologische Psychotherapie [German: Psycholytic therapy: deep psychology psychotherapy supported by hallucinogens]. In: A. Dittrich, C. Scharfetter, (eds.), Ethnopsychotherapie. Psychotherapie mittels aussergewöhnlicher Bewusstseinszustände in westlichen und indigenen Kulturen. Stuttgart, Germany: Enke, pp.151-161.

Lewin, K. (1911). Das Erhaltungsprinzip in der Psychologie [German: The conservation principle in psychology]. (Aus dem Nachlass). In A. Mertaux (Ed.), (1981), Kurt-Lewin-Werkausgabe vol 1. Bern, Swizerland: Huber, pp. 81-86

Lewin, K. (1926). Vorsatz, Wille und Bedürfnis. Untersuchungen zur Handlungs- und Affekt-Psychologie, I. Vorbemerkungen über die psychischen Kräfte und Energien und über die Strukturen der Seele [German: Intent, will and need. Investigations on action- and affect-psychology, I. Preliminary remarks on the psychic powers and energies and on the structures of the soul]. Zeitschrift Psychologische Forschung, 7, pp. 330-386.

Lewin, L. (1924). Phantastica, die betäubenden und erregenden Genussmittel [German: Phantastica, the numbing and exciting stimulants]. Berlin,

Germany: Verlag von Georg Stilke. Retrieved January 15, 2018, Web site: https://archive.org/details/b29822270

Lewin, L. (1929). Banisteria Caapi, ein neues Rauschgift und Heilmittel [German: Banisteria Caapi, a new drug and remedy]. Beitrag zur Giftkunde Heft 3. Berlin, Germany: Verlag von Georg Stilke.

Liester, M. B., Prickett, J. I. (2012). Hypotheses Regarding the Mechanisms of Ayahuasca in the Treatment of Addictions. Journal of Psychoactive Drugs 44(3), pp. 200-208.

Lindquist, G. (1997). Internalization: Core Shamanism. In: G. Lindquist. Shamanic Performance on the Urban Scene: Neo-Shamanism in Contemporary Sweden. Stockholm Studies in Social Anthropology. Stockholm, Sweden: Socialantropologiska institutionen, ISBN 91-7153-691-4.

Lindstrom, B., Eriksson, M. (2007). Antonovsky's sense of coherence scale and its rela on with quality of life: a systema c review. Journal of Epidemiology and Community Health, 61.

Loizaga-Velder, A., Loizaga Pazzi, A. (2014). The therapeutic value of ayahuasca for addiction treatment from psychotherapeutic perspective. In B. C. Labate, C. Cavnar (eds.), The therapeutic use of ayahuasca. Heidelberg, Germany: Springer, pp. 133-152.

Loizaga-Velder, A., Verres, R. (2014). Therapeutic effects of ritual ayahuasca use in the treatment of substance dependence - qualitative results. Journal of Psychoactive Drugs, 46(1), pp. 63-72, DOI: 10.1080/02791072.2013.873157

Losonczy, A.-M., Mesturini, S. (2010). La Selva Viajera: Rutas del chamanismo ayahuasquero entre Europa y América. [Portuguese: The travelling Jungle: Routes of ayahuasquero shamanism between Europe and America]. Religião & Sociedade, 30(2), pp. 164-183. Retrieved January 6, 2015, DOI: 10.1590/S0100-85872010000200009, Retrieved January 10, 2015, Web site: http://www.scielo.br/scielo.php?script=sci_arttext&pid=S0100-85872010000200009&lng=es&tlng=es

Löwer, W. (2011). Freiheit in Forschung und Lehre. In D. Merten, H.-J. Papier (eds.), Handbuch der Grundrechte in Deutschland und Europa. Band IV Grundrechte in Deutschland: Einzelgrundrechte I. Heidelberg, Germany: C. F. Müller Verlag, p. 729.

Lichtenberg, J. D. Lachmann, F. M., Fosshage, J. L. (2016 [2009]). The interpretative Sequence. In Self and Motivational Systems: Towards A Theory of Psychoanalytic Technique. NY, USA: Routledge, pp. 96-121.

Lifton, R. J. (1988). Ärzte im dritten Reich. Stuttgart: Klett-Cotta.

Lüddeckens, D., Walthert, R. (2010). Fluide Religion, Neue religiöse Bewegungen im Wandel, Theoretische und empirische Systematisierungen [German: Fluide Religion, New Religious Movements in Transition, Theoretical and

Empirical Systematizations]. Bielefeld, Germany: transcript Verlag, ISBN: 978-3-8376-1250-9

Ludwig, A. M., Levine, J., Stark, L., Lazar, R. (1969). A clinical study of LSD treatment in alcoholism. American Journal of Psychiatry, 126(1).

Luna, L. E. (1984). The concept of plants as teachers among four mestizo shamans of Iquitos, northeast Peru. Journal of Ethnopharmacology 11(2), pp. 123-133.

Luna, L. E. (1986a). Apéndices. América Indígena 46(1), pp. 241-251.

Luna, L. E. (1986b). Vegetalismo: Shamanism among the Mestizo Population of the Peruvian Amazonas. Acta Universitatis Stockholmensis, Stockholm Studies in Comparative Religion. No. 27. Stockholm, Sweden: Almquist and Wiksell International.

Luna, L. E., Amaringo, P. (1999). Ayahuasca Visions: The Religious Iconography of a Peruvian Shaman. Berkley, USA: North Atlantic Books.

Luna, L. E. (2003). Ayahuasca: Shamanism Shared Across Cultures. Cultural Survival Quarterly 27(2), pp. 20-23. retrieved August 18, 2016, Web site: https://www.culturalsurvival.org/publications/cultural-survival-quarterly/ayahuasca-shamanism-shared-across-cultures.

Luna, L. E. (2004). Ayahuasca Ritual Use. In E.J. Neumann Fridman, M. N. Walters, (eds.), Shamanism: An Encyclopedia of World Beliefs, Practices and Cultures. Santa Barbara, Denver, Oxford: ABC-CLIO, pp. 378-382.

Luna, L. E. (2006). Traditional and syncretic Ayahuasca rituals. In H. Jungaberle, R. Verres, F. DuBois (eds.), Rituale erneuern. Giessen, Germany: Psychosozial Verlag, pp. 319-337.

Luna, L. E. (2010). Ayahuasca and the Concept of Reality. Ethnographic, Theoretical, and Experimental Considerations. In R. Ascott, Garvik & Jahrman (eds.), Making Reality Really Real. Consciousness Reframed. Trondheim, Norway: TEKS Publishing. retrieved August 17, 2016, Web site: http://www.wasiwaska.org/research/wasi-research/article-1.

Lundberg, O., Nyström, P. (1994). Sense of coherence, social structure and health: Evidence from a population survey in Sweden. European Journal of Public Health, Vol. 4(4), pp. 252-257, https://DOI.org/10.1093/eurpub/4.4.252

Mabberley, D. J. (1997). A Portable Dictionary of the Higher Plants. Cambridge, UK: Cambridge Univ. Press. The Plant Book, p. 858.

MacCannell, D. (1973). Staged Authenticity: Arrangements of Social Space in Tourist Settings. American Journal of Sociology, 79(3), pp. 589-603. Retrieved July 7, 2017, Web site: http://www.jstor.org/stable/2776259

MacDonald, D. C., LeClair, L., Holland, C. J., et al. (1995). A survey of measures of transpersonal constructs. Journal of Trancepersonal Psychology 27, pp. 171-235.

MacLean, J., MacDonald, D., Byrne, U., Hubbard, A. (1961). The use of LSD-25 in the treatment of alcoholism and other psychiatric problems. Quarterly Journal of Studies on Alcohol, 22.

MacLean, K. A., Johnson, M. W., Griffiths, R. R. (2011). Mystical experiences occasioned by the hallucinogen psilocybin lead to increases in the personality domain of openness. Journal of Pychopharmacology 25(11), pp. 1453-1461, DOI: 10.1177/0269881111420188

Masters, R., Houston, J. (2001 [1966]). The Varieties of Psychedelic Experience. Rochester, Vermont: Park Street Press [Dell Publishing].

Marais, A., Stuart, A. D. (2005). The role of temperament in the development of post- traumatic stress disorder amongst journalists. South African Journal of Psychology, 35(1).

Martin, W. R., Sloan, J. W., Sapira, J. D., Jasinski, D. R. (1971). Physiologic, subjective, and behavioral effects of amphetamine, methamphetamine, ephedrine, phenmetrazine, and methylphenidate in man. Clin Pharmacol Ther. 1971;12, pp. 245-58. PMID: 5554941

Mattila, A. (2001). Seeing Things in a New Light" – Reframing in Therapeutic Conversation. Rehabilitation Foundation, Research Reports 67/2001. Helsinki, Finland: University Press. Retrieved November 2, 2018, Website: https://onlinelibrary.wiley.com/DOI/pdf/10.1046/j..1992.00449.x

Mayring, P. (2015). Qualitative Inhaltsanalyse. Grundlagen und Techniken. (12th rev. ed.). Weinheim, Germany: Beltz.

McGlothlin, W., Cohen, S., McGlothlin, M. S. (1967). Long Lasting Effects of LSD on Normals. Arch Gen Psychiatry. 1967;17(5), pp. 521-532, DOI: 10.1001/archpsyc.1967.01730290009002.

McKenna, D., Towers, G., and Abbott, F. (1984). Monoamine-oxidase inhibitors in south-american hallucinogenic plants - tryptamine and beta-carboline constituents of ayahuasca. J Ethnopharmacol, 10(2), pp. 195-223, DOI: 10.1016/0378-8741(84)90003-5

McKenna, D. J., Towers, G. H. (1984). Biochemistry and pharmacology of tryptamines and beta-carbolines: A mini-review. Journal of Psychoactive Drug. 16(4), pp. 347-358. PMID: 6394730, DOI: 10.1080/02791072.1984.10472305

McKenna, D.J., Callaway, J.C., Grob, C. S. (1998). The scientific investigation of ayahuasca: a review of past and current research. The Heffter Review of Psychedelic Research, Vol 1, pp 65-77.

McKenna, D. J. (1999). Ayahuasca: An Ethnopharmacologic History. In R. Metzner (Ed.), Ayahuasca: Human Consciousness and the Spirit of Nature. New York: Thunder's Mouth Press.

McKenna, D. J. (2007). The healing vine: Ayahuasca as medicine in the 21st century. in M. J. Winkelman, T. B. Roberts (eds.), Psychedelic medicine:

New evidence for hallucinogenic substances as treatments (Vol. 1). Westport, CT, USA: Praeger, pp. 21-44.

McKenzie, K., Patel, V., Araya, R. (2004). Learning from low income countries: Mental health. British Medical Journal, 329 (7475), pp. 1138-40.

Manske, R. H. F. (1931). A Syntesis of the methyltryptamines and some derivates. Canadian Journal of Research, 1931, 5(5), pp. 592-600. DOI: 10.1139/cjr31-097

McKenna, D., Riba, J. (2015). New World Tryptamine Hallucinogens and the Neuroscience of Ayahuasca. Curr. Top. Behav. Neurosci. Advance online publication. DOI: 10.1007/7854_2015_368

Mello, S. M., Soubhia, P. Ch., Silveira, G., et al. (2018). Effect of Ritualistic Consumption of Ayahuasca on Hepatic Function in Chronic Users. Journal of psychoactive drugs, pp. 1-9, DOI: 10.1080/02791072.2018.1557355

Metzner, R. (1993). Letter from Ralph Metzner. Newsletter of the Multidisciplinary Association for Psychedelic Studies MAPS. 4(1), retrieved August 23, 2016, Web site: http://www.maps.org/news-letters/v04n1/04143met.html

Metzner, R. (1994). Therapeutische Anwendung veränderter Bewußtseinszustände [German: Thereapeutic use of altered states of consciousness]. In A. Dittrich (Ed.), Welten des Bewußtseins. Berlin, Germany: Verlag Wissenschaft und Bildung.

Mihaljevic, S., Aukst-Margetic, B., Karnicnik, S., Vuksan-Cusa, B., Milosevic, M. (2016). Do spirituality and religiousness differ with regard to personality and recovery from depression? A follow-up study. Compr Psychiatry. 2016 Oct;70, pp. 17-24, DOI: 10.1016/j.comppsych.2016.06.003.

Miller, H. (1987). How to Build a Magnet Church. Nashville, TN USA: Abingdon Press.

dimethyltryptamine (DMT) and harmala alkaloids. Addiction, 102, pp. 24-34, DOI: 10.1111/j.1360-0443.2006.01652.x. Retrieved July 25, 2016, Web site: https://www.iceers.org/docs/science/ayahuasca/ayahuasca-paper-addiction-ja07.pdf

Miller-Weisberger, J. S. (2000). A Huaorani myth of the first Miiyabu. In L. E. Luna, S. White (eds.), Ayahuasca reader: Encounters with the Amazon's Sacred Vine. Santa Fe: Synergetic Press.

Mitchell, S. W. (1896). Mescaline,' British Medical Journal. in Smythies, J. (1953). The mescaline phenomena. British Journal for the Philosophy of Science 3(12), pp. 339-347.

Mithoefer, M. C. (2008). MDMA bei der Behandlung posttraumatischer Belastungsstörungen (PTBS). In H. Jungaberle, P. Gasser, J. Weinhold, R. Verres (eds.), Therapie mit psychoaktiven Substanzen, Praxis und Kritik der Psychotherapie mit LSD, Psilocybin und MDMA. Bern, Switzerland: Hogrefe.

Mithoefer M. C., Wagner, M. T., Mithoefer, A. T., et al. (2010). The safety and efficacy of 3,4-methylenedioxymethamphetamine- assisted psychotherapy in subjects with chronic, treatment-resistant posttraumatic stress disorder: the first randomized controlled pilot study. J Psychopharmacology 0(0) 1-14, DOI: 10.1177/0269881110378371. Retrieved August 23, 2016, Web site: http://www.maps.org/research-archive/mdma/ptsdpaper.pdf

Mithoefer, M. C., Wagner, M. T., Mithoefer, A. T., et al. (2012). Durability of improvement in posttraumatic stress disorder symptoms and absence of harmful effects or drug dependency after 3,4-methylenedioxymethamphetamine-assisted psychotherapy: a prospective long-term follow-up study. J Psychopharmacol 0(0) 1-12, DOI: 10.1177/0269881112456611. Retrieved August 24, 2016, Web site: http://www.maps.org/research-archive/mdma/mithoefer_etal_2012_ltfu.pdf

Mithoefer, M. C. (2013). A Manual for MDMA-Assisted Psychotherapy in the Treatment of Posttraumatic Stress Disorder. Multidisciplinary Association for Psychedelic Studies (MAPS). Retrieved August 24, 2016, Web site: http://www.maps.org/research-archive/mdma/MDMA-Assisted_Psychotherapy_Treatment_Manual_Version_6_FINAL.pdf

Mittelmark, B, Sagy, S., Erikson, M., et al. (2017). Handbook of Salutogenesis. Switzerland: Springer, p. 268, DOI: 10.1007/978-3-319-04600-6

Morris, B. (2006). Neoshamanism. Religion and Anthroplogy, a critical introduction. Cambridge, UK: Cambridge University Press.

Mors, W. B., Ribeiro, O. (1957). Ocurrence of scopoletin in genus Brunfelsia. Journal of Organic Chemistry 22, pp. 978-979.

Narby, J., Huxley, F. (2001). Introduction: Five Hundred Years of Shamans and Shamanism. In J. Narby, F. Huxley (eds.). Shamans Through Time: 500 Years on the Path to Knowledge. London, UK: Thames & Hudson.

National Institute of Mental Health (2016). Schizophrenia. retrieved March 23, 2016, Web site: http://www.nimh.nih.gov/health/statistics/prevalence/schizophrenia.shtml.

Neuendorf, K. A. (2002). The content analysis guidebook. Thousand Oaks, CA, USA: Sage.

Neumeister, A., Normandin, M. D., Pietrzak, R. H., et al. (2013). Elevated brain cannabinoid CB1 receptor availability in post-traumatic stress disorder: A positron emission tomography study. Molecular Psychiatry, 18, pp. 1034-1040, DOI: 10.1038/mp.2013.61.

Nichols, D. (1986). Differences Between the Mechanism of Action of MDMA, MBDB, and the Classic Hallucinogens. Identification of a New Therapeutic Class: Entactogens. J. Psychoactive Drugs. 18(4), pp. 305-13. DOI:10.1080/02791072.1986.10472362.

Nichols, D., Yensen, R., Metzner, R. (1993). The Great Entactogen - Empathogen Debate. Newsletter of the Multidisciplinary Association for Psychedelic Studies MAPS. 4(2), pp. 47-49. Retrieved August 23, 2016, Web site: http://www.maps.org/news-letters/v04n2/04247eed.html.

Nimea Kaya Healing Center (2016). Ayahuasca Testimonial – Healing Physical Disease in the Body. Youtube. Retrieved October 2, 2018, Web site: https://www.youtube.com/watch?v=eGqd_NNq3Hw

Nour, M. M., Evans, L, Carhart-Harris, R. L. (2017). Psychedelics, Personality and Political Perspectives. Journal of Psychoactive Drugs 49(3), pp. 182-191.

Ogalde, J. P. Arriaza, B. T., Soto, E. C. (2009): Identification of psychoactive alkaloids in ancient Andean human hair by gas chromatography/mass spectrometry. Journal of Archaeological Science, 36(2), pp. 467-472. Retrieved May 17, 2016, Web site: http://www.unap.cl/docs/quimicafarmacia/2009/3.pdf. In Beyer, S. V. (2012). On the Origins of Ayahuasca. Online article retrieved May 17, 2016, Web site: http://www.singingtotheplants.com/2012/04/on-origins-of-ayahuasca/

Osório, Fde L., Sanches R. F., Macedo, L. R., et al. (2015). Antidepressant effects of a single dose of ayahuasca in patients with recurrent depression: a preliminary report. Revista Brasileira psicuiatria. Jan-Mar;37(1), pp. 13-20, DOI: 10.1590/1516-4446-2014-1496.

Ott, J. (1994). Ayahuasca Analogues: Pangæan Entheogens (1st ed.). Kennewick, WA, USA: Natural Products, pp. 81-3. ISBN 978-0-9614234-5-2.

Ott, J. (1996). Pharmacotheon, Entheogenic drugs, their plant sources and history. Kennewick, WA, USA: Natural Products, pp. 174-176.

Ott, J. (1998). Pharmahuasca, anahuasca and vinho da jurema: human pharmacology of oral DMT plus harmine. In Müller-Ebeling, C. Special: Psychoactivity. Yearbook for Ethnomedicine and the Study of Consciousness. 6/7 (1997/1998). Berlin, Germany: VWB. ISBN 3-86135-033-5

Ott, J. (2011). Psychonautic Uses of „Ayahuasca" and its Analogues. in B.C. Labate, H. Jungaberle (eds.), The Internationalization of Ayahuasca. Zürich, Switzerland: LIT.

Pachter, I. J, Zacharias, D.E, Ribeir, O. (1959). Indole Alkaloids of Acer saccharinum (the Silver Maple), Dictyoloma incanescens, Piptadenia colubrina, and Mimosa hostilis. J. Org. Chem. 24, pp. 1285-7.

Pallant, J. F., Lae, L. (2002). Sense of coherence, well-being, coping and personality factors: Further evaluation of the sense of coherence scale. Personality and Individual Differences, 33(1).

Palhano-Fontes, F., Andrade, K. C., Tofoli, L. F., Santos, A. C., Crippa, J. A. S., Hallak, J. E. C., de Araujo, D. B. (2015). The Psychedelic State Induced by

Ayahuasca Modulates the Activity and Connectivity of the Default Mode Network. PLoS ONE, 10(2), e0118143. Retrieved August 13, 2016, Web site: http://DOI.org/10.1371/journal.pone.0118143

Passie, T. (1996/97). Hanscarl Leuner: pioneer of hallucinogen research and psycholytic therapy. Multidisciplinary Association for Psychedelic Studies Bulletin 7(1) (1997), pp. 46-49.

Passie, T. (2006). Psychische Wirkungen von Halluzinogenen. Objektive und subjektive Perspektiven. in Emrich, H. M. & U. Schneider, U. (Ed.). Facetten der Sucht. Stuttgart, Leipzig: Peter Lang.

Passie, T., Halpern, J. H., Stichtenoth, D. O., Emrich, H. M., Hintzen, A. (2008). The Pharmacology of Lysergic Acid Diethylamide: A Review. CNSNeuroscience & Therapeutics 14(2008), pp. 295-314, DOI: 10.1111/j.1755-5949.2008.00059.x. Retrieved August 22, 2016, Web site: http://www.maps.org/research-achive/w3pb/2008/2008_Passie_23067_1.pdf

Passie, T. (2012). Healing with Entactogens – Therapist and Patient Perspectives on MDMA-Assisted Group Psychotherapy. Santa Cruz, CA: MAPS, p. 64.

Passie, T., Emrich, H. M., Brandt, S. D., Halpern, J. H. (2012). Mitigation of post-traumatic stress symptoms by Cannabis resin: A review of the clinical and neurobiological evidence. Drug Testing and Analysis, 4, pp. 649-659. DOI: 10.1002/dta.1377.

Patiño, V. M. (1968). Guayusa, a neglected stimulant from eastern Andean foothills. Economic Botany 22(3). pp. 310-316.

Patton, M. Q. (2002). Qualitative evaluation and research methods (3rd ed.). Thousand Oaks, CA: Sage Publications, Inc.

Pawlowsky, G. (2009). Alloplastisch/autoplastisch. In G. Stumm, A. Pritz (eds.), Wörterbuch der Psychotherapie. Wien, Austria: Springer.

Pearce, P. (1988). The Ulysses factor: Evaluing Visitors in Tourist Settings. New York, USA: Springer. Mentioned in Vester H.-G. (1993). Authentizität. In H. Hahn, H.-J. Kagelmann (eds.). Tourismuspsychologie und Tourismussoziologie: Ein Handbuch zur Tourismuswissenschaft, München, Germany, p. 122-124.

Pedrero-Pérez, E. J. (2006). Diferencias de personalidad entre adictos a sustancias y población general. Estudio con el TCI-R de casos clínicos con controles emparejados. Adicciones 18, pp. 135-148.

Peluso, D. M., Alexiades, M. N. (2006). For Export Only: Ayahuasca Tourism and Hyper-Traditionalism. Traditional Dwellings and Settlements Review: Hypertraditions. Journal of the International Association for the study of Traditional Environments. TDSR Vol. XVIII, No 1, pp. 73-74.

Peruecologico (2016). Toé. Retrieved July 20, 2016, Web site: http://www.peruecologico.com.pe/med_toe.htm

Petrie, K., Brook, R. (1992). Sense of coherence, self-esteem, depression and hopelessness as correlates of reattempting suicide. British Journal of Clinical Psychology, 31(3).

Pfitzner, F. (2008). Amazonische Heilkunde in der Behandlung der Drogensucht. Eine explorative Studie. Saarbrücken, Germany: VDM Verlag.

Piedmont, R. L. (1999). Does spirituality represent the sixth factor of personality? Spiritual transcendence and the Five-Factor Model. Journal of Personality, 67(6), pp. 985-1013. http://dx.DOI.org/10.1111/1467-6494.00080

Piron, H. (2003). Meditation und ihre Bedeutung für die seelische Gesundheit. Oldenburg, Germany: BIS-Verlag 2003: pp. 198-356.

Plowmann, T. C. (1977). Brunfelsia in ethnomedicine. Botanical Museum Leaflets. Harvard University 25(10), pp. 289-320.

Poisson J. (1965). Note sur le "Natem", boisson toxique péruvienne et ses alcaloïdes [Note on "Natem", a toxic Peruvian beverage, and its alkaloids]. Annales Pharmaceutiques Françaises, 23, pp. 241–4. ISSN 0003-4509. PMID 14337385.

Polewka, A., Chrostek-Maj, J., Kroch, S., Mikołaszek-Boba, M., Ryn, E., Datka, W., Rachel, W. (2001). The sense of coherence and risk of suicide attempt. Przeglad Lekarski, 58(4).

Presser-Velder, A. (2012). Treating substance dependencies with psychoactives: A theoretical and qualitative empirical study on the therapeutic use of ayahuasca. Dissertation, Ruprecht-Karls-University, Heidelberg, Germany.

Raup, J., Vogelsang, J., (2009). Medienresonanzanalyse, Eine Einführung in Theorie und Praxis. [German: Media Resonance Analysis, An Introduction to Theory and Practice]. Wiesbaden, Germany: VS Verlag für Sozialwissenschaften. ISBN: 978-3-531-16000-9

Reichel-Dolmatoff, G. (1972). The cultural context of an aboriginal hallucinogen: Banisteriopsis Caapi. In P. Furst (Ed.), Flesh of the Gods – The Ritual Use of Hallucinogens. Prospect Heights, IL, USA: Waveland Press. In Metzner R.. Ayahuasca: Human Consciousness and the Spirit of Nature. New York: Thunder's Mouth Press, p. 11.

Reichel-Dolmatoff, G. (1975). The Shaman and the Jaguar: A Study of Narcotic Drugs among the Indians of Colombia. Philadelphia, USA: Temple University Press. Also in Schultes, R. E. (1978). El Chaman y el Jaguar: Estudio de las Drogas Narcoticas entre los Indios de Colombia. Mexico City: Siglo Veintiuno. pp. XI-XIV

Resolución Ministerial 836 del INC (2008). El peruano diario oficial. normas legales. Retrieved August 19, 2016, Web site: http://www.sunat.gob.pe/legislacion/nor_graf/2008/julio/nl20080712.pdf

Riba, J., Rodriguez-Fornells, A., Urbano, G., Morte, A., Antonijoan, R., Montero, M., Callaway, J. C., Barbanoj, M. J. (2001). Subjective effects and tolerability of the south american psychoactive beverage ayahuasca in healthy volunteers. Psychopharmacology (Berl), 154(1), pp. 85-95. PMID: 11292011.

Riba, J. (2003). Human Pharmacology of Ayahuasca. dissertation, Barcelona, Spain: Autonomous University of Barcelona. Retrieved August 20, 2016, Web site: https://www.researchgate.net/publication/246400389_Human_Pharmacology_of_Ayahuasca.

Riba, J., Barbanoj, N. J. (2005). Bringing Ayahuasca to the clinical research laboratory. J. Psychoactive Drugs 2005, 37, p. 219.

Riba, J., Barbanoj, M. J. (2006). Ayahuasca. In J. C. Peris, J. C Zurián, G. C. Martínez, G. R. Valladolid (eds.), Tratado SET de Transtornos Adictivos. Madrid, Spain: Ed. Médica Panamericana.

Richter, P., Hacker, W. (1998). Belastung und Beanspruchung. Streß, Ermüdung und Burnout im Arbeitsleben [German: Load and stress. Stress, fatigue and burnout in working life]. Heildelberg: Asanger. In Udris, I., Frese, M. (1999). Belastung und Beanspruchung. In C. Hoyos, D. Frey, D. (eds.), Arbeits- und Organisationspsychologie. Weinheim: Beltz, p. 431.

Rivier, L., Lindgren, J.-E. (1972). Ayahuasca, the South American hallucinogenic drink: An ethnobotanical and chemical investigation. Economic Botany 26(1), pp. 101-129. In Ott, J. (1996). Pharmacotheon, Entheogenic drugs, their plant sources and history. Kennewick, WA, USA: Natural Products.

Rodd, R. (2002). Snuff synergy: Preparation, use and pharmacology of yopo and Banisteriopsis caapi among the Piaroa of southern Venezuela. Journal of Psychoactive Drugs 34(3), pp. 273-279.

Roitman, P., Mechoulam, R., Cooper-Kazaz, R., et al. (2014). Preliminary, open-label, pilot study of add-on oral Δ9-tetrahydrocannabinol in chronic posttraumatic stress disorder. Clinical Drug Investigation, 34, pp. 587-591, DOI: 10.1007/s40261-014-0212-3.

Roediger, E. (2011). Praxis der Schematherapie [German: Practice of Schema Therapy]. Stuttgart, Germany: Schattauer, p.67.

Roediger, E. (2015). Das Modus- bzw. Teilemodell [German: The model of modes and parts] Germany. Retrieved May 3, 2016, Web site: http://www.schematherapie-roediger.de/down/Modus%20Teilemodell.pdf

Rogers C. R. (1965). Client Centered Therapy. New York, USA: Houghton Mifflin.

Rosengarten, H., Friedhoff, A. J. (1976). "A review of recent studies of the biosynthesis and excretion of hallucinogens formed by methylation of neurotransmitters or related substances" (PDF). Schizophrenia Bulletin 2(1), pp. 90-105. DOI:10.1093/schbul/2.1.90. PMID 779022

Ross, S. (2012). Serotonergic hallucinogens and emerging targets for addiction pharmacotherapies. Psychiatric Clinics of North America, 35, pp. 357-374.
Roth, K.-H. (2000). Strukturen, Paradigmen und Mentalitäten in der luftfahrtmedizinischen Forschung des „dritten Reichs" 1933-1941: Der Weg ins Konzentrationslager Dachau [German: Structures, paradigms and mentalities in aviation medical research of the "Third Reich" 1933-1941: The road to the Dachau concentration camp]. 1999 - Zeitschrift für Sozialgeschichte des 20. Jahrhunderts 15, pp. 49–77.
Rotter, J. B. (1966). Generalized expectancies of internal versus external control of reinforcements. Psychological Monographs. 80(609), DOI: 10.1037/h0092976.
Rouhier A. (1927). Le Peyotl – La Plante Qui Fait Les Yeux Émerveillés [French: The Peyote - the plant that makes the eyes wonder]. Paris, France: Gaston DOIn.
Rush, B. (2015). May 2015. The Effectiveness of Ayahuasca for the Treatment of Addictions in Latin America: Ayahuasca Treatment Outcome Project. Unpublished ATOP report from May 2015.
Ruf, M., Schauer, M. (2012). Facing childhood trauma. Narrative Exposure Therapy within a Cascade Model of Care. In: J. Murray (Ed.), Exposure Therapy. New Developments. New York, USA: Nova Science Publishers, pp. 229–261.
Russo, E. B. (1992). Headache treatment by native peoples of the Ecuadorian Amazon: A preliminary cross-disciplinary assessment. Journal of Ethnopharmacology 36(3), pp. 193-206.
Sanchez-Ramos, J. R. (1991). Banisterine and Parkinson's disease. Clin Neuropharmacol. 1991 Oct;14(5), pp. 391-402. PMID: 1742748.
Sandison, R. (1954): Psychological Aspects of the LSD Treatment of Neurosis. Journal of Mental Science 100, pp. 508-518.
Santos, R. G., Landeira-Fernandez, J., Strassman, R. J., et al. (2007). Effects of ayahuasca on psychometric measures of anxiety, panic-like and hopelessness in Santo Daime members. J Ethnopharmacol 112, pp. 507-513. Retrieved June 5, 2016, Web site: http://www.maps.org/images/pdf/ayahuasca-jep.pdf
Saum-Aldehoff, T., Trebes, S. (1994). Psychotherapie mit einer Modedroge [German: psychotherapy with a fashon drug]. Psychologie heute, 21, pp. 56-61.
Schenberg, E. E. (2013). Ayahuasca and cancer treatment. SAGE Open Medicine, 1, 2050312113508389. Retrieved October 2, 2018, Web site: http://DOI.org/10.1177/2050312113508389
Schenberg, E. E., de Castro Comis, M. A., Morel Alexandre, J. F., et al. (2017). Treating drug dependence with the aid of ibogaine: A qualitative study.

Journal of Psychedelic Studies 1(1), pp. 10-19, DOI: 10.1556/2054.01.2016. 002

Scheuch, K., Schröder, H. (1990). Mensch unter Belastung [German: Human under stress]. Berlin, Germany: Deutscher Verlag der Wissenschaften.

Schütz, A. (1971). Gesammelte Aufsätze [collected essays]. vol. 1. The Hague, Netherlands: Nijhoff.

Schmid, J. T. (2010). Selbst-Behandlungsversuche mit der psychoaktiven Substanz Ayahuasca: Eine qualitative Studie über subjektive Theorien zu Krankheit, Gesundheit und Heilung [German: Self-treatment experiments with the psychoactive substance ayahuasca: A Qualitative Study of Subjective Theories on Disease, Health, and Healing]. Doctoral dissertation. Saarbrücken, Germany: Südwestdeutscher Verlag für Hochschulschriften (SVH).

Schmid, J. T. (2014). Healing with Ayahuasca: Notes on Therapeutic Rituals and Effects in European Patients Treating Their Diseases. in B. C. Labate, C. Cavnar (eds.), The Therapeutic Use of Ayahuasca. Springer-Verlag Berlin, pp. 77-93.

Schonecke, O. W., Hermann, J. M. (1986). Psychophysiologie. Uexküll – Psychosomatische Medizin, chapter 8.3. München, Germany: Urban & Schwarzer, p. 151.

Schönpflug, W. (1987). Beanspruchung und Belastung bei der Arbeit – Konzepte und Theorien [German: Stress and strain at work - concepts and theories]. In U. Kleinbeck, J. Rutenfranz (eds.), Arbeitspsychologie. Enzyklopädie der Psychologie, Themenbereich D, Serie III, Band 1, p. 130-184. Göttingen, Germany: Hogrefe.

Schreier, M. (2012). Qualitative content analysis in practice. London, UK: Sage.

Schröder, H. (1996). Intervention zur Gesundheitsförderung für Klinik und Alltag [Intervention for the health improvement for clinic and everyday life]. Regensburg, Germany: Roderer

Schröder, H. (1997). Persönlichkeit, Ressourcen und Bewältigung [German: Personality, resources and coping]. In R. Schwarzer (Ed.), Gesundheitspsychologie, ein Lehrbuch. Göttingen, Germany: Hogrefe.

Schröder, H. (2008). Gesundheit. In H. Berth, F. Balck, E. Brähler (eds.), Medizinische Psychologie und Medizinische Soziologie von A bis Z.. Göttingen, Germany: Hogrefe.

Schultes, R. E. (1957). The identity of the malpighiaceous narcotics [sic] of South America. Botanical Museum Leaflets Harvard University 18(1), pp. 1-56. Reprinted in May 1968.

Schultes R. E., Raffauf R. F. (1960). Prestonia: An Amazon narcotic or not?. Botanical Museum Leaflets, Harvard University 19(5), pp. 109-122. ISSN 0006-8098.

Schultes, R. E. (1972). De plantis toxicariis e mundo novo tropicale commentationes XI.. The ethnotoxicological significance of additives to New World hallucinogens. Plant Science Bulletin 18, pp. 34-41.

Schultes, R. E. (1983). Richard Spruce: An early ethnobotanist and explorer of the northwest amazon and northern andes. J. Ethnobiol. 3(2), pp. 139-147. Retrieved August 10, 2016, Web site: https://ethnobiology.org/sites/default/files/pdfs/JoE/3-2/Schultes1983.pdf

Schultes, R. E., Hofmann, A. (1979). Plants of Gods: Origins of Hallucinogenic Use., New York, USA: McGraw-Hill.

Schultes, R. E., Hofmann, A. (1980). The Botany and Chemistry of Hallucinogens. Revised and enlarged second edition. Springfield, USA: Charles C. Thomas Pub Ltd.

Schultes, R. E., Raffauf, R. F. (1990). The Healing Forrest: Medicinal and Toxic Plants of the Northwest Amazonia. Historical, Ethno-& Economic Botany (Volume 2). Portland, USA: Dioscorides Press.

Schultes, R. E., Raffauf, R. F. (1992). Vine of the Soul: Medicine Men, their Plants and Rituals in the Colombian Amazon. Synergetic Press, Oracle.

Schütz, A. (1971). Begriffs- und Theoriebildung in den Sozialwissenschaften [German: concept and theory building in the social sciences]. In A. Schütz, Gesammelte Schriften Bd, I, pp. 55-76. Den Haag, Netherlands: Nijhoff.

Selye, H. (1946). The general adaptation syndrom and the disease of adaptation. Journal of clinical endocrinology. 6, pp. 117-230.

Selye, H. (1951). The General-Adaptation-Syndrome. Annual Review of Medicine. Vol. 2, p. 327, DOI: 10.1146/annurev.me.02.020151.001551. Retrieved May 24, 2016, Web site: https://www.annualreviews.org/doi/abs/10.1146/annurev.me.02.020151.001551

Selye, H. (1953). Einführung in die Lehre vom Adaptationssyndrom [German: Introduction to the theory of adaptation syndrome]. Stuttgart, Germany: Georg Thieme Verlag.

Selye, H. (1976). The stress of life. New York, USA: McGraw Hill.

Semmer, N. (1984). Streßbezogene Tätigkeitsanalyse [German: Stress related analysis of action]. Weinheim: Beltz. In Udris, I., Frese, M. (1999). Belastung und Beanspruchung. In C. Hoyos, D. Frey (eds.). Arbeits- und Organisationspsychologie. Weinheim, Germany: Beltz. p. 331.

Sessa, B., Nutt, D. (2015). The British Journal of Psychiatry Jan 2015, 206(1), pp. 4-6, DOI: 10.1192/bjp.bp.114.152751.

Seymour, R. B. (1986). MDMA. San Francisco, CA, USA: Haight Ashbury Publications.

Shafranske, E. P., Gorsuch, R. L. (1984). Factors associated with the perception of spirituality in psychotherapy. Journal of Transpersonal Psychology 16(2), pp. 231-243.

Shallice, T. (1982) Specific impairments of planning. Phil Trans R Soc Lond 298, pp. 199-209.
Shanon. B. (2002). The Antipodes of the Mind. Charting the Phenomenology of the Ayahuasca Experience. Oxford, UK: Oxford University Press.
Shanon, B. (2003). Altered states and the study of consciousness: The case of ayahuasca. The Journal of Mind and Behavior. 24(2), pp. 125-154.
Shanon, B. (2014). Moments of insights, Healing, and Transformation: A Cognitive Phenomenological Analysis. In B. C. Labate, C. Cavnar (eds.), The Therapeutic Use of Ayahuasca. Heidelberg, Germany: Springer.
Shemluck, M. J. (1979). The flowers of Ilex guayusa. Botanical museum Leaflets harvard university 27(5-6). pp. 155-160.
Shen. H. W., Jiang. X. L., Yu. A. M. (2009). Development of a LC-MS/MS method to analyze 5-methoxy-N,N-dimethyltryptamine and bufotenine, and application to pharmacokinetic study. Bioanalysis (1), pp. 87-95, DOI: 10.4155/bio.09.7. PMC 2879651. PMID 20523750.
Shore, B. 1996. Culture in Mind: Cognition, Culture, and the Problem of Meaning. Oxford, UK: Oxford University Press.
Shulgin A. T., Nichols D. E. (1978). Characterization of three new psychotomimetics. In R. C. Stillman, R. E. Willette (eds.). The psychopharmacology of the hallucinogens. New York, USA: Pergamon Press, pp. 74-83.
Silberer, H. (1909): Bericht über eine Methode, gewisse symbolische Halluzinationserscheinungen hervorzurufen und zu beobachten. Jahrbuch für psychoanalytische und psychopathologische Forschungen 1, pp. 302ff.
Silberer, H. (1912): Symbolik des Erwachens und Schwellensymbolik überhaupt. Jahrbuch für psychoanalytische und psychopathologische Forschungen 3, p. 621 ff.
Singer, S., Brähler, E. (2014). Die "Sene of Coherence Scale" – Testhandbuch zur deutschen Version. Göttingen, Germany: Vandenhoeck & Ruprecht.
Sisley, S., Vandrey, R., Bonn-Miller, M., Riggs, P.. Marijuana for Symptoms of PTSD in U.S. Veterans. Retrieved May 27, 2016, Web site: http://www.maps.org/index.php?option=com_content&view=category&id=248&Itemid=593.
Skrzypińska, K. (2014). The Threefold Nature of Spirituality (tns) in a Psychological Cognitive Framework. Archive for the Psychology of Religion, 36(3), pp. 277-302. DOI: 10.1163/15736121-12341293
Smart, R. G., Storm, T., Baker, E. F. W., Solursh, L. (1966). A controlled study of lysergide in the treatment of alcoholism. Quarterly Journal of Studies on Alcohol, 27(3).
Smith, R. L., Canton, H., Barrett, R. J., Sanders-Bush, E. (1998). Agonist properties of N,N-dimethyl- tryptamine at serotonin 5-HT2A and 5-HT2C receptors. Pharmacol Biochem Behav 1998 (61), pp. 323-330. PMID: 9768567

Sobiecki, J. F. (2014a). The intersection of culture and science in South African traditional medicine. Indo-Pacific Journal of Phenomenology, 14(1), p. 219.
Sobiecki, J. F. (2014b). Psychoactive plants: A neglected area of ethnobotanical research in Southern Africa (review). Studies of Ethno-Medicine, 8(2), pp. 165-172.
Späth, E. (1920): Über die Anhalonium Alkaloide: I. Anhalin und Mezcalin. [German: About the anhalonium alcaloids: I. Anhaline and Mescaline]. Monatshefte für Chemie 40, pp. 129-154.
Stace, W. T. (1960). Mysticism and Philosophy. London, UK: MacMillan & Co.
Stangl, W. (2018). NEO-5-Faktoren Inventar (NEO-FFI) nach Costa und McCrae. Werner Stangls Arbeitsblätter-News. Retrieved April 13, 2018, Web site: http://arbeitsblaetter-news.stangl-taller.at/neo-5-faktoren-inventar-neo-ffi-nach-costa-und-mccrae/
Steinke, I. (2003). Gütekriterien qualitativer Forschung [German: Quality criteria of qualitative research]. In U, Flick, U., E. v. Kardorff, I. Steinke (eds.), Qualitative Forschung – Ein Handbuch, 4.7. Hamburg, Germany: Rowohlt Verlag.
Stern. D.N. [1985] (1992). Die Lebenserfahrung des Säuglings [German: Life experience of the infant]. Stuttgart, Germany: Klett-Cotta.
Sternberg, S. (1966). High-speed scanning in human memory. Science 153, pp. 652-654.
Stolaroff, M. J. (1997). The Secret Chief – Conversations with Leo Zeff, pioneer in the underground psychedelic therapy movement. Sarasota, FL, USA: MAPS. Retrieved August 24, 2016, Web site: http://www.maps.org/images/pdf/books/scr/scr.pdf
Strassman (1992). Subjective effects of DMT and the development of the Hallucinogen Rating Scale. Newsletter of the Multidisciplinary Association for Psychedelic Studies MAPS - Volume 3 Number 2 Spring 1992. Retrieved July 24, 2016, Web site: http://www.maps.org/news-letters/v03n2/03208dmt.html
Strassman, R. J., Qualls, C. R., Uhlenhuth, E. H., Kellner, R. (1994). Dose-response study of N,N-dimethyltryptamine in humans. II. Subjective effects and preliminary results of a new rating scale. Arch Gen Psychiatry. 1994 Feb;51(2), pp. 98-108, PMID: 8297217.
Strassman R. J., Qualls C. R., Berg L. M. (1996). Differential tolerance to biological and subjective effects of four closely spaced doses of N,N-dimethyltryptamine in humans. Biol Psychiatry 1994; 39: pp. 784-95. Retrieved August 24, 2016, Web site: http://www.maps.org/research-archive/w3pb/1996/1996_Strassman_22710_1.pdf

Studerus, E., Gamma, A., Vollenweider, F. X. (2010). Psychometric Evaluation of the Altered States of Consciousness Rating Scale (OAV). PLoS ONE 5(8): e12412. DOI: 10.1371/journal.pone.0012412

Styk, J. (2008). Integration und Krisenintervention. in Jungaberle, H., Gasser, P., Weinhold, J., Verres, R. (2008). Therapie mit psychoaktiven Substanzen, Praxis und Kritik der Psychotherapie mit LSD, Psilocybin und MDMA. Bern, Switzerland: Hogrefe.

Sullivan, G. C. (1993). Towards clarification of convergent concepts: Sense of coherence, will to meaning, locus of control, learned helplessness and hardiness. Journal of Advanced Nursing, 18(11).

Surtees, P. G., Wainwright, N. W. J., & Khaw, K.-T. (2006). Resilience, misfortune, and mortality: Evidence that sense of coherence is a marker of social stress adaptive capacity. Journal of Psychosomatic Research, 61(2).

Szabo, A., Kovacs A., Frecska, E., Rajnavolgyi, E. (2014). Psychedelic N,N-Dimethyltryptamine and 5-Methoxy-N,N-Dimethyltryptamine Modulate Innate and Adaptive Inflammatory Responses through the Sigma-1 Receptor of Human Monocyte-Derived Dendritic Cells. PLoS ONE 9(8): e106533, DOI: 10.1371/journal.pone.0106533. PMID 25171370.

Tanne, J. H. (2004). Humphry Osmond. BMJ: British Medical Journal, 328(7441), p. 713.

Tanner, C. (2015). Personal communication. October 3, 2015. Lima, Peru.

Taubert, S., Förster, Ch. (2005). Sinnfindung, Krankheitsverarbeitung und Lebensqualität von Tumorpatienten im perioperativen Verlauf [German: Sense finding, disease processing and quality of life of tumor patients in the perioperative course]. Zeitschrift für Gesundheitspsychologie 13(4).

Torres, C. M., Repke, D. B., Chan, K., et al. (1991). Snuff powders from pre-Hispanic San Pedro de Atacama: Chemical and contextual analysis. Current Anthropology, 32(5), pp. 640-649. Retrieved August 30, 2016, Web site: http://www2.ups.edu/faculty/bdasher/Chem361/Review_Articles_files/Snuff%20Powders,%20Schultes.pdf.

Torres, C. M. (1996). Archelogical Evidence for the Antiquity of Psychoactive Plant Use ind the Central Andes. Annali dei Musei Civici-Rovereto, 11, pp. 291-326. Retrieved May 17, 2016, Web site: http://www.cyjack.com/cognition/art10[1].pdf

Torres, C. M., & Repke, D. B. (2006). Anadenanthera: Visionary plant of ancient South America. New York: Haworth Herbal. In Beyer S. V. (2012). On the Origings of Ayahuasca. Online article recived May 17, 2016, Web site: http://www.singingtotheplants.com/2012/04/on-origins-of-ayahuasca/

Tuck, I., Alleyne, R., Thinganjana, W. (2006). Spirituality and stress management in healthy adults. J Holist Nurs. 2006 Dec;24(4), pp. 245-53; discussion pp. 254-5, PMID: 17098877, DOI: 10.1177/0898010106289842

Tupper, K. W. (2009). Ayahuasca Healing beyond the Amazon: The Globalization of a Traditional Indigenous Entheogenic Practice. Global Networks: A Journal of Transnational Affairs, 9(1), pp. 117-136.

Turner, V (1969). The ritual process: structure and anti-structure. New Brunswick, USA: Transaction Publishers, Reprint from 2008.

Tylš, F., Páleníček, T., Horáček, J. (2013). Psilocybin – Summary of knowledge and new perspectives. European Neuropsychopharmacology (2014) 24, pp. 342-356, DOI: http://dx.DOI.org/10.1016/j.euroneuro.2013.12.006. Retrieved August 10, 2016, Web site: http://whereareyouquetzalcoatl.com/Xochipilli_TylsEtAll2014.pdf

Udenfriend, S., Witkop, B., Redfield, B., Weissbach, H., (1958). Studies with the reversible inhibitors of monamine oxidase: harmaline and related compounds. Biochemical Pharma- cology 1(2), pp. 160-165, DOI: 10.1016/0006-2952(58)90025-X

Callaway, J. C., McKenna, D. J. Grob, C. S., et al. (1999). Pharmacokinetics of Hoasca alkaloids in healthy humans. Journal of Ethnopharmacology 65(1999). pp. 243-256.

Udris, I., Frese, M. (1999). Belastung und Beanspruchung [German: Load and stress]. In C. Hoyos, C. & D. Frey (eds.). Arbeits- und Organisationspsychologie. Weinheim: Beltz, pp. 429-445.

Udris, I., Kraft, U., Mussmann, C., Rimann, M. (1992). Arbeiten, gesund sein und gesund bleiben: Theoretische Überlegungen zu einem Resourcenkonzept [German: Work, be healthy and stay healthy: Theoretical considerations on a resource concept]. In I. Udris (Ed.). Arbeit und Gesundheit. Psychosozial, Band 52, pp. 9-22.

UNWTO (2014). Glossary of tourism terms. Retrieved August 18, 2016, Web site: http://cf.cdn.unwto.org/sites/all/files/Glossary-of-terms.pdf

Urry, J. (1990). The Tourist Gaze: Leisure and Travel in Contemporary Societies. London, UK: Sage, p. 100 et seqq.

Van Gennep, A. (1986). Übergangsriten (les rites de passage) [German translation from French: Rites of passage]. Frankfurt, Germany): Campus Verlag.

Vaughan, F. (1991). Spiritual issues in psychotherapy. Journal of Transpersonal Psychology, 23(2), pp. 105-119.

Varendonk, J. (1922). Über das vorbewußte phantasierende Denken [German: About the preconscious imaginative thinking]. Leipzig, Germany: IPV.

Veigl, F. X. (1798). Vormaliger Mißionar der Gesellschaft Jesu. Gründliche Nachrichten über die Verfassung der Landschaft von Maynas in Süd-Amerika bis zum Jahre 1768. Zweytes Buch. Beschreibung der Landschaft von Maynas in Rücksicht auf die Erzeugungen der Natur, und Beschaffenheit der Sitten [German: Former missionary of the Society of Jesus. Thorough news about the constitution of the landscape of Maynas in South America until the year 1768. Second book. Description of the landscape of Maynas in respect of the generations of nature, and constitution of the customs]. Nürnberg, Germany: Zeh. p. 189. Retrieved August 17, 2016, Web site: http://digital.slub-dresden.de/id330590324.

Verdejo-García, A., Lawrence, A. J., Clark, L. (2008). Impulsivity as a vulnerability marker for substance-use disorders: review of findings from high-risk research, problem gamblers and genetic association studies. Neurosci Biobehav Rev 32: pp. 777-810.

Vester H.-G. (1993). Authentizität [German: Authenticity]. In H. Hahn, H.-J. Kagelmann (eds.). Tourismuspsychologie und Tourismussoziologie: Ein Handbuch zur Tourismuswissenschaft, München, Germany, p. 122-124.

Verres, R. (1986). Krebs und Angst. Subjektive Theorien von Laien über Entstehung, Vorsorge, Früherkennung, Behandlung und die psychosozialen Folgen von Krebserkrankungen [German: Cancer and anxiety. Subjective theories of lay people on the origin, prevention, early detection, treatment and the psychosocial consequences of cancer]. Berlin, Germany: Springer.

Verres, R. (1989). Zur Kontextabhängigkeit subjektiver Krankheitstheorien [German: About the context dependency of subjective theories about diseases]. In: C. Bischoff, H. Zenz (eds.), Patientenkonzepte von Körper und Krankheit. Bern-Stuttgart-Toronto, Huber.

Verres, R. (2008). Die Beeinflussung substanz-induzierter veränderter Bewußtseinszustände durch Musik [German: Influencing substance-induced altered states of consciousness through music]. In Jungaberle, H., Gasser, P., Weinhold, J., Verres, R. (2008). Therapie mit psychoaktiven Substanzen, Praxis und Kritik der Psychotherapie mit LSD, Psilocybin und MDMA. Bern, Switzerland: Hogrefe.

Vickers, W. T., Plowmann, T. C. (1984). Useful plants of the Siona and Secoya Indians of eastern Ecuador. Fieldiana 15, pp. 1-63.

Volanen, S.-M. (2011). Sense of Coherence: Determinants and Consequences. Dissertation, Faculty of Medicine, University of Helsinki Helsinki, Finland. retrieved October 5, 2016, Web site: http://urn.fi/URN:ISBN:978-952-10-6588-0

Vollenweider, F. X., Kometer, M. (2010). The neurobiology of psychedelic drugs: implications for the treatment of mood disorders. Nat Rev Neurosci. 2010 Sep;11(9), pp. 642-51. DOI: 10.1038/nrn2884.

Von Schrenck-Notzing, A. (1892) (2016). Die Bedeutung narkotischer Mittel für den Hypnotismus: mit besonderer Berücksichtigung des indischen Hanfes [German: The importance of narcotic agents for hypnotism: with special regard to Indian hemp]. Germany: Edition Geheimes Wissen. ISBN: 978-3-902974-77-8

Walsh, R. & Vaughan, F (1993). On transpersonal definitions. Journal of Transpersonal Psychology, 25 (2), pp. 125-182.

Wasson, R. G. (1957). Seeking the magic Mushroom. Life Magazine June 10, 1957.

Weis, J. (1998). Krankheitsverarbeitung und subjektive Krankheitstheorien – Theoretische Konzepte, Forschungsmethodik und Forschungsergebnisse [German: Disease Processing and Subject Disease Theories - Theoretical Concepts, Research Methodology, and Research Results]. In U. Koch, J. Weis, J. (Edts), Krankheitsbewältigung bei Krebs und Möglichkeiten der Unterstützung. Stuttgart, Germany: Schattauer.

Weiss, S. (2018). People Are Drinking Ayahuasca to Treat Physical Illnesses: Could the psychedelic be changing people's perception of pain?. Tonic Vice. Internet magazine article. Retrieved October 2, 2018, Web site: https://tonic.vice.com/en_us/article/neknyx/drinking-ayahuasca-to-treat-pain-illness

WHO (1948). Preamble to the Constitution of the World Health Organization as adopted by the International Health Conference, New York, USA, 19-22 June, 1946; signed on July 22, 1946 by the representatives of 61 States (Official Records of the World Health Organization, no. 2, p. 100) and entered into force on 7 April 1948.

WHO Expert Committee on Drug Dependence (1985): World Health Organization Technical Report Series 729. Geneva, Switzerland: WHO 1985.

WHO (2000). General Guidelines for Methodologies on Research and Evaluation of Traditional Medicine, p. 1. Retrieved August 17, 2017, Web site: http://whqlibdoc.who.int/hq/2000/WHO_EDM_TRM_2000.1.pdf?ua=1

Wilbert, J. (1987). Tobacco and Shamanism in South America. In R. E. Schultes, R. F. Raffauf (eds.). Psychoactive Plants of the World. New Haven, USA: Yale Univ. Press.

Wilbert, J. (1991). Does pharmacology corroborate the nicotine therapy practices of South American Shamans?. Journal of Ethnopharmacology 32(1-3). pp. 179-186. PMID: 1881155.

Winkelmann, M. (2005). Drug Tourism or spiritual Healing? Ayahuasca Seekers in Amazonia. Journal of Psychoactive Drugs. Vol 37(2), June 2005.

Witzel, A. (2010). Längsschnittdesign [German: Longitudinal design]. In G. Mey, K. Mruck (eds.), Handbuch Qualitative Forschung in der Psychologie. Wiesbaden 2010: VS Verlag, p. 291.

WMA (2013). Declaration of Helsinki –Ethical Principles for Medical Research Involving Human Subjects. Retrieved October 3, 2016, Web site: https://www.wma.net/wp-content/uploads/2016/11/DoH-Oct2013-JAMA.pdf

Wolff, T. J. (2015). Biodanza und seine Wirkung auf den alltäglichen Umgang mit Musik: Eine Zielgruppenanalyse und kulturvergleichende Untersuchung [German: Biodanza and its effect on the everyday use of music: a target group analysis and cross-cultural examination]. Hamburg: Diplomica

Wolff, T. J. (2018). Ayahuasca-Tourismus in Südamerika [German: ayahuasca tourism in South America]. In R. Feustel, H. Schmidt-Semisch, U. Bröckling (eds.), Handbuch Drogen in sozial- und kulturwissenschaftlicher Perspektive [German: Handbook on Drugs in Social and Cultural Studies Perspective]. Wiesbaden, Germany: Springer VS, pp. 555-575.

Wolff, T. J., Passie, T. (2018). Motivational structure of ayahuasca drinkers in social networks. Journal of Pychedelic Studies, vol. 2, issue 2, pp. 89-96, DOI: 10.1556/2054.2018.010

Wolff, T. J., Ruffell, S., Netzband, N., Passie, T. (2019). A phenomenology of subjectively relevant experiences induced by ayahuasca in Upper Amazon vegetalismo tourism. Journal of Pychedelic Studies, online publication, DOI: 10.1556/2054.2019.007

Wang, Y.-H., Samoylenko, V., Tekwani, B. L., et al. (2010). Composition, Standardization and Chemical Profiling of Banisteriopsis caapi, a Plant for the Treatment of Neurodegenerative Disorders Relevant to Parkinson's Disease. J Ethnopharmacol. 2010 Apr 21; 128(3), pp. 662–671. Online publication, DOI: 10.1016/j.jep.2010.02.013

Yalom, I. D. (1980). Existential psychotherapy. USA, NY: Basic Books.

Yancey, W. L., Erickson, P., Juliani R. N. (1976). Emergent Ethnicity: A Review and Reformulation. American Sociological Review, 41(3), pp. 391-403.

Yensen, R. (1994). Perspectives on LSD and Psychotherapy: The Search for a new paradigma. In A. Pletscher, D. Ladewig (eds.), 50 Years of LSD: Current Status and Perspectives of Halluzinogenes. New York, USA.

Yensen, R., Dreyer, D. (1994). Dreißig Jahre psychedelische Forschung: Das Spring Grove Experiment und seine Folgen [German: Thirty years of psychedelic research: The Spring Grove Experiment and Its Consequences]. In: A. Dittrich, A. Hofmann, H. Leuner (eds.), Welten des Bewusstseins, Band 4 Bedeutung veränderter Bewusstseinszustände für die Psychotherapie. Berlin, Germany: Verlag für Wissenschaft und Bildung, pp. 155-187.

Yong W. G., Sukanlaya Sawang, Tian P. S. Oei (2010). The Revised Transactional Model (RTM) of Occupational Stress and Coping: An Improved Process Approach. The Australian and New Zealand Journal of Organisational Psychology, 3, pp. 13-20, DOI: 10.1375/ajop.3.1.13.

Zacharias, S. (2005). Das psychotherapeutische Wissen und die Behandlung psychischer Erkrankungen innerhalb des mexikanischen Curanderismus – eine qualitative einzelfallorientierte Studie [German: Psychotherapeutic knowledge and treatment of mental illness within Mexican curanderism - a qualitative case-by-case study]. Dissertation, University of Leipzig, Leipzig, Germany.

Zinberg, N. (1983). Soziale Kontrollmechanismen und soziales Lernen im Umfeld des Rauschmittelkonsums [German: Social control mechanisms and social learning in the context of intoxicant use]. In D. Letteri, R. Welz (eds.), Drogenabhängigkeit – Ursachen und Verlaufsformen: Ein Handbuch. Weinheim: Beltz.

Zinberg, N. (1986). Drug, Set, And Setting: The Basis For Controlled Intoxicant Use. USA: Yale University Press. ISBN 0-300-03634-5.

Znamenski, A. A. (2007). The Beauty of the Primitive: Shamanism and the Western Imagination. Oxford, UK: University Press.

Zografos, C., Kenrick, J. (2005). Negotiating 'Indigenousness' through Ecotourism in the Amazonian Ecuador. Tourism Vol. 53(3), pp. 205-215.

Zwingmann, C. (2004). Spiritualität/Religiosität und das Konzept der gesundheitsbezogenen Lebensqualität: Definitionen, empirische Evidenz, Operationalisierungen [German: Spirituality/religiosity and the concept of health-related quality of life: definitions, empirical evidence, operationalisations]. In C. Zwingmann, H. Moosbrugger (eds.), Religiosität: Messverfahren und Studien zu Gesundheit und Lebensbewältigung: Neue Beiträge zur Religionspsychologie. Münster, Germany: Waxmann, pp. 215-237.